Depression

For a catalogue of publications available from ACP–ASIM, contact:

Customer Service Center
American College of Physicians–American Society of Internal Medicine
190 N. Independence Mall West
Philadelphia, PA 19106-1572
215-351-2600
800-523-1546, ext. 2600

Visit our Web site at www.acponline.org

Depression

■ ■ ■

James L. Levenson, MD
Professor of Psychiatry, Medicine, and Surgery
Chair, Division of Consultation-Liaison Psychiatry
Vice-Chair, Department of Psychiatry
Medical College of Virginia–Virginia Commonwealth University
Richmond, Virginia

A|C|P

American College of Physicians
Philadelphia, Pennsylvania

Clinical Consultant: David R. Goldmann, MD
Manager, Book Publishing: David Myers
Administrator, Book Publishing: Diane McCabe
Production Supervisor: Allan S. Kleinberg
Production Editor: Scott Thomas Hurd
Developmental Editor: Victoria Hoenigke
Copy Editor: Karen Christine Nolan
Acquisitions Editor: Mary K. Ruff
Editorial Assistant: Alicia Dillihay
Indexer: Nelle Garrecht
Interior Design: Kate Nichols
Cover Design: Elizabeth Swartz

Printed in the United States of America
Composition by Fulcrum Data Services, Inc.
Printing/binding by Versa Press

American College of Physicians (ACP) became an imprint of the American College of Physicians–American Society of Internal Medicine in July 1998.

Library of Congress Cataloging-in-Publication Data

Depression / [edited by] James Levenson.
   p. cm.
   Includes bibliographical references.
   ISBN 0-943126-85-1
   1. Depression, Mental. I. Levenson, James L.
   [DNLM: 1. Depressive Disorder–diagnosis–Case Report. 2. Depressive Disorder–therapy–Case Report. WM 207 E96 2000]
   RC537.E97 2000
   616.85'27—dc21   99-057889

00 01 02 03 04 / 9 8 7 6 5 4 3 2 1

In memory of Mary Beth Levenson

Contributors

George S. Alexopoulos, MD
Professor of Psychiatry
Department of Psychiatry
Weill Medical College of Cornell University
White Plains, New York

Douglas Dale Brink, BS Pharm, PharmD, BCPP
Clinical Pharmacy Specialist for Psychiatry
Department of Psychiatry Services
Assistant Clinical Professor of Pharmacy and Psychiatry
Medical College of Virginia–Virginia Commonwealth University
Richmond, Virginia

Christopher C. Colenda, MD, MPH
Professor and Chair
Department of Psychiatry
Michigan State University
East Lansing, Michigan

Caroline Carney Doebbeling, MD, MS
Assistant Professor of Psychiatry and Internal Medicine
Director, Combined Internal Medicine/ Psychiatry Training Program
University of Iowa College of Medicine
Iowa City, Iowa

Charles DeBattista, MD
Department of Psychiatry and Behavioral Sciences
Stanford University School of Medicine
Stanford, California

Robert N. Glenn, PhD
Department of Consultation-Liaison Psychiatry
Medical College of Virginia–Virginia Commonwealth University
Richmond, Virginia

Yvonne M. Greene, MD
Wesley Woods Health Center
Emory University School of Medicine
Atlanta, Georgia

Ira R. Katz, MD, PhD
Professor of Psychiatry
Director, Section of Geriatric Psychiatry
Department of Psychiatry
University of Pennsylvania
Philadelphia, Pennsylvania

John W. Klocek, PhD
Director, Clinical Psychology Center
Department of Psychology
University of Montana
Missoula, Montana

Susan G. Kornstein, MD
Associate Professor of Psychiatry and Obstetrics and Gynecology
Chair, Division of Ambulatory Care Psychiatry
Director, Women's Psychiatric Services
Medical College of Virginia–Virginia Commonwealth University
Richmond, Virginia

Kurt Kroenke, MD
Professor of Medicine,
Indiana University School of Medicine;
Senior Scientist
Regenstrief Institute of Health Care
Indianapolis, Indiana

James L. Levenson, MD
Professor of Psychiatry, Medicine, and Surgery
Chair, Division of Consultation-Liaison Psychiatry
Vice-Chair, Department of Psychiatry
Medical College of Virginia–Virginia Commonwealth University
Richmond, Virginia

J. Stephen McDaniel, MD
Associate Professor of Psychiatry and Behavioral Sciences
Emory University School of Medicine
Atlanta, Georgia

William M. McDonald, MD
Associate Professor of Psychiatry
Emory University School of Medicine;
Director, Fuqua Center for Late-Life
  Depression
Wesley Woods Health Center
Atlanta, Georgia

Anthony L. Pelonero, MD
Medical Director
Trigon Behavioral Healthcare
Trigon Blue Cross and Blue Shield
Richmond, Virginia;
Clinical Associate Professor of Psychiatry
Medical College of Virginia–Virginia
  Commonwealth University
Richmond, Virginia

Charles F. Reynolds III, MD
Professor of Psychiatry, Neurology,
  and Neuroscience
Western Psychiatric Institute and Clinic
University of Pittsburgh School of
  Medicine
Pittsburgh, Pennsylvania

Michael J. Roy, MD, MPH
Associate Professor
Department of Medicine
Uniformed Services University of the
  Health Sciences
Bethesda, Maryland

Alan F. Schatzberg, MD
Chairman
Department of Psychiatry and
  Behavioral Sciences
Stanford University School of Medicine
Stanford, California

Lon S. Schneider, MD
Professor of Psychiatry, Neurology,
  and Gerontology
Department of Psychiatry and the
  Behavioral Sciences
University of Southern California
Los Angeles, California

Robert K. Schneider, MD
Departments of Psychiatry and
  Internal Medicine
Division of Consultation-Liaison Psychiatry
Medical College of Virginia–Virginia
  Commonwealth University
Richmond, Virginia

David L. Smith, MD
Department of Psychiatry and
  Behavioral Sciences
Stanford University School of Medicine
Stanford, California

Aradhana A. Sood, MD
Associate Professor of Psychiatry
Medical College of Virginia–Virginia
  Commonwealth University
Richmond, Virginia

Rakesh K. Sood, MD
Associate Professor
Department of Psychiatry
Director, Sleep Disorders Center
Medical College of Virginia–Virginia
  Commonwealth University
Richmond, Virginia

**Michele Lynn Thomas, BS Pharm,
PharmD**
Post-Doctoral Fellow in Psychiatric
  Pharmacy Practice
Medical College of Virginia–Virginia
  Commonwealth University
Richmond, Virginia

Barbara A. Wojcik, MD
Resident in Psychiatry
Medical College of Virginia–Virginia
  Commonwealth University
Richmond, Virginia

Thomas S. Zaubler, MD, MPH
Assistant Professor
Department of Psychiatry
Georgetown University Medical Center
Washington, District of Columbia

Contents

Clinical Vignettes

Foreword

■　■　■

Over the past two decades, remarkable progress has been made in our understanding of the epidemiology of depression in all patient populations. We also have witnessed a tremendous expansion in our therapeutic armamentarium, with exciting new advances in antidepressant medication, psychotherapy, electroconvulsive therapy, and light therapy.

The selective serotonin-reuptake inhibitors revolutionized the treatment of depression and have heralded the development of many other novel antidepressants. Several psychotherapies (e.g., cognitive-behavioral, interpersonal, and problem-solving therapies) have been developed and proved effective in randomized trials. The Agency for Health Care Policy and Research (AHCPR) published guidelines on the epidemiology and treatment of depression in 1993 (1), which were followed rapidly by guidelines from the American Psychiatric Association and the American Psychological Association. An update of the AHCPR guidelines was published in 1998 (2), and several studies funded by the National Institute of Mental Health have demonstrated effective ways to implement these guidelines in primary care. This increase in epidemiologic and treatment findings coincided with the acceptance of depression as a valid medical diagnosis. Studies on depression are appearing regularly in major medical journals such as the *Journal of the American Medical Association, British Medical Journal, Annals of Internal Medicine, Archives of Internal Medicine,* and *Archives of Family Medicine.*

Now, James L. Levenson—a clinician and researcher who has been at the forefront of psychiatric medicine for almost two decades—brings us *Depression,* a superbly edited text that lucidly reveals the exciting advances in current depression research. Case studies are effectively integrated to amplify and crystallize key educational points, and Clinical Vignettes are included to offer sample patients and their problems for reader diagnosis. In sum, *Depression* provides state-of-the-art knowledge to internists, other primary care physicians, and medical specialists.

Wayne Katon, MD

■   ■   ■

REFERENCES

1. **Public Health Service Agency for Health Care Policy and Research.** *Depression in Primary Care: Treatment of Major Depression.* Rockville, MD: U.S. Department of Health and Human Services; 1993 [AHCPR Publication No. 93-051].
2. **Schulberg HC, Katon W, Simon G, Rush AJ.** Treating major depression in primary care practice: an update of the AHCPR practice guidelines. *Arch Gen Psychiatry.* 1998;55:1121–7.

Preface

■   ■   ■

Depression is not the soul's annihilation; men and women who have recovered from the disease—and they are countless—bear witness to what is probably its only saving grace: it is conquerable.

—William Styron, *Darkness Invisible*

Depression is a "key disease" for internists and other nonpsychiatric physicians because it is the most common medical diagnosis in primary care settings—surpassed only by hypertension in some populations—and because most patients who are depressed initially seek treatment from their primary care physicians. Although progress has been made in helping the primary care practitioner recognize and treat depression, the ongoing need for improvement in this area has been demonstrated in numerous studies conducted in practice settings. The diagnosis of depression is still frequently missed, and even when it is recognized, treatment is often inadequate or not given at all. This is a sad irony at a time when a wide range of pharmacologic and psychological treatments has been empirically demonstrated to be effective.

Like the other books in the ACP-ASIM Key Diseases series, *Depression* is designed to be useful in clinical practice. Its purpose is to help physicians develop a more thorough and systematic approach to the diagnosis and treatment of depression in the same way they learn to manage other illnesses. Because the chapters have been written by a diverse collection of psychiatric and nonpsychiatric clinicians—including psychiatrists, psychologists, general internists, and pharmacists—this book provides guidance from multiple points of view on the recognition of and the interventions for depression in the wide variety of patients encountered in medical care settings. The key points found at the end of each chapter reflect consensus among the experts.

Depression, however, is not intended to be a comprehensive review of all the relevant literature. When recommendations are evidence-based, the authors have indicated this and have cited the appropriate studies. Even though a great deal of research has been devoted to the diagnosis and treatment of depression, not all findings are able to be generalized between different settings and populations (e.g., mental health patients vs. primary care patients; adults vs. children).

Chapter 1 examines the relationship between depression and medical illness and its impact on health care. Major depression causes as much (or even more) impairment of physical and social functioning as other chronic disorders, including arthritis, diabetes, and hypertension. Depression increasingly occurs with many chronic medical disorders and has a variety of undesirable consequences, including lack of treatment adherence, unnecessary medical use, increased costs, impaired quality of life, amplification of physical distress symptoms, adverse health behaviors, and suicide. Independent of other risk factors, depression appears responsible for increased morbidity and mortality in diseases such as diabetes mellitus and coronary artery disease.

Chapter 2 reviews epidemiology, risk factors, and prevention. The lifetime prevalence of depression is currently 5% in the community at large, 5% to 10% in medical outpatients, and 10% to 14% in medical inpatients. Women are at increased risk for depression, as are individuals with chronic medical illness, a family history of depression, chronic sleep disorders, or stressful life events.

Chapter 3 covers diagnosis. Major depression is but one of a spectrum of depressive disorders, all of which are associated with impairment in functioning and may cause unexplained physical complaints. Compared with mental health settings, diagnosis of depression in primary care is more difficult because depressed patients are more likely to present with physical rather than emotional complaints—just one reason why the diagnosis is frequently missed.

Chapter 4 reviews general considerations in the management of depression, including how to handle suicidal patients, when to refer to a mental health specialist, and ethical and risk-management issues. Adjunctive interventions also are reviewed, including exercise, nutrition, hydration, sleep hygiene, reduction of psychoactive substance abuse, relaxation techniques, religious involvement, support groups, patient education, light therapy, and alternative medicine.

Chapters 5 through 7 cover specific treatments and address the question, "Which is the most appropriate initial treatment—antidepressant medication, psychotherapy, or a combination of the two?" In keeping with the fact that a clear consensus has yet to emerge, the authors of these chapters differ in their views about exactly what the right answer is. However, all of them would agree that the choice of initial treatment should be guided by each patient's preferences and individual characteristics.

Chapter 5 reviews the antidepressants currently available in the United States, including the selective serotonin-reuptake inhibitors (fluoxetine, sertraline, paroxetine, citalopram, and fluvoxamine), the 5HT-2 antagonists (nefazodone and trazodone), venlafaxine, bupropion, mirtazapine, the tricyclic antidepressants, the monoamine oxidase inhibitors, and the stimulants. Although all antidepressants are of approximately equal efficacy, the choice of a particular drug should be based on safety, side-effect profile, age, comorbid medical illness, other medications, history of response, and patient preference.

Chapter 6 focuses primarily on those psychotherapies that have been empirically demonstrated to be efficacious for depression. The questions of who provides psychotherapy and how and to whom patients should be referred are also addressed, as are brief psychotherapeutic techniques that primary care physicians can use in the management of depressed patients.

Chapter 7 addresses the complex array of options available for treatment-resistant depression. Up to 40% of patients do not respond to an initial course of antidepressant treatment, and 10% to 15% of patients remain chronically depressed despite continued treatment. The most common reason for treatment failure is inadequacy of therapy in dose or duration due to patient nonadherence or inadequate follow-up by the physician. Unrecognized comorbid medical illness, other psychiatric illness, substance abuse, and social pathology also may account for the failure of standard treatment. This chapter discusses switching antidepressants, combining two antidepressants, augmentation strategies, psychotherapy, and electroconvulsive therapy—the most effective and yet widely underused treatment for severe depressions.

Chapters 8 through 11 review the phenomenology, diagnosis, and treatment of depression in special populations, including the elderly (Chapter 8), women (Chapter 9), children and adolescents (Chapter 10), and the terminally ill (Chapter 11). Chapter 9 gives special consideration to depression caused by menstrual cycling, pregnancy, childbirth, and menopause. Chapter 11 includes important sections on evaluating the competency of patients to make medical decisions and on patient requests for assisted suicide.

Chapter 12 is devoted to the application of practice guidelines to the treatment of depression, focusing on those provided by the Agency for Health Care Policy and Research and the American Psychiatric Association.

Chapter 13 provides a succinct description of clinically significant interactions between antidepressants and other medications.

Finally, the eleven Clinical Vignettes test the reader's knowledge and show how experts approach commonly encountered clinical dilemmas.

With depression, as with other diseases, primary care physicians vary in their levels of interest, comfort, experience, and skill. All physicians should know about the key aspects of diagnosis and treating depression, but each must choose which responsibilities to assume and which patients to refer to a psychiatrist or other mental health professional. Our hope is that, after reading this book, the primary care physician will recognize and treat depression with more confidence and familiarity and will regard it as they would any other illness that requires the integration of educational, behavioral, and pharmacologic interventions.

James L. Levenson, MD

1

■ ■ ■

Depression, Medical Illness, and Health Care

J. Stephen McDaniel, MD

"Some days I felt like the hypochondriac from Hell. Some days I knew I was dying. . . . Everything felt wrong."

Major depression is a serious illness in the United States. It is a clearly recognizable, eminently treatable syndrome affecting 20% to 30% of patients with comorbid medical illnesses (1–3). Once thought of as a short-term problem, major depression is now considered a recurrent or long-term condition for many patients (4). If a patient has a first episode, there is a 50% chance that a second episode will occur; after a second episode, the chances of a third episode rise to between 80% and 90% (5). Recent research also has documented that occurrences of major depression are increasing with each successive decade, that is, earlier onset and higher rates (6,7). Moreover, the disorder is associated with substantial medical, personal, social and economic costs, particularly in the medically ill and the elderly (8,9).

This chapter will focus on some of the general consequences and correlates of major depression in the medically ill and the more direct impact of depression on certain medical disorders. The commonly intertwined relationship of depression and somatization are described, as well as those medical disorders and medications that can cause depressive syndromes.

Hopefully, clarifying the effects of major depression on the medical setting will improve awareness of the need to adequately diagnose and aggressively treat depression in the medically ill.

Prevalence and Underdiagnosis of Depression

Major depression is the most common clinical psychiatric problem seen in primary care settings, and the prevalence of depression is generally higher in severely medically ill patients (10). Increasing numbers of patients are receiving treatment for depression in primary care settings: one study of psychotropic medication prescribing trends among medical specialties, Pincus and coworkers (11), showed that between 1984 and 1994 patient visits to primare care providers for the treatment of depression doubled. Medical illness is thought to be a factor in recurrent episodes of major depression. For example, a 5-year recurrence rate of 92% has been documented in patients with major depression and diabetes mellitus (12).

After many years of research documenting the failure to detect major depression and the suboptimal use of antidepressant medications in primary care settings, the disorder remains underdiagnosed and undertreated (13). For example, in a 1994 study that examined patients who received care at a variety of primary care and specialist care offices, only 29% of those with depression of high severity received an antidepressant (14). In another study that examined distressed individuals who were high users of primary care services, 45% were diagnosed with depression and in need of treatment; however, only 1 in 9 received adequate dose and duration of antidepressant treatment (15). Table 1.1 lists common explanations for these high rates of underdiagnosis and undertreatment. Recently, physician and patient education efforts have been undertaken in an effort to increase recognition and adequate treatment of depression in primary care (16).

Table 1.1   Reasons for Underdiagnosis and Undertreatment of Depression in Medically Ill Patients

- Emphasis on somatic symptoms rather than cognitive and mood complaints

- Reluctance to stigmatize patients with psychiatric diagnosis

- Mild or nonspecific symptoms of depression

- Fear of antidepressant side effects

- Mistaken notion that reactive depressions are not pathological (e.g., "She should be depressed; she has cancer.")

- Time limitation in primary care

- Inadequate training of primary care physicians in psychiatry

---

Republished with permission from Rouchell et al. Depresssion. In Rundell JR, Wise MG, eds. *Textbook of Consultation-Liaison Psychiatry.* Washington, DC: American Psychiatric Press; 1996:310-1345.

General Consequences of Major Depression

The presence of depression in the medically ill patient can result in a range of unfavorable consequences for the patient, his or her family, health care providers, and even society. Although most extreme outcomes can be lethal, including suicide and increased medical-illness mortality, other negative effects of depression may be more long-term and insidious (e.g., impaired daily functioning, reduced quality of life). A number of common adverse consequences are outlined in Table 1.2.

Nonadherence to Treatment

Noncompliance with medical treatment can have profound effects on overall medical outcome. Depressed medically ill patients are more likely to be uncooperative with medical treatment (17,18). Depression may prevent or delay patients from seeking care (e.g., neglecting a self-discovered breast lump), and it may decrease patients' motivation to care adequately for an existing medical illness, which can lead to additional medical complications. This is a well-documented finding in depressed patients with diabetes mellitus and coronary artery disease (19,20). Depressed patients with coronary artery disease are also less likely to adhere to cardiac exercise programs (20).

Depression also has a negative effect on the doctor-patient relationship. Decreased adherence is partly caused by reduced communication between doctor and patient. For example, a depressed patient may ask fewer questions, leading the treating physician to presume falsely that he or she understands the treatment plan when, in fact, the patient is too depressed to

---

Table 1.2   Consequences of Major Depression in the Medically Ill

Amplification of physical symptoms

Impaired functioning

Impaired quality of life

Increased medical morbidity and mortality

Increased health care use

Increased financial and social costs

Adverse health behaviors (including "high-risk" lifestyle behaviors)

Lack of treatment adherence

Suicide

participate in treatment decisions. Prominent depressive symptoms such as decreased energy, pessimism, and diminished self-care may be "contagious," causing the physician to become unnecessarily pessimistic and passive with such patients.

Some interventions have treated depression aggressively to improve adherence. For example, aggressive treatment of depression in patients with HIV infection has improved compliance with complex antiretroviral treatment regimens (21). The same has been found for patients with multiple sclerosis receiving interferon therapy: active treatment of depression is associated with increased medical treatment adherence (22). It is necessary to recognize and treat depression in medically ill patients whose treatment adherence is critical, and it is appropriate to suspect depression among nonadherent patients (Case 1.1).

CASE 1.1   *Uncontrolled diabetes mellitus*

A woman 57 years of age with previously stable insulin-dependent diabetes mellitus was followed regularly by her primary care physician. In recent months, her blood glucose levels were increasingly difficult to normalize, even with a more stringent diet and frequent insulin adjustments. During one follow-up visit, the patient was tearful and appeared sad when discussing her condition. On further questioning, her physician ascertained a 3-month history of progressive symptoms of major depression. The patient admitted feeling unmotivated about self-care and dietary restrictions.

Antidepressant treatment was initiated, and the patient's depressive symptoms were resolved over several weeks as her motivation to adhere to her treatment increased, after which her blood glucose levels stabilized.

Amplification of Physical Symptoms

Untreated depression may increase or amplify physical symptoms. These physical symptoms may be associated with diagnosed medical illnesses (e.g., increased pain perception after a myocardial infarction), or they may be undiagnosed symptoms. Symptoms that may be amplified by depression include chest pain, fatigue, dizziness, and headache (23). Katon and Walker (23) have studied medically unexplained physical symptoms in primary care settings and have found a significant linear relationship between the number of medically unexplained symptoms patients have experienced over their lifetimes, the number of anxiety and depressive disorders they have experienced currently and over their lifetimes, and the degree of current functional impairment. Their findings suggest 1) that clinicians should have a high index of suspicion for depression when patients present with physical symptoms that cannot be explained by a medical condition, and 2) that depression should be a prominent consideration in the differential diagnosis when physical symptoms persist despite seemingly successful medical intervention.

Increased Health Care Use

In their review of 26 outcome studies that evaluated the effects of psychiatric comorbidity on length of hospital stay, Saravay and Lavin (25) concluded that depression was a significant variable that predicted prolonged hospital stays and increased use of other health resources after discharge (25). In a retrospective study of hospitalized medical patients with secondary diagnoses of major depression, patients treated with antidepressants had significantly shorter hospital stays compared with those patients not treated with antidepressants (13.8 days vs. 45.6 days) (26). These findings are important for both their impact on individual patients and for health care systems in general. A number of studies have documented that somatic complaints associated with depression often increase medical use. Unexplained somatic symptoms often produce unnecessary hospitalizations, physician visits, diagnostic tests, and prescriptions. Patients with undiagnosed and/or untreated depression are three times more likely than nondepressed patients to use HMO physical health services, three to four times more likely to use emergency room services, and four to five times more likely to call their provider about health problems or for medication changes (27–29), thus placing a significant burden on health care services.

Increased Costs

Negative economic consequences that extend beyond health care use occur when depression complicates the course of medical care. By combining direct costs such as inpatient and outpatient care and pharmaceuticals, a recent study estimated the cost of depression to be more than $43 billion annually. Some have criticized this estimate as being too low because of the exclusion of such factors as underdiagnosis and increased medical morbidity associated with depression (30,31). From a practical standpoint, it is important to note that most studies that seek to examine health-related costs do not consider diminished quality of life or out-of-pocket expenses incurred by families of depressed patients for services such as child care (32). These costs are, however, significant and highlight how the social and economic burden of depression extends far beyond the personal toll of the illness.

Impaired Quality of Life and Functional Ability

Depression often has a marked effect on how patients perceive their quality of life, health, social and vocational performance, and physical activities (10,33). Major depression can cause severe functional disabilities. To illustrate this impairment, Wells and coworkers (34) compared physical and social functioning and debilitations in patients with arthritis, diabetes, hypertension, and no chronic medical illness to patients with major depression. They found that not only is the social functioning of depressed patients significantly more impaired than that found in the three illness groups, but the *physical* functioning of depressed patients was significantly more impaired as well. The secondary social and physical disabilities that can accompany a diagnosis of major depression are complications that often lag considerably behind the improvement in treated depressive symptoms (35).

Adverse Health Behaviors

Psychological factors often play a major role in risks associated with medical illnesses, such as cigarette smoking, obesity, physical inactivity, overuse of analgesics, alcohol and substance use, poor nutrition, poor sleep hygiene, and hazardous sexual practices (36). Depression has been found to increase many of these adverse health behaviors. For example, depressed smokers are 40% less likely to quit smoking when attempting cessation compared with nondepressed smokers (37). Untreated depression is also associated with increased HIV-risk behaviors (e.g., injection-drug use, unsafe sexual practices) in both "at risk" individuals and known HIV-positive persons (38–40). The contribution of untreated depression to adverse health behaviors has important implications for both preventative medical care and public health.

Suicide

Suicide is the most serious risk associated with major depression; in severe depression, the risk of death by suicide is 15% (41). Even this may be an underestimate because the true number of deaths from suicide may be three times higher than in coroners' reports (32). Suicide rates are increased significantly among medically ill, depressed patients (42,43). Illness has been implicated as a primary risk factor in 10% of younger suicide victims and in up to 70% of suicides among the elderly (44,45). Depression and chronic medical illness, especially when accompanied by chronic pain, account in part for the highest rates of completed suicide occurring in the elderly.

In two extensive literature reviews of completed suicides, rates of suicide among medically ill patients accounted for 34% to 43% of all reported suicides (46,47). A number of medical illnesses, often comorbid with major depression, have been documented to specifically increase suicide risk: HIV infection, cancers such as central nervous system cancer, and specific neurologic conditions like multiple sclerosis (43). In one study of 200 terminally ill inpatients who were evaluated for suicidal ideation and major depression, 8.5% of patients acknowledged a pervasive desire to die; the prevalence of major depression among these patients was 59%, highlighting the high rates of untreated comorbid depression among terminally ill patients (48).

Specific Medical Conditions and Depression

Depression may precede other signs and symptoms of some medical conditions, particularly endocrine diseases (e.g., Cushing's disease, thyroid disease) and some neurological illnesses (e.g., Huntingdon's disease). In other circumstances, depression is a common comorbid condition, co-occuring at rates as high as 67% (49). Common medical illnesses associated with depression include coronary artery disease, cancer, HIV infection, neurologic disorders, and endcrine disorders (50–57). Table 1.3 provides an overview of studies that identified depression rates by using stardardized interview methods with patients who have co-existing medical illnesses (for a review, *see* reference 49). For clinicians treating patients with these medical conditions, a high suspicion for the presence of depression will allow early diagnosis and treatment and hopefully offset the numerous adverse consequences of untreated depression.

Relationship of Specific Medical Illnesses and Depression

When major depression is comorbid with other medical illnesses, it affects mortality, morbidity, and cost (58–61). Numerous studies have documented increased risk for morbidity and mortality in depressed medically ill patients; proposed mechanisms to explain this have ranged from the behavioral (e.g., treatment nonadherence) to the biological (e.g., neuroendocrine and neuroimmune alterations associated with depression) (62). Although the exact pathophysiologies have eluded the field, increased morbidity and mortality associated with depression in the medically ill warrant attention and intervention in many patient populations. For example, the survival rate for depressed nursing home patients is 10% less at 6 months and 15% less at 1 year compared with nondepressed patients (63). A number of medical illnesses have been the subject of extensive research linking depression and medical complications; some of these are described in more detail below.

Table 1.3   Rates of Depression in Patients with Medical Illness

Medical Illness	Prevalence of Major Depression (%)*
Alzheimer's dementia	11–22
Cancer	6–39
Chronic fatigue syndrome	17
Congestive heart failure	36.5
Coronary artery disease	8–44
Diabetes mellitus	11
End-stage renal disease	5
Fibromyalgia	18
HIV/AIDS	4–35
Multiple sclerosis	54
Myocardial infarction	15–20
Parkinson's disease	10–32
Rheumatoid arthritis	12.5
Stroke	22–50
Traumatic brain injury	27

* Prevalence is reported as a range of rates when more than one study is available for review.
Adapted with permission from McDaniel et al. Depression in patients with cancer: Diagnosis, biology, and treatment. *Arch Gen Psychiatry.* 1995;52:89-99.

Coronary Artery Disease

Depression is common in the setting of coronary artery disease (CAD), with prevalence estimates as high as 20% after a myocardial infarction (64). Depression is also a known risk factor for developing CAD, even after correcting for other risk factors (55,65). A number of classic CAD risk factors are affected negatively by depression (e.g., smoking, obesity, sedentary lifestyle) (20). Likewise, CAD has been shown to be a risk factor for the development of depression, particularly for patients who experience a myocardial infarction (66). Moreover, some risk factors contribute significantly to both depression and CAD (e.g., living alone, bereavement, life stress, low education, low socioeconomic status); thus, the two conditions are linked in numerous ways that increase their rates of comorbidity.

Frasure-Smith and coworkers (67–69) have reported that depression during hospitalization for an acute myocardial infarction significantly increases the subsequent risk of mortality and that the increased risk is largely independent of cardiac disease severity and gender. In earlier research examining the relationship of CAD and depression, the presence of major depression was the best predictor of myocardial infarction, angioplasty, and death in the 12 months after cardiac catheterization; this effect was independent of other well-known predictors such as CAD severity, left ventricular ejection fraction, and smoking (70). One possible explanation may be the exaggerated platelet aggregation documented recently in depressed patients compared with control subjects (71). To date, these reports offer compelling evidence that patients who develop depression after a myocardial infarction are at greater risk for death than medically comparable post–myocardial infarction patients who are not depressed (72).

The clinical implications of these findings suggest that early diagnosis and aggressive treatment of depression is critical for patients with CAD, particularly those who have recently experienced a myocardial infarction. Although antidepressant treatment in general has been shown to be efficacious in this patient population, newer antidepressant agents such as selective serotonin reuptake inhibitors offer effective antidepressant treatment without the cardiac side effects (e.g., delayed cardiac conduction) of tricyclic antidepressants (73).

Cancer
Depression frequently occurs in patients with cancer; however, the prevalence varies widely depending on such variables as tumor type and disease stage. For cancers that originate in the pancreas and the oropharynx, the prevalence approaches 50% (62). Knowledge of known predictors of depression in patients with cancer can help with early detection and treatment. Severity of medical illness, presence of pain, deficits in social support, and the perception of poor quality of life have been found to be frequently associated with the co-occurrence of depression and cancer (74,75). A number of clinical trials that have included patients with various cancer types have found that antidepressant treatment is well-tolerated and efficacious and that the treatment results in improved quality of life (53). Moreover, adjunctive antidepressant treatment is sometimes helpful in treating pain and anorexia associated with cancer (76) and in controlling symptoms of chemotherapy such as restlessness and insomnia. Because some chemotherapeutic agents may also cause depression (e.g., vincristine, vinblastine, procarbazine, L-asparaginase, interferon, tamoxifen), the differential diagnosis for depression in patients with cancer should include a careful examination of current medications.

HIV Infection
Depression is a common psychiatric complication seen in patients with HIV infection. Depressive symptoms are particularly prevalent as infection progresses to AIDS; fatigue and insomnia, common complaints, are frequently neurovegetative symptoms of HIV-related depression and should

not be attributed automatically to HIV infection itself (77,78). Numerous controlled clinical trials have documented the efficacy and tolerability of antidepressants in patients with HIV infection, including those with advanced disease (52,79). Sudies have also documented enhanced quality of life as a result of HIV-related depression treatment (52).

Treatment of depression is critical in patients with HIV infection for a number of reasons. Depression has been associated with early disease progression and mortality; untreated depression has been associated with increased HIV-related risk behaviors; and depressed patients are less likely to adhere to complex regimens of antiretroviral medications (40,80,81). Lack of adherence not only renders medical treatment ineffective but may also give rise to new strains of HIV with viral resistance (82). In patients with HIV infection in which underrecognition and undertreatment of comorbid depression pose so many complications, diagnosis and treatment of depression are critical components of comprehensive care.

Stroke

Depression has been associated with a wide range of neurological disorders, with the depression that occurs after stroke being the one most commonly studied. Estimates of the prevalence of depression in poststroke patients ranges form 30% to 50% (83–86). Patients studied at 6 months after a stroke have been shown to have a higher prevalence of depression compared with patients initially hospitalized, suggesting that the early months of post-stroke recovery are a particularly vulnerable time for the development of depression. Lesion location is probably a significant factor in depression associated with stroke; higher frequency and severity of depression have been reported in patients with left hemisphere versus right-hemisphere lesions, and higher frequency has been associated with left anterior lesions (83–85). A number of studies, including double-blind trials, have shown that antidepressants are effective in the treatment of post-stroke depression. Like many other medical conditions, depression is associated with increased mortality among patients who experience a stroke. Morris and coworkers (87) reported that depressed patients were 3.4 times more likely to die during a 10-year period than patients without depression; among their depressed patients, those with fewer social contacts were particularly vulnerable, with a mortality rate as high as 90%.

Chronic Pain

Chronic pain syndromes are frequently associated with comorbid depression, including low back pain, headaches, post-traumatic pain, and neuropathic pain syndromes. The prevalence of depression in patients with chronic pain syndromes has been documented to be as high as 43% (88). A significant portion of these patients concurrently abuse psychoactive substances and have a previous history of depression and substance abuse predating the onset of their pain syndromes. Denial and masking of depressive symptoms with narcotics and benzodiazepines may obscure depression in patients who have chronic pain; however, diagnosis and treatment are critical because these patients are at significantly increased risk of suicide compared with other depressed patients (89,90). A number of controlled trials have documented that patients with chronic pain and depression generally respond to therapeutic interventions, including antidepressant medications and psychotherapy; treatment response includes both alleviation of depressive symptoms and better pain management (91).

Major Depression and Somatization

Major depression and somatization are linked in numerous ways in medically ill patients. Up to 50% of patients who present in primary care settings have no diagnosable medical illness (34). Only 41% of patient problems are attributed to clear organic diagnoses, and the most common single "diagnosis" in primary care settings is nonsickness (92). Although patients with physical complaints but no medical diagnosis are often considered the "worried well" by primary care providers, many studies demonstrate that these patients have a high prevalence of undiagnosed anxiety and depressive disorders (93).

More than 50% of primary care patients with psychiatric illness have been shown to present with somatic complaints, and researchers have demonstrated that somatization is the main reason for misdiagnosis of psychiatric illness in primary care settings (94,95). Patients with major depression have significantly more somatic complaints on a medical review of systems, even when controlling for medical illness, and this is especially true for pain symptoms (10). Depression is a frequent comorbid condition in patients with chronic fatigue syndrome and fibromyalgia (51). In general, there appears to be a linear relationship between the number of unexplained physical symptoms and the chance that a patient is depressed (24,96).

Clinicians unaware of these common somatized presentations may fail to recognize and properly treat depression. Often, depression leads to amplification of physical symptoms associated with chronic medical conditions by manifesting as physical complaints, which can cause both patients and clinicians to pursue unnecessary laboratory tests and medication changes. Numerous controlled trials show that antidepressant medications are effective in reducing somatic symptoms that accompany depression (Case 1.2). However, there is also evidence that a high level of somatization is a marker of more severe depression and a predictor of less likelihood of response to treatment (97). These findings indicate the importance of major depression as a possible differential diagnosis for patients with unexplained somatic complaints, rather than as a diagnosis of exclusion.

CASE 1.2   *Depression and somatic symptoms*

A man 36 years of age with no previous significant medical history began making frequent office visits to his primary care physician with vague complaints of abdominal cramping, diarrhea, and nervousness. After dietary changes and antidiarrheal medications failed to relieve his symptoms, a gastroenterology consultation was obtained that included endoscopy and an extensive battery of radiography and laboratory studies. All of the patient's tests were normal; however, the gastroenterology consultant noted that the patient seemed unusually nervous and irritable. On further evaluation by his primary care physician, the patient revealed a 2-month history of increasing symptoms of depression, irritability, inability to experience pleasure, insomnia, and fatigue accompanying his vague abdominal symptoms. The patient was educated about symptoms of depression and started on an antidepressant, and his psychological and physical symptoms resolved during the next 4 to 6 weeks as he was titrated to a therapeutic dosage.

Medical Causes of Depression

In some cases, depression in medically ill patients does not simply co-occur but is a pathophysciological manifestation of a specific medical condition or side effect of a medication; in such cases the depression is considered a mood disorder caused by the medical condition or the psychoactive substance (98). This condition differs from the earlier described depressive states that commonly co-occur with specific medical illnesses because depression caused by medical conditions or medications can be explained by the underlying causative factor; in other words, treating the medical condition or discontinuing the medication usually results in resolution of the depressive symptoms (Case 1.3).

A number of scenarios should lead clinicians to suspect an underlying medical etiology in depressed patients. For example, vegetative symptoms vastly disproportionate to mood disturbance (e.g., 50-lb weight loss with only moderate dysphasia), objective signs of neurological dysfunction (e.g., presence of Babinski reflex), cognitive dysfunction on mental status examination, and most importantly failure to respond to antidepressants treatment. Generally, clinicians should suspect an underlying medical etiology for depression in any patient over 45 years of age with no previous psychiatric history (99).

Various medical illnesses (e.g., endocrinopathies, stroke, chronic viral infections), medications (e.g., beta blockers, alpha-methyldopa, reserpine, chemotherapeutic agents, corticosteroids), and recreational drugs (e.g., cocaine, alcohol) have been linked causally to depressive syndromes (13,100–103). A comprehensive list of medical illnesses and substances commonly reported to be associated causally with depression is given in Table 1.4.

Table 1.4   Medical Illness and Substances That Commonly Cause Depression

Medical Illnesses	Substances
• Cancer (especially pancreatic cancer)	• Acyclovir
• Cerebrovascular disease (stroke)	• Alcohol
• Collagen-vascular disease (systemic lupus erythematosus)	• Amphotericin B
• Endocrinopathies (Cushing's syndrome, Addison's disease, hyperthyroidism, and hypothyroidism)	• Anabolic steroids
	• Analgesics (codeine, oxycodone)
	• Antihypertensives (reserpine, methyldopa, propranolol)
• End-stage renal disease	• Baclofen
• Head injury	• Barbiturates
• Lead poisoning	• Chemotherapeutic agents (vincristine, vinblastine, procarbazine, L-asparaginase, interferon, tamoxifen)
• Metabolic disorders (calcium, potassium, sodium, magnesium, phosphate, uremia)	• Cimetidine
• Movement disorders (Parkinson's disease, Huntington's disease)	• Clonidine
• Multiple sclerosis	• Corticosteroids
• Normal pressure hydrocephalus	• Cocaine
• Pernicious anemia (B_{12} deficiency)	• Cycloserine
• Postencephalitis	• Dapsone
• Viral illnesses (HIV/AIDS, hepatitis, mononucleosis, influenza, Epstein-Barr virus)	• Diazepam
	• Digitalis
	• Disopyramide
	• Disulfiram
	• Estrogens
	• Ethionamide
	• Fluoroquinoline antibiotics
	• Guanethidine
	• Histamine antagonists
	• Isotretinoin
	• Levodopa
	• Marijuana
	• Mefloquine
	• Methyldopa
	• Metoclopramide
	• Metrizamide
	• Metronidazole
	• Narcotics
	• Nonsteroidal anti-inflammatory drugs
	• Pergolide
	• Phencyclidine hydrochloride (PCP)
	• Phenylpropanolamine
	• Progestins
	• Sedative-hypnotics
	• Sulfonamides
	• Thiazide diuretics

Republished with permission from McDaniel et al. Assessment of depression and grief reactions in the medically ill. In Stoudemire A, Fogel BS, Greenberg D, eds. *Psychiatric Care of the Medical Patient*, 2nd edition. New York: Oxford University Press; (in press).

CASE 1.3 *Medical causes of major depression*

A woman 47 years of age with no previous psychiatric history reported to her primary care physician that she was "struggling with depression." After a thorough evaluation revealed no recent psychosocial stressors and no previous history of major depression, her physician inquired about physical symptoms in search of an underlying medical etiology. The patient revealed she had gained 20 pounds during the past 3 months, felt lethargic much of the time, and had experienced difficulty sleeping. Routine laboratory testing revealed that the patient was hypothyroid (TSH = 20 µIU/L, T_4 = 1.8 µg/dL). Within 6 to 8 weeks after thyroid replacement therapy, the patient's depressive symptoms resolved without the need for antidepressant medication.

Conclusions

This chapter has outlined the frequent occurrence of major depression in medically ill patients, and it has highlighted numerous potential adverse consequences of depression. Early detection and adequate treatment of depression among medically ill patients must be made a high priority to avoid the associated negative consequences.

Efficacious treatments for major depression are widely available. Through controlled studies, treatment of major depression has been clearly documented to be effective in medically ill patient (104,105). Treating depressed medically ill patients improves physical, mental, and social functioning, and aggressive approaches toward recognition, diagnosis, and treatment are warranted to minimize suffering, improve overall function and quality of life, promote treatment adherence, limit inappropriate use of health care resources, and diminish morbidity and mortality.

Recommendations

- Clinicians should maintain a high index of suspicion for major depression in patients with medical illnesses, because many illnesses cause or co-occur with depression and many medications that are used to treat medical illnesses can cause depression.
- Depression should be considered in the differential diagnosis of unexplained somatic symptoms, not merely as a diagnosis of exclusion.

▦ ▦ ▦

Key Points

- Depression is a common condition in the medically ill.

- Numerous negative consequences are associated with depression, including nonadherence, medical treatment, increased use of health care services, and suicide.

- In some medically ill patients (e.g., those who have experienced a recent myocardial infarction), depression is associated with increased morbidity and mortality.

- Inexplicable symptoms are often presentations of major depression, particularly in medically ill and geriatric patients.

- Some medical conditions and medications cause depressive syndromes.

▦ ▦ ▦

REFERENCES

1. **Boswell EB, Stoudemire A.** Major depression in the primary care setting. *Am J Med.* 1996;101(Suppl 6A):3S-9S.
2. **Brody DS, Thompson TL, Larson DB, et al.** Recognizing and managing depression in primary care. *Gen Hosp Psychiatry.* 1995;17:93-107.
3. **Crum RM, Cooper-Patrick L, Ford D.** Depressive symptoms among general medical patients: prevalence and one year outcome. *Psychosom Med.* 1994;56:109-117.
4. **Glass RM.** Treating depression as a recurrent or chronic disease. *JAMA.* 1999; 281:83-84.
5. **Kupfer DJ.** Long-term treatment of depression. *J Clin Psychiatry.* 1991;52(suppl 5):28-34.
6. **Cassem EH.** Depressive disorders in the medically ill: an overview. *Psychosomatics.* 1995;36:S2-S10.
7. **Cross-National Collaborative Group.** The challenging rate of major depression. *JAMA.* 1992;268:3098-3115.
8. **Lebowitz BD, Pearson JL, Schneider LS, et al.** Diagnosis and treatment of depression in late life: consensus statement update. *JAMA.* 1997;278:1186-1190.
9. **Cole MG, Bellavance F.** Review: Few elderly inpatients who are depressed improve. *CMAJ.* 1997;157:1055-1060.
10. **Katon WJ, Sullivan MD.** Depression and chronic medical illness. *J Clin Psychiatry.* 1990;51(6 Suppl):S3-S11.
11. **Pincus HA, Tanielian TL, Marcus SC, et al.** Prescribing trends in psychotropic medications: primary care, psychiatry, and other medical specialties. *JAMA.* 1998;279:526-531.

12. **Lustman PJ, Griffith LS, Freedland KE, Clouse RE.** The course of major depression in diabetes. *Gen Hosp Psychiatry.* 1997;19:138-143.

13. **Rouchelle AM, Pounds R, Tierney JG.** Depresssion. In Rundell JR, Wise MG, eds. *Textbook of Consultation-Liaison Psychiatry.* Washington DC: American Psychiatric Press; 1996:310-345.

14. **Wells KB, Katon W, Rogers B, Camp P.** Use of minor tranquilizers and antidepressant medications by depressed outpatients: results from the medical outcome study. *Am J Psychiatry.* 1994;151:694-700.

15. **Katon W, Schulberg H.** Epidemiology of depression in primary care. *Gen Hosp Psychiatry.* 1992;14:237-247.

16. **Depression Guideline Panel.** Clinical Practice Guideline Number 5: Depression in Primary Care. Volume 2: Treatment of Major Depression. Rockville, MD: US Dept of Health and Human Services, Agency for Health Policy and Research; 1993. AHCPR publication 93-0550.

17. **Fulop G, Strain JJ, Vita J, et al.** Impact of psychiatric co-morbidity on length of hospital stay for medical/surgical patients: a preliminary report. *Am J Psychiatry.* 1987;144:878-882.

18. **Stoudemire A, Thompson TL.** Medication noncompliance: systematic approaches to evaluation and intervention. *Gen Hosp Psychiatry.* 1983;5:233-239.

19. **Surridge DHC, Williams-Erdahl DL, Lawson JS, et al.** Psychiatric aspects of diabetes mellitus. *Br J Psychiatry.* 1984;145:269-276.

20. **Blumenthal JS, Williams RS, Wallace AG, et al.** Physiological and psychological variables predict compliance to prescribed exercise therapy in patients recovering from myocardial infarction. *Psychosom Med.* 1982;44:519-527.

21. **Singh N, Squier C, Sivek C, et al.** Determinanats of compliance with antiretroval therapy in patients with human immunodeficiency virus: prospective assessment with implications for enhancing compliance. *AIDS Care.* 1996;8;261-269.

22. **Mohr DC, Goodkin DE, Likosky W, et al.** Treatment of depression improves adherence to interferon beta-1b therapy for multiple sclerosis. *Arch Neurology.* 1997;54:531-533.

23. **Katon WJ, Walker EA.** Medically unexplained symptoms in primary care. *J Clin Psychiatry.* 1998:59(Suppl 20);15-21.

24. **Saravay SM, Lavin M.** Psychiatric comorbity and lenth of stay in the general hospital: a critical review of outcome studies. *Psychosomatics.* 1994;35:233-252.

25. **Jonsson B, Bebbington PE.** What price depression? The cost of depression and the cost-effectiveness of pharmacological treatment. *Br J Psychiatry.* 1994;164:665-673.

26. **Verbosky LA, Franco K, Zrull JP.** The relationship between depression and length of stay in general hospital patients. *J Clin Psychiatry.* 1993;54:177-181.

27. **Gerber PD, Barrett JE, Barrett JA, et al.** The relationship of presenting physical complaints to depressive symptoms in primary care patients. *J Gen Intern Med.* 1992;2:170-173.

28. **Katon WJ, VonKorff M, Lin E, et al.** Distressed high utilizers of medical care. DSM-III-R diagnoses and treatment needs. *Gen Hosp Psychiatry.* 1990;12:355-362.

29. **Keller MB, Klerman G, Lavori P, et al.** Treatment received by depressed patients. *JAMA.* 1982;248:1848-1855.

30. **Greenberg PE, Stiglin LE, Finkelstein SN, Berndt ER.** The economic burden of depression in 1990. *J Clin Psychiatry.* 1993;54:405-418.

31. **Panzarino PJ.** The costs of depression: direct and indirect; treatment versus non-treatment. *J Clin Psychiatry.* 1998;59(Suppl 20):S11-S14.

32. **Hall RCW, Wise MG.** The clinical and financial burden of mood disorders: cost and outcome. *Psychosomatics.* 1995;36:S11-S18.

33. **Kroenke K, Spitzer RL, Williams JBW, et al.** Physical symptoms in primary care: predictors of psychiatric disorders and functional impairment. *Arch Fam Med.* 1994;3:774-779.

34. **Wells KB, Stewart A, Hays RD, et al.** The functioning and well-being of depressed patients: results from the Medical Outcomes Study. *JAMA.* 1989;262:914-919.

35. **Mintz J, Mintz LI, Arruda MH, Hwang S.** Treatments of depression and the functional capacity to work. *Arch Gen Psychiatry.* 1992;49:761-768.

36. **Levenson JL, McDaniel JS, Stoudemire A, Moran M.** Psychological factors affecting medical conditions. In Hales RE, Yudofsky SC, Talbot JA, eds. *American Psychiatric Press Textbook of Psychiatry,* Third Edition. Washington, DC: American Psychiatric Press; 1999:635–61.

37. **Stoudemire A, McDaniel JS.** History, classifacation, and current trends in psychosomatic medicine. In Kaplan HI, Saddock BJ, eds. *Comprehensive Textbook of Psychiatry/VII,* Seventh Edition. Baltimore: Williams and Wilkins; 2000:1765–74.

38. **Joe GW, Knezek L, Watson D, Simpson DD.** Depression and decision-making among intravenous drug users. *Psychol Rep.* 1991;68:339-347.

39. **Stiffman AF, Dore P, Earles F, Cunningham R.** The influence of mental health problems on AIDS-related risk behaviors in young adults. *J Nerv Ment Dis.* 1992; 180:314-320.

40. **Kelly JA, Murphy DA, Bahr GR, et al.** Factors associated with severity of depression and high-risk sexual behavior among persons with human immunodeficiency virus infection. *Health Psychol.* 1993;12:215-219.

41. **Hirschfeld RMA, Keller MB, Panico S, et al.** The National Depressive and Manic-Depressive Association concensus statement on the undertreatment of depression. *JAMA.* 1997;277:333-340.

42. **Marzuk PM, Tardiff K, Leon AC, et al.** HIV seroprevalence among suicide victims in New York City, 1991-1993. *Am J Psychiatry.* 1997;154:1720-1725.

43. **Hughes D, Kleespies P.** *Suicide in the Medically Ill.* Paper presented at the National Suicide Prevention Conference, Reno, Nevada, 1998.

44. **Conwell Y.** Management of suicidal behavior in the elderly. *Psychiatr Clin North Am.* 1997;20:667-683.

45. **Rimer Z, Rutz W, Pihlgren H.** Depression and suicide in Gotland: an intensive study of all suicides before and after a depression-training program for general practitioners. *J Affective Dis.* 1995;35:147-152.

46. **Whitlock F.** Suicide and physical illness. In Ray A, ed. *Suicide.* Baltimore: Williams and Wilkins; 1986.

47. **MacKenzie T, Polkin M.** Medical illness and suicide. In Blumenthal S, Kupfer D, eds. *Suicide over the Life Cycle: Risk Factors, Assessment, and Treatment of Suicidal Patients.* Washington, DC: American Psychiatric Press; 1990.

48. **Chochinov HM, Wilson KG, Enns M, Lander S.** "Are you depressed?" Screening for depression in the terminally ill. *Am J Psychiatry.* 1997;154:674-676.

49. **Cohen-Cole SA, Kaufman KG.** Major depression in physical illness: diagnosis, prevalence, and antidepressant treatment (a ten-year review: 1982-1992). *Depression.* 1993;1:181-204.

50. **Stoudemire A, ed.** *Psychological Factors Affecting Medical Conditions.* Washington, DC: American Psychiatric Press; 1995.

51. **Jorge CM, Goodnick PJ.** Chronic fatigue syndrome and depression: biological differentiation and treatment. *Psychiatr Ann.* 1997;27:365-371.

52. **Stober DR, Schwartz JAJ, McDaniel JS, Abrams RF.** Depression and HIV disease: prevalence, correlates, and treatment. *Psychiatr Ann.* 1997;27:353-359.

53. **McDaniel JS, Musselman DL, Nemeroff CB.** Cancer and depression: theory and treatment. *Psychiatr Ann.* 1997;27:360-364.

54. **Goodnick PJ.** diabetes mellitus and depression: issues in theory and treatment. *Psychiatr Ann.* 1997;27:353-359.

55. **Shapiro PA, Lidagoster L, Glassman AH.** Depression and heart disease. *Psychiatr Ann.* 1997;27:353-359.

56. **Maldonado JL, Fernanadez F, Trevino-Garza ES, Levy JK.** Depression and its treatment in neurological disease. *Psychiatr Ann.* 1997;27:347-352.

57. **Koenig HG.** Depression in hospitalized older patients with congestive heart failure. *Gen Hosp Pschiatry.* 1998;20:29-43.

58. **Malzberg B.** Morality among patients with involution melancholia. *Am J Psychiatry.* 1937;93:1231-1238.

59. **Kessler LG, Clearly PD, Burke JD.** Psychiatric disorders in primary care: results of a follow-up study. *Arch Gen Psychiatry.* 1985;42:583-587.

60. **Shapiro S, Skinner EA, Kessler LG, et al.** Utilization of health and mental health services: three Epidemologic Catchment Area sites. *Arch Gen Psychiatry.* 1984;41:971-978.

61. **Wuslin LR, Vaillant GE, Wells VE.** A systematic review of morality of depression. *Psychosom Med.* 1999;61:6-17.

62. **McDaniel JS, Musselman DL, Porter MR, et al.** Depression in patients with cancer: diagnosis, biology, and treatment. *Arch Gen Psychiatry.* 1995;52:89-99.

63. **Rovner BW, German PS, Brant LJ, et al.** Depression and morality in nursing homes. *JAMA.* 1991;265:993-996.

64. **Evans DL, Staab JP, Petitto JM, et al.** Depression in the medical setting: biopsychosocial interactions and treatment considerations. *J Clin Psychiatry.* 1999;60 (Suppl 4):40-55.

65. **Goldstein MG, Niaura R.** Cardiovascular disease, Part I: coronary artery disease and sudden death. In: Stoudemire A, ed. *Psychological Factors Affecting Medical Conditions.* Washington, DC: American Psychiatric Press; 1995:19-38.

66. **Dwight MM, Stoudemire A.** Effects of depressive disorders on coronary artery disease: a review. *Harvard Rev Psychiatry.* 1997;5:115-122.

67. **Frasure-Smith N, Lesperance F, Juneau M, et al.** Gender, depression, and one-year prognosis after myocardial infarction. *Psychosom Med.* 1999;61:26-37.

68. **Frasure-Smith N, Lesperance F, Talajic M.** Depression following myocardial infarction: impact on six-month survival. *JAMA.* 1993;270:1819-1825.

69. **Frasure-Smith N, Lesperance F, Talajic M.** Depression and 18-month prognosis following myocardial infarction. *Circulation.* 1995;91:999-1005.

70. **Carney RM, Rich MW, Freedland KE, et al.** Major depressive disorder predicts cardiac events in patients with coronary artery disease. *Psychosom Med.* 1988;50:627-633.

71. **Musselman Dl, Tomer A, Manatunga AK, et al.** Exaggerated platelet reactivity in major depression. *Am J Psychiatry.* 1996;153:1313-1317.

72. **Glassman AH, Shapiro PA.** Depression and the course of coronary artery disease. *Am J Psychiatry.* 1998;155:4-11.

73. **Roose SP, Laghrissi-Thode F, Kennedy JS, et al.** Comparison of paroxetine and nortriptyline in depressed patients with ischemic heart disease. *JAMA.* 1998;279:287-291.

74. **Noyes R, Kathol RG.** Depression and cancer. *Psychiatr Dev.* 1986;2:77-100.

75. **Godding PR, McAnulty RD, Wittrock DA, et al.** Predictors of depression among male cancer patients. *J Nerv Ment Dis.* 1995;183:95-98.

76. **Lesko LM, Massie MJ, Holland J.** Oncology. In Stoudemire A, Fogel B, eds. *Psychiatric Care of the Medical Patient.* New York: Oxford University Press; 1993: 565-590.

77. **Lyketsos CG, Hoover DR, Guccione M, et al.** Changes in depressive symptoms as AIDS develops. *Am J Psychiatry.* 1996:153;1430-1437.

78. **Perkins DO, Leserman J, Stern RA, et al.** Somatic symptoms and HIV infection: relationship to depressive symptoms and indicators of HIV disease. *Am J Psychiatry.* 1995;152:1776-1781.

79. **Schwartz JAJ, McDaniel JS.** A double-blind comparison of fluoxetine and desipramine in the treatment of depressed women with advanced HIV disease: a pilot study. *Depression and Anxiety.* In press.

80. **Evans DL, Leserman J, Perkins DO, et al.** Severe life stress as a predictor of early disease progression in HIV infection. *Am J Psychiatry.* 1997;154:603-634.

81. **Mayne TJ, Vittinghoff E, Chesney MA, et al.** Depressive affect and survival among gay and bisexual men infected with HIV. *Arch Intern Med.* 1996;156:2233-2238.

82. **Voelker R.** Protease inhibitors bring new social, clinical uncertainties to HIV care. *JAMA.* 1997;277:1182-1184.

83. **Robinson RG, Price TR.** Post-stroke depressive disorders: a follow up study of 103 patients. *Stroke.* 1982;13:635-641.

84. **Robinson RG, Starr LB, Kubos KL, Price TR, et al.** A two year longitudinal study of post-stroke mood disorder: findings during the initial evaluation. *Stroke.* 1983;14:736-741.

85. **Robinson RG, Kubos KL, Starr LB, et al.** Mood disorders in stroke patients–importance of lesion location. *Brain.* 1984;107:81-93.

86. **Robinson RG, Bolduc P, Price TR.** A two-year longitudinal study of poststroke depression: diagnosis and outcome at one and two year follow-up. *Stroke.* 1987;18:837-843.

87. **Morris PL, Robinson RG, Andrzejewski P, et al.** Association of depression with 10 year post-stroke mortality. *Am J Psychiatry.* 1993;150:124-129.

88. **Katon W, Egan K, Miller D.** Chronic pain: lifetime psychiatric diagnoses and family history. *Am J Psychiatry.* 1985;142:1156-1160.

89. **Bouckoms AJ.** Chronic pain: neuropsychopharmacology and adjunctive psychiatric treatment. In: Rundell JR, Wise MG, eds. *Textbook of Consultation-Liaison Psychiatry.* Washington DC: American Psychiatric Press; 1996:1006-1037.

90. **Breibart W.** Suicide risk and pain in cancer and AIDS patients. In: Chapman CR, Foley KM, eds. *Current and Emerging Issues in Cancer Pain: Research and Practice.* New York: Raven Press. 1993:49-66.

91. **Sullivan MJ, Reesor K, Mikail S, Fisher R.** The treatment of depression in chronic low back pain: review and recommendations. *Pain.* 1992;50:5-13.

92. **Brown JW, Robertson LS, Kosa J, Alpert JJ.** A study of general practice in Massachusetts. *JAMA.* 1971;216:301-306.

93. **Katon WJ, Walker EQ.** Medically unexplained symptoms in primary care. *J Clin Psychiatry.* 1998;59(Suppl 20):15-21.

94. **Wilson DR, Widmer RB, Cadoret RJ, Judiesch K.** Somatic symptoms: a major feature of depression in a family practice. *J Affect Disord.* 1983;5:199-207.

95. **Bridges KW, Goldberg DP.** Somatic presentation of DSM-III psychiatric disorders in primary care. *J Psychosom Res.* 1985;29:563-569.

96. **Simon GE, Katon W, Rutter C, et al.** Impact of improved depression treatment in primary care on daily functioning and disability. *Psychol Med.* 1998;28:693-701.

97. **McDaniel JS, Brown FW, Cole SA.** Assessment of depression and grief reactions in the medically ill. In Stoudemire A, Fogel BS, Greenberg D, eds. *Psychiatric Care of the Medical Patient,* 2nd edition. New York: Oxford University Press; 2000:149–64.

98. **American Psychiatric Association.** *Diagnostic and Statistical Manual of Mental Disorders,* Fourth Edition. Washington, DC: American Psychiatric Press; 1995.

99. **Pies RW.** Medical mimics of depression. *Psychiatr Ann.* 1994;24:519-420.

100. **Maricle RA, Kinzie JD, Lewinsohn P.** Medication-associated depression: a two and one-half year follow-up of a community sample. *Int J Psychiatry Med.* 1988; 18:283-292.

101. **Patten SB.** Propanolol and depression: evidence from the antihypertensive trials. *Can J Psychiatry.* 1990;35:257-259.

102. **Abromowics M.** *Medical Letter.* 1998;40:1020.

103. **Brown TM, Stoudemire A.** *Psychiatric Side Effects of Prescription and Over-the-Counter Medications: Recognition and Management.* Washington DC: American Psychiatric Press; 1998.

104. **Schulbert HC, Katon W, Simon GE, Rush J.** Treating major depression in primary care: a update of the agency for health care policy and practice guidelines. *Arch Gen Psychiatry.* 1998;55:1121-1127.

105. **Lyketsos CG, Taragano F, Treisman CG, Paz J.** Major depression and its response to sertraline in primary care vs. psychiatric office practice patients: results of an open-label trial in Argentina. *Psychosomatics.* 1999;40:70-75.

KEY REFERENCES

Cohen-Cole SA, Kaufman KG. Major depression in physical illness: diagnosis, prevalence, and antidepressant treatment (a ten-year review: 1982-1992). *Depression.* 1993;1:181–204.

This systematic review of the literature examines issues of diagnosis, prevalence, and antidepressant treatment trials in patients with major depression and co-occurring medical illness.

Depression Guideline Panel. Clinical Practice Guideline Number 5: Depression in Primary Care. Volume 2: Treatment of Major Depression Rockville, MD: US Dept of Health and Human Services, Agency for Health Policy and Research; 1993. AHCPR publication 93-0550.

This document offers well-defined, evidence-based guidelines for the diagnosis and management of depression in primary care settings.

Katon WJ, Sullivan MD. Depression and chronic medical illness. *J Clin Psychiatry.* 1990;51(6 suppl):S3–11.

This review is a critical evaluation of the prevalence and correlates of depression in patients with chronic medical conditions.

Rouchell AM, Pounds R, Tierney JG. Depression. In Rundell JR, Wise MG, eds. *Textbook of Consultation-Liaison Psychiatry.* Washington, DC: American Psychiatric Press; 1996:310–1345.

This comprehensive review of depression among medical and surgical patients is outlined in textbook format for consultation-liaison psychiatrists.

Stoudemire A, ed. *Psychological Factors Affecting Medical Conditions.* Washington, DC: American Psychiatric Press; 1995.

A thorough review of the range of psychological factors that affect medical conditions, including the role of depression in numerous medical illnesses.

2

■ ■ ■

Epidemiology, Risk Factors, and Prevention

Caroline Carney Doebbeling, MD, MS

"Depression superimposes itself over a particular being with a particular family history, gene pool, temperament, and set of values."

Prevalence Studies

Classification of Depression

The classification of depressive symptoms in the United States dates to the 1880 census in which melancholia was one of seven categories of mental illness recorded in the population. In 1952, the first *Diagnostic and Statistical Manual of Mental Disorders* (DSM) was published, establishing criteria by which mental disorders could be diagnosed and studied more uniformly. The DSM is currently in its fourth edition (DSM-IV) (1). The manual classifies mood disorders into the following broad categories: 1) major depressive disorder, 2) dysthymic disorder, 3) bipolar disorders, 4) mood disorders caused by general medical conditions or substances, and 5) adjustment disorder with depressed mood. Use of diagnostic criteria is of utmost importance in studying depressive disorders. DSM diagnostic criteria, much like case definitions for rheumatic fever or chronic fatigue syndrome, seek to ensure that clinicians and researchers speak the same language about the same condition. For instance, one must determine if the condition is episodic major depression, minor or subsyndromal depression, or the chronic persistent state of depression known as dysthymia. The correct classification of affective symptoms provides the essential foundation for the study of these disorders, regardless of the setting.

In the past, major depression was subdivided into "reactive" and "endogenous" depressions. Endogenous depressions were considered to be those that occur as a result of a spontaneous neurobiological "imbalance" or a genetic predisposition. Reactive depressions were thought to be those that occur after a stressful life event such as death, divorce, or loss of employment. This descriptive dichotomy, however, assumed that the apparent difference in origin translated into differences in evaluation and treatment. Epidemiologic and clinical studies have not supported the distinction as being meaningful. Stressful life events, genetic predisposition, and other psychosocial and biological factors may contribute in varying degrees to the development of a depressive episode, but reactive depressions are not fundamentally different than endogenous depressions in phenomenology or treatment response. Clinicians should consider the role that life events and other factors play in the development of major depression and dispense with the notion that two forms of the disorder exist.

Limitations of Prevalence Studies

The determination of prevalence (the proportion of individuals in a given population who have a particular disease at a point in or during an interval of time) and incidence (the number of new cases that develop in a population of individuals at risk during a specified time interval) in depression is problematic. Despite advances in diagnostic criteria, prevalence studies are still limited by the lack of uniformity in the selection of instruments by researchers to survey study populations. Currently, there is a variety of statistically reliable and valid screening (e.g., PRIME-MD) and diagnostic (e.g., Structured Clinical Interview for DSM-III-R) instruments for major depression and other psychiatric disorders. The instruments range from patient-administered self-report instruments to surveys that must be administered by trained clinicians. Additionally, the instruments may be applied in clinical or research settings.

When critically evaluating the literature on prevalence and incidence, one must first understand that the definition of depression in research is not always standardized. For instance, researchers may: 1) use different instruments (e.g., Center for Epidemiological Studies Depression Scale [CES-D] or Beck Depression Inventory [BDI]; 2) include subthreshold or minor depression; or 3) survey only a demographically limited sample of subjects. Most studies, for instance, have been performed on select clinical samples; therefore, one may not be able to compare different studies given the different sample populations. Surveys conducted in one population may not be able to be generalized to other populations that differ in composition (e.g., in the number of medically ill, minority, or elderly subjects studied), so the external validity can be affected.

History of Prevalence Studies

Two major studies have been conducted to determine the prevalence of mental disorders in the general population in the United States: the Epidemiological Catchment Area (ECA) study and the National Cormorbidity Survey (NCS). Both provided significant advances in surveying the general population for psychiatric syndromes. Additional studies have evaluated the prevalence of depression in both medical and psychiatric clinical samples.

Before the ECA study, prevalence studies were widely disparate in their results, likely the result of differences in methodology and case definition (2). Earlier international studies using instruments such as the Present State Exam (PSE) and the ICD-9 criteria showed point prevalence per 100 individuals ranging from 3.6 to 4.9 in men and 4.3 to 10.2 in women (3). With the publication of the *Diagnostic and Statistical Manual of Mental Disorders*, Third Edition (DSM-III) (3a), criteria for defining mental disorders became more uniform, making a large-scale epidemiologic survey like the ECA feasible. The sample was composed of community-dwelling individuals 18 to 65 years of age or older in five "catchment areas": New Haven, Baltimore, Durham, Los Angeles, and St. Louis. The samples were weighted to take into account age, gender, and ethnicity in the United States based on the 1980 national population census (4). The overall response rate was approximately 75% (n = 18,571).

After the ECA study, the U.S. Congress mandated the NCS, a study designed to evaluate the prevalence, risk factors, and comorbidity of mental disorders in the noninstitutionalized population of the country. The NCS advanced the study of the epidemiology of mental disorders by basing diagnoses on DSM-III-R criteria, studying risk factors for mental disorders, and examining a sample of the entire country instead of the five catchment areas surveyed in the ECA (5,6). Interviews were conducted between September 1990 and February 1992. Overall, the investigators achieved a response rate of 82.6% (n = 8098). Age, gender, race, educational achievement, marital status, region of residence, and urban habitation closely approximated that of the U.S. population based on the National Health Interview Survey in 1989.

Prevalence

In 1988, the findings for 2-week, 1-month, 6-month, 1-year, and lifetime prevalence were published for all five catchment areas in the ECA study (7). Mean rates were as follows: 2-week, 1.5%; 1-month, 1.6%; 6-month, 2.2%; 1-year, 2.6%; lifetime, 4.4% (Table 2.1). Lifetime rates for dysthymia were 3.1% (range 2.1%–4.2%).

Table 2.1   Prevalence of Major Depression in the General Population

Study Site	Year Published	1 Year (%)	Lifetime (%)
U.S. ECA	1994	2.6	4.4
U.S. NCS	1998	4.9	17.1
Canada	1988	3.2*	8.6
Puerto Rico	1987	3.0*	4.6
Italy	1990	5.2	—
Korea	1987	—	3.4
New Zealand	1990	5.3	12.6
Switzerland	1984	7.0	—
Belgium	1997	5.0*	—
France	1997	9.1*	—
Germany	1997	3.8*	—
Netherlands	1997	6.9*	—
Spain	1997	6.2*	—
United Kingdom	1997	9.9	—
Taiwan	1996	0.8	1.5
Lebanon	1996	5.8	19.0

* Six-month prevalence.
ECA = Epidemiological Catchment Area study; NCS = National Comorbidity Survey.
Adapted from Lepine et al. (12); Paykel (3); Weissman (22).

The NCS results were slightly different, showing a higher prevalence than the ECA study (5,6). Overall, 4.9% (*n* = 394) of subjects (men and women, all races and ages) met criteria for a current (30-day) major depressive episode. Of these, major depression was the only diagnosis in 172 respondents. The remaining 222 had major depression occurring with another psychiatric syndrome. Other syndromes commonly included generalized anxiety disorder, substance and alcohol abuse, and panic disorder.

The NCS study's overall 1-month and lifetime rates were markedly higher than those reported in the ECA study: 17.1% of the sample reported a lifetime episode of major depression. Importantly, the lifetime rates were similar in those subjects 15 to 24 years of age and in subjects 45 to 54 years of age, suggesting either a recall bias, with older subjects failing to remember and report previous episodes of depression, or a cohort effect, with younger individuals having higher lifetime rates of depression (8).

Angst (9) published a comprehensive review of 17 studies that had used operationalized diagnostic criteria for depression. He found 1-year prevalence rates for major depressive disorder (DSM-III criteria) ranging between 2.6% and 6.2% and lifetime rates between 4.4% and 19%. Angst also conducted a prospective study with four waves of interviews conducted over 10 years in Zurich, Switzerland (10). Evaluated prospectively, the 10-year prevalence rates for subjects 20 to 30 years of age were 14.4% for major depression and 0.9% for dysthymia (11). Prospective lifetime rates of major depression in the Zurich study ranged from 16% to 20%. Prospective methodology may be more accurate in determining lifetime prevalence because recall bias and forgetfulness are less likely to influence symptom reports from subjects (11).

The Depression Research in European Society (DEPRES) study was conducted to assess the prevalence of depression in six European countries: Belgium, Germany, France, the Netherlands, Spain, and the United Kingdom (12). The sample was composed of 78,463 adults. Depression defined as major depression, minor depression, and depressive symptoms was found in 13,359 (17%) subjects. Overall, 6.9% of study respondents met criteria for current major depression. Minor depression was noted in 1.8% and depressive symptoms in 8.3%. Women outnumbered men for both major depression and depressive symptoms, which is consistent with other studies.

The Diagnostic Interview Schedule (DIS), the instrument in the ECA study, has been used in a variety of international settings, with results similar to those reported in the United States for affective disorders (3). The 1-year rate per 100 adults ranged from 5.2 to 7.0. Interestingly, the 1-year prevalence was markedly lower in Taiwan (0.6–1.1) than in most other countries.

Depression and Psychiatric Comorbidity

Comorbidity is common in psychiatric disorders. The NCS study revealed that, although 52% of the sample population had no psychiatric diagnosis, 21% had one, 13% had two, and 14% had three or more diagnoses. Women, Hispanics, low socioeconomic groups, major metropolitan inhabitants, and individuals in the 15- to 24-year-old age group seemed to be at higher risk for the presence of three or more disorders (5,6). Clinicians should be aware that when an individual presents with depressive symptoms, the likelihood of another psychiatric disorder being present is quite high.

Alcohol Abuse or Dependency

When evaluating a patient with substance abuse and depressive symptoms, clinicians are often faced with the task of trying to determine which condition is the patient's primary problem. Longitudinal evaluations of individuals with primary depression reveal that alcoholism develops in less than 5% of the patients, a figure similar to the prevalence of alcoholism in the general population (13). The situation changes, however, for individuals with primary alcoholism. At least 24 separate studies support the finding that 10% to 30% of alcoholics develop depressive disorders. The odds ratio (OR) for the development of depression in an alcoholic is 1.7 (13). Women have a higher likelihood of having coexistent depression and alcoholism. The presence of depression in an alcoholic may predict a poorer outcome for the alcoholism. Even in nonalcoholic women, quantity of alcohol consumption is a significant predictor for depressive symptoms and depression (14). Conversely, depression also may predict quantity of consumption in women. The clinician should always inquire about the presence of depressive symptoms in alcoholic patients and the presence of alcohol use in depressed patients.

Depression and Anxiety Disorders

The presence of an anxiety disorder may result in greater medical use, help-seeking behaviors, and medication use. The NCS study revealed lifetime prevalence for panic disorder to be 3.5% and generalized anxiety disorder to be 5.1% (5,6). The presence of any anxiety disorder, which would include phobic disorders, was 24.9%. Thus, anxiety disorders are extremely common in the general population. The ECA study showed that the OR for 6-month comorbidity of panic disorder and depression in the same subject was 21.3 (7) compared with individuals with no mental disorder, whereas the NCS was 14.4.

An analysis using the NCS data that specifically evaluated the relationship between panic attacks, panic disorder, and depression showed that a primary depressive episode predicted the development of panic attacks (15). Conversely, primary panic attacks predicted the development of subsequent major depressive episodes. The OR for panic attacks with depression was 6.2 and for panic disorder with depression 6.8. Kessler and coworkers (6) stressed that primary panic attack is a marker, not a risk factor, for a subsequent primary depressive episode. The clinician should be aware that both panic disorder and depression may commonly occur in the same patient. Treatment options for both conditions are similar.

Prevalence in the Medically Ill

The increased prevalence of major depression in the medically ill has been described frequently (Table 2.2). Primary care providers evaluate and treat a substantial number of patients with depressive symptoms in the United

Table 2.2   Prevalence of Depression in Select Medical Populations

Medical Population	Point Prevalence Range (%)
General outpatients	5–15
Coronary artery disease patients	16–19
Cancer patients	6–39
Stroke patients	22–50
Diabetes mellitus patients	11–24
HIV patients	4–30
Parkinson's disease patients	25–37

States (16). The prevalence of depression and depressive symptoms increases as one moves from the general community to the outpatient and inpatient medical settings (17). Prevalence estimates for major depression range from 5% to 10% of primary care outpatients to 10% to 14% of inpatients. There are two to three times as many patients with depressive symptoms that fall short of major depression criteria and who are considered to have either minor depression or dysthymia (17).

The prevalence rate of depression in the medically ill varies with the medical condition and the methodology selected to define cases. Cohen-Cole and coworkers (18) recently reviewed studies using either structured or semistructured interviews for diagnosis. Prevalence rates for major depression have ranged from as low as 0% for patients with spinal cord injury to 54% in multiple sclerosis (18). This review did not consider the prevalence of dysthymic disorder, minor depression, or depressive symptoms. Winokur (19) suggested that the presentation of depression could be different in individuals with a primary depressive syndrome than in those with depression secondary to a medical illness. Patients presenting with depression secondary to a medical illness compared with patients with primary psychiatric illness generally exhibit the following characteristics: older age of onset, fewer suicidal thoughts and attempts, family history with lower rates of depression and alcohol abuse, physical signs on the mental status examination (e.g., confusion, fatigue, memory deficits), and increased likeliness to respond to (and to improve as a result of) electroconvulsive therapy (19).

The strong role of health and functional ability in the prevalence of depression was observed in the Alameda County study (20), a study of 2417 elderly patients (mean age = 65). A multivariate analysis revealed that the initial apparent age effect was due almost entirely to chronic health problems and functional impairments. The authors concluded that healthy, normally functioning older adults are at no greater risk of depression than are younger adults.

Onset

Mean age of onset of major depression in the ECA study was 27.2 years with no significance differences in age of onset between genders (7). Age of onset differed only slightly by catchment area. The NCS study showed that women in the age group of 10 to 14 years had the highest relative hazard of onset of depression (OR 12.3) (21). A review of 10 international epidemiologic surveys reported that mean age of onset ranged from 24.8 to 34.8 years (22). Clinicians should be aware that depression is a disorder with an early age of initial onset, often first presenting in teenagers. For individuals presenting with first onset of depression in mid- or late-life, the clinician should attempt to elicit a history of previous depressive episodes. The presence or absence of previous episodes may influence duration of treatment or need for a medical evaluation.

Gender Differences

It has long been observed by clinicians that depression occurs more frequently in women than in men. In clinical populations, however, women may be overrepresented because of differences in willingness to seek and accept care. Epidemiologic research supports the perception that the prevalence is higher in women. Data from the ECA study strongly suggested a gender difference in both the prevalence and incidence of major depression (7). At all age ranges and in all five sites, the prevalence was higher in women than in men (female-to-male ratio range 1.9–5.0). Similarly, incidence rates were also nearly two times greater in women than in men (24). The age of onset of major depression was not different between the genders. Klerman and coworkers (24) also reported a similar age of onset for major depression in men and women. Similar to major depression, the lifetime rates for dysthymia were significantly higher in women (female-to-male ratio range 1.5–3.0) (7).

Similar to the ECA study, significant gender differences in the prevalence of major depression were noted in the NCS (5,6). The female-to-male ratio was also approximately 2 to 1 at nearly every age level for both current and lifetime episodes. The higher prevalence in women was noted for whites, blacks, and Hispanics.

The Zurich study also examined gender differences in the prevalence of mood syndromes and DSM III criteria for major depression (10). Across the spectrum from dysphoric mood to full-criteria major depression, the rate of mood syndromes was greater for women than for men. Over time, the level of reporting of women's symptoms remained constant, whereas men had a decreased level of symptom reporting, enhancing gender differences. For major depression, however, the female-to-male ratio remained constant at 2 to 1, similar to studies conducted in the United States (25). Because the sex ratio increased significantly with time after the interview, the authors suggested that women remember past mood fluctuations better than do men. Overall, women with depression reported more avoidant behavior and somatic symptoms, including decreased libido, insomnia, and binge eating, than did men. Work impairment was similar between the two groups for major depression.

Postulated reasons for the gender differences observed in depression have centered on social and biological differences between the sexes. Some authors have postulated that biological changes associated with puberty and onset of menses account for the higher risk of onset for the first episode of depression in female adolescents. This higher risk appears in late adolescence (~10 years of age) and continues through adulthood (26). The difference in adolescents may be enhanced by decreasing rates of depression in adolescent boys. In addition to hormonal factors contributing to the higher risk in women, societal roles may contribute to this as well. Depressed women may worry about their problems more than do men when depressed, thereby amplifying the severity and duration of symptoms (27). Social roles in which women have little autonomy also have been associated with depressive symptoms. Frank (28) has reported that that women have a greater expressivity of symptoms at the same level of severity than do men, thereby making them more likely to meet criteria for diagnosis in a clinical encounter.

Other postulated factors for the differences in prevalence include the longer lengths and frequent recurrences of episodes (prevalence = incidence × length of episode) experienced by women (11).

Cultural Differences

Overall, the ECA study did not find any differences between non-Hispanic whites, Hispanics and non-Hispanic blacks in the prevalence of depression (29). In the NCS study, non-Hispanic blacks had lower current and lifetime prevalence of affective disorders than other groups. Generally, non-Hispanic blacks have lower rates of suicide than non-Hispanic whites. Hispanics had a higher prevalence of depression than all other groups in the NCS. Although previous research indicated that non-Hispanic blacks reported higher levels of distress than non-Hispanic whites, the differences between the two groups were lost when the analysis was controlled for socioeconomic status.

Weissman and coworkers (22) reported the rates of major depression in 10 countries: the United States, Canada, Puerto Rico, France, West Germany, Italy, Lebanon, Taiwan, Korea, and New Zealand (*see* Table 2.1). The lifetime prevalence differed widely, ranging from 1.5 cases per 100 adults in Taiwan to 19.0 cases per 100 adults in Lebanon. Differences in the prevalence of depression among racial and social groups may be related to different cultural expressions of symptoms. In Weissman's review, the symptoms of insomnia and loss of energy were consistent across countries. In some cultures, depressive symptoms may manifest primarily as nonspecific somatic complaints instead of psychological complaints such as low mood or excessive guilt. Additionally, individuals in some cultures may not express mood symptoms openly. This may explain the apparent lower prevalence of depression in the Taiwanese study. In Taiwan, physicians and patients are more likely to attribute depressive symptoms to neurasthenia (30,31). Revaluation of patients given a diagnosis of neurasthenia using Westernized concepts of depressive symptoms showed that the majority suffered from an affective syndrome. A study using the Zung Self-Rating Depression Scale compared elderly Canadian and Japanese men and women (32). The study showed that the Canadians expressed depressed moods more clearly and spontaneously than did the Japanese. Although most studies evaluating Asian populations have reported higher rates of somatization symptoms and lower rates of depression than in non-Asian countries, a recent study using the CES-D in the elderly found no differences between Asian, North American, and European cultures (33). When evaluating depressive symptoms in a patient with potential cultural barriers, clinicians may need to rely on interpretation of symptoms in the context of change in ability to function, collateral history, and lack of objective physical and laboratory examination findings supporting a medical explanation for the symptoms. Additionally, the CES-D may be an effective instrument for evaluating depression in elder Asians.

Cohort Effect

The cohort effect describes the condition in which successive generations have had a higher prevalence of depression. Whether or not a cohort effect truly exists is controversial (34). Many investigators have reported that the prevalence of major depression has increased since World War II (6,35–39). Possible causes include social or environmental factors such as changes in nutrition, urbanization, family structure, the role of women, occupational patterns, or unknown chemical or biological agents (37). Others believe that the apparent cohort effect is an artifact of bias caused by age and memory effects, changes in the meaning and labeling of and attitudes toward emotional phenomena across different birth cohorts, differential mortality and/or institutionalization rates, changing diagnostic criteria, increased recognition and labeling of psychological symptoms, and selective migration (34,40,41). Clinical observations of increased incidence and prevalence of depression may be based in greater recognition and attribution of nonspecific somatic complaints to depressive disorders. More long-term, prospective studies are needed to determine whether or not a cohort effect actually exists (34).

Risk Factors

Commonly cited risk factors for the development of major depression include medical illness, death of a parent during childhood, young age, female gender, divorced or separated marital status, low socioeconomic status, residence in urban settings, previous personal history of depression, and family history of depression (42).

The NCS study delineated several risk factors for the development of depression (8). ORs were calculated for many factors, including age, gender, race, education, income, marital status, employment, religious affiliation, household composition, region of the United States, and urban residence. For depression without other psychiatric comorbidity, the following risk factors emerged with statistically significant ORs: female gender (OR 1.56), employment listed as homemaker (OR 2.83), and nonmarried cohabitation (OR 1.83). Risk factors for depression accompanied by other psychiatric disorders were slightly different and included age 15 to 24 years (OR 3.0), age 35 to 44 years (OR 2.8), female gender (OR 1.56), Hispanic ethnicity (OR 2.31), education 0 to 11 years (OR 6.82), education 12 years (OR 3.45), education 13 to 15 years (OR 3.79), employment listed as homemaker (OR 2.61), and nonmarried cohabitation (OR 2.16). Poverty seems to have a significant negative impact on the development of depression in the United States (43). Socioeconomic status also may influence the prevalence of anxiety disorders (6). Given that socioeconomic status and level of education are closely related, it is difficult to determine which risk factor primarily predisposes to depression. Protective factors may include marital status (8) and working for pay (44). Ethnicity findings have not been consistent between studies (34).

Factors related to depression in adult mothers include socioeconomic disadvantage, single motherhood, and lack of social support (45–47). Adolescent mothers (15–19 years of age) experience high rates of depressive symptoms relative to adult mothers. The effect of age diminishes, however, when factors including income and marital status are controlled (48). Inner-city mothers who self-report poor financial or health status or activity limitation because of illness have been found to have high levels of depressive symptoms (49). Mothers of children with attention deficit–hyperactivity disorder (ADHD) may be at substantially higher risk than other mothers surveyed in the primary care setting. Mothers of children with ADHD had a 17.9% prevalence of major depression and a 20.5% prevalence of minor depression compared with population norms of 4% to 6% and 6% to 14%, respectively (50). Clinicians should screen patients in these groups for depression.

Stressful Life Events

Stressful life events (e.g., the death of loved ones, financial pressures, changes in personal habits or routines) are associated with the subsequent development of depressive episodes (51–53). Stressful life events may be considered either independent or dependent. The former events are those that occur because of factors outside an individual's control, such as a major meteorologic phenomenon (e.g., a tornado) or freak event (e.g., school shootings). Dependent events are those that occur because the individual has placed himself or herself into situations with a high probability of becoming stressful life events (e.g., marriage to a known substance abuser) (54,55). Although both independent and dependent life events contribute to the development of a subsequent depressive episode, genetically influenced traits may predispose individuals to select exposure to stressful life events and therefore episodes of depression (56). The clinician should evaluate the stressful life event in the context of the individual's life, recognizing that similar events result in different levels of stress for different individuals. For example, the death of a pet may be more traumatic than the death of a family member for some patients.

Socioeconomic Status

Multiple studies have suggested that people who are unemployed, divorced, or impoverished have higher rates of depression. Working for pay has been associated with a lower risk of depression (44).

Sleep Disturbances

Sleep disturbances seem to increase the risk for major depression. In a longitudinal study of young adults (21–30 years of age), the relative risk for new onset of major depression was 4.0 for individuals with baseline insomnia and 2.9 for those with hypersomnia. Other studies confirm sleep disturbances as risk factors for depression (57). Given that sleep complaints are also common symptoms of depression, a sleep disturbance may herald the first onset of depression or relapse in remitted depressed patients. The relationship between sleep apnea and depressive and anxiety symptoms remains controversial (58–61). Sleep deprivation may play a role in precipitating postpartum depression. Lack of sleep may be especially common in mothers of infants with disturbed sleeping patterns, improving when infants sleep in regular overnight patterns (62). Thus, what seems to be postnatal depression may show significant improvement when childhood sleep disturbances are corrected. Individuals who work swing shifts (e.g., factory workers, nurses) or extended-hour shifts (e.g., resident physicians) also may develop mood disturbance and cognitive impairment (63,64).

Genetic Risk

In determining the genetic contribution to the onset of mood disorders, one must keep in mind that the pathway from genotype to phenotype is complex and probably heterogeneous (65). Overall, the risk of any mood disorder in a child of a parent with bipolar disorder is 12% and any mood disorder in a child of a parent with major depression is 7% (65). These numbers have been estimated from genetic studies using many research methodologies.

Research methods including family, twin, association, and linkage studies all support a genetic contribution to the development of mood syndromes. Family studies evaluating the risk of bipolar disorder and major depression among relatives of probands with bipolar disorder compared with controls revealed that the relative risk (RR) for the development of bipolar disorder ranged from 3.7 to 17.7 (average RR 11.0) and the relative risk of major depression ranged from 1.6 to 9.7 (average RR 3.4). Relatives of probands with major depressive disorder compared with controls have relative risks ranging from 1.2 to 11.0 (average RR 5.5) for the development of bipolar disorder and 1.5 to 18.9 (average RR 5.0) for major depression. Although family studies demonstrate a familial aggregation of mood disorders, neither the mode of transmission nor the effect of environment is clear. Twin studies have revealed that, compared with major depression, bipolar disorder exhibits a greater degree of involvement of genetic factors. When one twin has bipolar disorder, the risk of the other twin also being affected is eightfold higher in monozygotic twins than in dizygotic twins, suggesting a strong genetic contribution in bipolar disorder. Adoption studies suggest that although genetic factors play a role in the development of mood disorders, environmental factors (e.g., a behavioral disturbance, death of an adoptive parent) play the significant role.

Serum Cholesterol

A possible relationship between serum cholesterol levels, depression, and violent behavior was first raised in large clinical trials directed at cardiovascular risk factors and death (66,67). In these studies, it was noted that, although cholesterol lowering was associated with a decrease in cardiac death, noncardiac mortality from suicide, accidental, and other violent deaths increased. Baseline low or lowered cholesterol has been implicated as a cause in increased mortality from suicide (68–70). Small studies (sample size range from n = 20s–40s) have suggested that low serum cholesterol levels are associated with major depression, suicide, and possibly even antisocial personality (71–73). However, in a study of 3490 veterans 31 to 45 years of age, men with depression had cholesterol levels similar to controls (74). Other researchers have reported no relationship of serum cholesterol to major depression or suicide (75–78), and none found that the higher risk of death was secondary to smoking-related malignancies or alcohol consumption (79,80). Definitive conclusions about the role of cholesterol in depression and suicide must await large, prospective epidemiologic studies designed to specifically address this question. Clinicians should be aware that low serum cholesterol or significant lowering of cholesterol may be a marker for risk of suicidal, accidental, or violent death in some individuals. Patients with risk factors for suicide may require careful monitoring.

Prevention

The morbidity associated with major depression in the United States is great. In 1996, the National Institute of Mental Health estimated that the 1-year financial burden of all mental disorders in the United States was $148 billion (81). This figure included costs for direct treatment and lost earning capacity. The DEPRES study conducted in Europe showed that individuals with depression make almost three times as many visits to general practitioners and lose four times as many working days as do nondepressed individuals (12). In addition to the financial burden, other "costs" associated with the depressive disorders (e.g., suicide), and the intangible costs of the illness for the patient, family, and society must be considered.

Because of the significant costs of the depressive disorders, in the past 15 years increasing attention has been paid to whether or not depression is preventable. The traditional preventive paradigms include primary, secondary, and tertiary prevention. Primary prevention to avert the onset of a first episode of depression could be directed either at the whole population or at those individuals with specific risk factors. Secondary prevention would involve methods for the early detection and treatment of a new incident depressive syndrome. Finally, tertiary prevention would aim to reduce the recurrence of depressive episodes in individuals with previous history of depression.

Primary Prevention

Harrington and Clark (82) have published a comprehensive review of prevention and early intervention for depression in adolescence and early adult life. The review notes that the additive effects of genetic vulnerability and environmental factors contribute to the overall risk for the development of depression. Therefore, preventive interventions should be directed ideally at more than one risk factor. Preventive measures may be universal or selective. Universal measures are directed at the general population and may be problematic to implement. Societal problems such as poverty, substance abuse, or familial dysfunction are extremely difficult to prevent. Whether improvements in the standard of living could actually prevent depression is controversial given that the increased standard of living after World War II has been accompanied by increasing incidence and prevalence of depression (82–84). Additionally, school-based programs directed at reducing depressive symptoms may not be effective (85). The U.S. Preventive Services Task Force has recommended against universal screening for asymptomatic individuals (86).

Selective interventions directed at at-risk populations have been studied. As previously mentioned, because early pregnancy is associated with depression, measures to educate minors and young adults about contraception and family planning could have a useful preventive effect (82).

Because children of parents who have experienced an affective disorder may be at higher risk for developing depression, interventions directed at promoting their resiliency and decreasing the impact of other risk factors have been tested. Clinician-directed educational interventions may be effective in increasing family communications about depression and promoting changes in behaviors and attitudes (87–89). Structured, psychoeducational groups such as Teaching Kids to Cope may provide short-term benefit, but long-term studies have not been conducted (90). Children, adolescents, and adults who have suffered traumatic experiences (e.g., abuse, bereavement) may benefit from interventions like debriefing (82).

Secondary and Tertiary Prevention

Secondary preventive methods have been evaluated in adolescents who report high levels of depressive symptoms on questionnaires (91,92). Early psychotherapeutic interventions may be beneficial in the short term to reduce symptoms and prevent a full depressive episode.

Tertiary prevention of major depression has been studied in both primary care and mental health settings (93–95). Risk factors predicting the development of relapse in both settings include a history of three or more depressive episodes, dysthymia, presence of another mental disorder, presence of a comorbid medical condition, older age of onset for the first episode, psychotic affective episodes, previous serious suicide attempt, positive family history of bipolar affective disorder, family history of suicide, severe functional impairment while depressed, and residual depressive symptoms after acute-phase treatment. Approximately 50% to 80% of individuals who experience a first episode of major depression will have at least one subsequent episode in their lifetime. The highest period of risk for relapse is within the first 4 to 6 months after the initial remission. Patients whose symptoms remit after 12 weeks of therapy should continue treatment with antidepressant medication for at least an additional 26 weeks to minimize the risk of relapse (total treatment time ~9 months) (96). The World Health Organization and the Agency for Health Care Policy and Research (AHCPR) recommend preventive maintenance pharmacotherapy for individuals with three or more depressive episodes and for those who do not fully recover from any given episode (13). Preventive maintenance pharmacotherapy also is recommended for individuals with two past episodes and vulnerability to future recurrences because of associated risk factors (97,98). Preventive agents include antidepressants and lithium.

Screening

The U.S. Preventive Services Task Force (USPSTF) stated in 1996 that there was insufficient evidence to recommend for or against the routine use of standardized questionnaires to screen for depression in asymptomatic primary care patients (86). Other organizations have made similar recommendations, generally suggesting that providers maintain a high index of suspicion for symptoms of depression (99,100). The USPSTF specifically recommends that clinicians should maintain an especially high index of suspicion for depressive symptoms in adolescent and young adults; individuals with a family or personal history of depression; those who perceive or have experienced a recent loss; and those with chronic illness, sleep disorders, chronic pain, or multiple unexplained somatic complaints (86). There was insufficient evidence to recommend for or against routine screening by primary care clinicians to detect suicide risk in asymptomatic individuals. Physicians, however, should ask patients routinely about their use of alcohol and other drugs (86).

Adolescents should be asked annually about behaviors or emotions that indicate recurrent or severe depression (101,102). When evaluating adolescents, there are four main categories in the clinical assessment (103): 1) exhibition of self-destructive behavior; 2) a loss as a precipitating factor (e.g., a parent's death, a divorce, parental inattention); 3) the adolescent's history of adjustment in school, family, and social activities (including his or her style of coping with stress); and 4) parent-child relationships and family environment (103). Chapter 3 provides a more in-depth discussion of screening and diagnosis.

▪ ▪ ▪

Key Points

- The lifetime prevalence for depression in the United States is approximately 4% to 17%.

- The prevalence of current depression in the community setting is approximately 5%. Prevalence estimates increase in medically ill individuals. The prevalence of depression in the outpatient clinic setting is approximately 5% to 10%, and in the inpatient medical setting it is approximately 10% to 14%.

- Common factors for depression include female gender, medical illness, family history, sleep disturbances, low socioeconomic status, and stressful life events.

- First-degree relatives of patients with mood disorders have an elevated relative risk for the development of major depression (average RR 5.0).

- The relationship between low cholesterol, depression, and suicide is controversial.

- Primary prevention should be directed toward individuals with risk factors. Tertiary prevention, which involves treatment of depressive episodes for at least 9 months, is essential in individuals who have had three or more episodes of depression.

▪ ▪ ▪

REFERENCES

1. **American Psychiatric Association.** *Diagnostic and Statistical Manual of Mental Disorders*, 4th ed. Washington, DC: American Psychiatric Press, 1994.

2. **Kramer M.** Cross national study of diagnosis of the mental disorders: origins of the problem. *Am J Psychiatry.* 1969;125(Suppl I-II).

3. **Paykel ES (ed).** *Handbook of Affective Disorders*, 2nd ed. New York: Guilford Press;1992.

3a. **American Psychiatric Association.** *Diagnostic and Statistical Manual of Mental Disorders*, 3rd ed. Washington, DC: American Psychiatric Press, 1994.

4. **Regier DA, Kaelber CT.** The Epidemiologic Catchment Area (ECA) Program: studying the prevalence and incidence of psychopathology. In: Tsuang MT, Tohen M, Zahner GEP (eds). *Textbook in Psychiatric Epidemiology.* New York: Wiley-Liss; 1995:135–55.

5. **Kessler RC, McGonagle KA, Nelson CB, et al.** Sex and depression in the National Comorbidity Study. Part II: Cohort effects. *J Affect Disord.* 1994;30:15–26.

6. **Kessler RC, McGonagle KA, Zhao S, et al.** Lifetime and 12-month prevalence of DSM-III-R psychiatric disorders in the United States: results from the National Comorbidity Survey. *Arch Gen Psychiatry.* 1994;51:8–19.

7. **Weissman MM, Leaf PJ, Tischler GL, et al.** Affective disorders in five United States communities. *Psychol Med.* 1988;18:141–53.

8. **Blazer DG, Kessler RC, McGonagle KA, Swartz MS.** The prevalence and distribution of major depression in a national comorbidity sample: the National Cormorbidity Survey. *Am J Psychiatry.* 1994;151:979–86.

9. **Angst J.** How recurrent and predictable is depressive illness? In Montgomery SA, Rouillon F (eds). *Progress in Psychiatry: The Long-Term Treatment of Depression.* vol. 3. Sussex, England: Wiley; 1990.

10. **Angst J, Dobler-Mikola A, Binder J.** The Zurich Study: a prospective epidemiological study of depressive, neurotic, and psychosomatic syndromes. Part I: Problem, methodology. *Eur Arch Psychiatry Neurol Sci.* 1984;234:13–20.

11. **Angst J.** Epidemiology of depression. *Psychopharmacology.* 1992;106(Suppl): 71–4.

12. **Lepine J-P, Gastpar M, Mendlewicz J, Tylee A.** Depression in the community: the first pan-European study DEPRES (Depression Research in European Society). *Int Clin Psychopharmacol.* 1997;12:19–29.

13. **Depression Guideline Panel.** *Depression in Primary Care,* vol. 1, no. 5. Rockville, MD: Department of Health and Human Services, Public Health Service, Agency for Health Care and Policy and Research [Pub no. 93-0550].

14. **Hartka E, Johnstone B, Leino EV, et al.** A meta-analysis of depressive symptomatology and alcohol consumption over time. *Br J Addict.* 1991;86:1283–98.

15. **Kessler RC, Stang PE, Wittchen H, et al.** Lifetime panic-depression comorbidity in the National Cormorbidity Survey. *Arch Gen Psychiatry.* 1998;55:801–7.

16. **Pincus HA, Tanielian TL, Marcus SC, et al.** Prescribing trends in psychotropic medications: primary care, psychiatry, and other medical specialties. *JAMA.* 1998;279:526–31.

17. **Katon W, Schulberg H.** Epidemiology of depression in primary care. *Gen Hosp Psychiatry.* 1992;14:237–47.

18. **Cohen-Cole SA, Brown FW, McDaniel JS.** Assessment of depression and grief reactions in the medically ill. In Stoudemire A, Fogel BS (eds). *Psychiatric Care of the Medical Patient.* New York: Oxford University Press;1993:53–70.

19. **Winokur G.** The concept of secondary depression and its relationship to comorbidity. *Psychiatr Clin North Am.* 1990;123:567–83.

20. **Roberts RE, Kaplan GA, Shema SJ, Strawbridge WJ.** Prevalence and correlates of depression in an aging cohort: the Alameda County Study. *J Gerontol.* 1997; 52(Suppl B):S252–8.

21. **Kessler RC, McGonagle KA, Swartz M, et al.** Sex and depression in the National Comorbidity Survey. Part I: Lifetime prevalence, chronicity, and recurrence. *J Affect Disord.* 1993;29:85–96.

22. **Weissman MM, Bland RC, Canino GJ, et al.** Cross-national epidemiology of major depression and bipolar disorder. *JAMA.* 1996;276:292–9.

23. **Eaton WW, Kramer M, Anthony JC, et al.** The incidence of specific DIS/DSM-III mental disorders: data from the NIMH epidemiologic Catchment Aria Program. *Acta Psychiatr Scand.* 1989;79:163–8.

24. **Klerman GL, Lavori PW, Rice J, et al.** Birth-cohort trends in rates of major depressive disorder among relatives of patients with affective disorder. *Arch Gen Psychiatry.* 1985;42:689–93.

25. **Ernst C, Angst J.** The Zurich Study. Part XII: Sex differences in depression—evidence from longitudinal epidemiological data. *Curr Arch Psychiatry Clin Neurosci.* 1992;241:222–30.

26. **Burke KC, Burke JD, Regier DA, et al.** Age at onset of selected mental disorders in five community populations. *Arch Gen Psychiatry.* 1990;47:511–18.

27. **Nolen-Hoeksema S.** Responses to depression and their effects on the duration of depressive episodes. *J Abnorm Psychol.* 1991;100:569–82.

28. **Frank E, Carpenter LL, Kupfer D.** Sex differences in recurrent depression: Are there any that are significant? *Am J Psychiatry.* 1988;145:41–5.

29. **Somervell PD, Leaf PJ, Weissman MM, et al.** The prevalence of major depression in black and white adults in five United States communities. *Am J Epidemiol.* 1989;130:725–35.

30. **Kleinman A.** Depression, somatization, and the "new cross-cultural psychiatry." *Soc Sci Med.* 1977;11:3.

31. **Kleinman A.** Neurasthenia and depression: a study of somatization and culture. *Culture Med Psychiatry.* 1982;6:117.

32. **Komahashi T, Ganesan S, Ohmori K, Nakano T.** Expression of depressed mood: a comparative study among Japanese and Canadian aged people. *Can J Psychiatry.* 1997;42:852–7.

33. **Mackinnon A, McCallum J, Andrews G, Anderson I.** The Center for Epidemiological Studies Depression Scale in older community samples in Indonesia, North Korea, Myanmar, Sri Lanka, and Thailand. *J Gerontol B Psychol Sci Soc Sci.* 1998;53:343–52.

34. **Burvill PW.** Recent progress in the epidemiology of major depression. *Epidemiol Rev.* 1995;17:21–31.

35. **Klerman GL.** The current age of youthful melancholia: evidence for increase in depression among adolescents and young adults. *Br J Psychiatry.* 1988;152:4–14.

36. **Hagnell O, Lanke J, Rorsman B, et al.** Are we entering an age of melancholy? Depresive illnesses in a prospective epidemiological study over 25 years: the Lundby Study, Sweden. *Psychol Med.* 1982;12:279–89.

37. **Klerman GL, Weissman MM.** Increasing rates of depression. *JAMA.* 1989;261:2229–35.

38. **Weissman MM, Bland R, Joyce PR, et al.** Sex differences in rates of depreesion: cross-national perspectives. *J Affect Dis.* 1993;29:77–84.

39. **Angst J, Merikangas K.** The depressive spectrum: diagnostic classification and course. *J Affect Dis.* 1997;45:31–40.

40. **Simon GE, VonKorff M.** Recall of psychiatric history in cross-sectional surveys: implications for epidemiologic research. *Epidemiol Rev.* 1995;17:221–7.

41. **Wickramaratne PJ, Weissman MM, Leaf PF, et al.** Age, period and cohort effects on the risk of major depression: results from five United States communities. *J Clin Epidemiol.* 1989;42:333–43.

42. **Weissman MM.** Advances in psychiatric epidemiology: rates and risks for depression. *Am J Public Health.* 1987;77:445–51.

43. **Bruce ML, Takeuchi DT, Leaf PJ.** Poverty and psychiatric status: longitudinal evidence from the New Haven Epidemiologic Catchment Area Study. *Arch Gen Psychiatry.* 1991:48:470–4.

44. **Anthony JC, Petronis KR.** Suspected risk factors for depression among adults 18–44 years old. *Epidemiology.* 1991;2:123–32.

45. **Orr ST, James S.** Maternal depression in an urban pediatric practice: implications for health care delivery. *Am J Public Health.* 1984;74:363–5.

46. **Reis J.** Correlates of depression according to maternal age. *J Genet Psychol.* 1988;149:535–45.

47. **Bromet EJ, Cornley PJ.** Correlates of depression in mothers of young children. *J Am Acad Child Psychiatry.* 1984;23:335–42.

48. **Deal LW, Holt VL.** Young maternal age and depressive symptoms: results from the 1988 national maternal and infant health survey. *Am J Public Health.* 1998;88: 266–70.

49. **Heneghan AM, Silver EJ, Bauman LJ, et al.** Depressive symptoms in inner-city mothers of young children: who is at risk? *Pediatrics.* 1998;102:1394–1400.

50. **McCormick LH.** Depression in mothers of children with attention deficit hyperactivity disorder. *Family Med.* 1995;27:176–9.

51. **Holmes TH, Rahe RH.** The Social Readjustment Rating Scale. *J Psychosom Res.* 1967;11:213–218.

52. **Paykel ES.** Contribution of life events to causation of psychiatric illness. *Psychol Med.* 1978;8:245–53.

53. **Kessler RC.** The effects of stressful life events to causation of psychiatric illness. *Annual Rev Psychol.* 1997;48:191–214.

54. **Paykel ES.** Methodology of life events research. *Adv Psychosom Med.* 1987;17: 13–29.

55. **Brown GW, Sklair F, Harris TO, Birley JLT.** Life events and psychiatric disorders. Part I: Some methodological issues. *Psychol Med.* 1973;3:74–87.

56. **Kendler KS, Karkowski LM, Prescott CA.** Causal relationship between stressful life events and the onset of major depression. *Am J Psychiatry.* 1999;156:837–41.

57. **Gillin JC.** Are sleep disturbances risk factors for anxiety, depressive, and addictive disorders. *Acta Psychiatr Scand Suppl.* 1998;393:39–43.

58. **Barbe, Pericas J, Munoz A, et al.** Automobile accidents in patients with sleep apnea syndrome: an epidemiological and mechanistic study. *Am J Respir Crit Care Med.* 1998;158:18–22.

59. **Briones B, Adams N, Srauss M, et al.** Relationship between sleepiness and general health status. *Sleep.* 1996;19:583–8.

60. **Pillat G, Lavie P.** Psychiatric symptoms in sleep apena syndrome: effects of gender and respiratory disturbance index. *Chest.* 1998;114:697–703.

61. **Enright PL, Newman AB, Wahl PW, et al.** Prevalence and correlates of snoring and observed apneas in 5201 older adults. *Sleep.* 1996;19:531–8.

62. **Armstrong KL, Van Haeringen AR, Dadds MR, Cash R.** Sleep deprivation or postnatal depression in later infancy: separating the chicken from the egg. *J Paediatr Child Health.* 1998;34:260–2.

63. **Leonard C, Fanning N, Attwood J, Buckley M.** The effect of fatigue, sleep deprivation, and onerous working hours on the physical and mental well-being of pre-registration house officers. *Irish J Med Sci.* 1998;167:22–5.

64. **Hart RP, Buchsbaum DG, Wade JB, et al.** Effect of sleep deprivation on first-year residents' response times, memory, and mood. *J Med Educ.* 1987;62:940–2.

65. **Merikangas KR, Kupfer DJ.** Mood disorders: genetic aspects. In Kaplan HI, Saddock BI (eds). *Comprehensive Textbook of Psychiatry,* 6th ed. Baltimore: Williams & Wilkins; 1995:1102–16.

66. **Muldoon MF, Manuck SB, Matthews KA.** Lowering cholesterol concentrations and mortality: a quantitative review of primary prevention trials. *Br Med J.* 1990; 301:309–14.

67. **Golomb BA.** Cholesterol and violence: is there a connection? *Ann Intern Med.* 1998;128:478–87.

68. **Golier JA, Marzuk PM, Leon AC, et al.** Low serum cholesterol level and attempted suicide. *Am J Psychiatry.* 1995;152:419–23.

69. **Gallerani M, Manfredini R, Caracciolo S, et al.** Serum cholesterol concentrations in parasuicide. *Br Med J.* 1995;310:1632–6.

70. **Zureik M, Courbon D, Ducimetiere P.** Serum cholesterol concentration and death from suicide in men: Paris prospective study. *Br Med J.* 1996;313:649–51.

71. **Maes M, Delanghe J, Meltzer HY, et al.** Lower degree of esterifciation of serum cholesterol in depression: relevance for depression and suicide research. *Acta Psychiatr Scand.* 1994;9022–8.

72. **Maes M, Smith R, Christophe A, et al.** Lower serum high-density lipoprotein cholesterol (HDL-C) in major depression and in depressed men with serious suicidal attempts: relationship with immune-inflammatory markers. *Acta Psychiatr Scand.* 1997;95:212–21.

73. **Agargun MY, Algun E, Sekeroglu R, et al.** Low cholesterol levels in patients with panic disorder: the association with major depression. *J Affect Disord.* 1998;50: 29–32.

74. **Freedman DS, Byers T, Barrett DH, et al.** Plasma lipid levels and psychologic characteristics in men. *Am J Epidemiol.* 1995;141:507–17.

75. **Oxenkrug GF, Branconnier RJ, Harto-Truax N, Cole JO.** Is serum cholesterol a biological marker for major depressive disorder? *Am J Psychiatry.* 1983; 140:920–1.

76. **Iribarren C, Reed DM, Wergowske G, et al.** Serum cholesterol level and mortality due to suicide and trauma in the Honolulu Heart Program. *Arch Intern Med.* 1995;155:695–700.

76a. **Iribarren C, Reed DM, Chen R, Yano K, Dwyer JH.** Low serum cholesterol and mortality: Which is the cause and which the effect? *Circulation.* 1995;92: 2396–403.

77. **Markovitz JH, Smith D, Raczynski JM, et al.** Lack of relations of hostility, negative affect, and high-risk behavior with low plasma lipid levels in the Coronary Artery Risk Development in Young Adults Study. *Arch Intern Med.* 1997;157: 1953–9.

78. **Law MR, Thompson SG, Wald NJ.** Assessing possible hazards of reducing serum cholesterol. *Br Med J.* 1994;308:373–9.

79. **Cullen P, Schulte H, Assmann G.** The Munster Heart Study (PROCAM): total mortality in middle- aged men is increased at low total and LDL cholesterol concentrations in smokers, but not in nonsmokers. *Circulation.* 1997;96:2128–36.

80. **Vartiainen E, Puska P, Pekkanen, et al.** Serum cholesterol and mortality from accidents, suicide, and other violent causes. *Br Med J.* 1994;309:445–7.

81. **National Institutes of Health, National Institute of Mental Health.** *A Plan for Prevention Research for the National Institute of Mental Health.* Bethesda, MD: National Institutes of Health; 1996.

82. **Harrington R, Clark A.** Prevention and early intervention for depression in adolescence and early adult life. *Eur Arch Psychiatry Clin Neurosci.* 1998;248:31–54.

83. **Diekstra RW.** The epidemiology of suicide and parasuicide. *Acta Psychiatr Scand.* 1993;371:S9–20.

84. **Fombonne E.** Depessive disorders: time trends and putative explanatory mechanisms. In Rutter M, Smith D (eds). *Psychosocial Disorders in Young People: Time Trends and Their Origins.* Wiley: Chichester, England; 1995:544–615.

85. **Clarke GN, Hawkins W, Murphy M, Sheeber L.** School-based primary prevention of depressive symptomatology in adolescents: findings from two studies. *J Adolesc Res.* 1993;8:183–204.

86. **U.S. Preventive Services Task Force.** *Guide to Clinical Preventive Services,* 2nd ed. Alexandria, VA: International Medical Publishing; 1996.

87. **Beardslee WR, Wright E, Rothberg PC, et al.** Response of families to two preventive intervention strategieis: long-term differences in behavior and attitude change. *J Am Acad Child Adolesc Psychiatry.* 1996;35:774–82.

88. **Beardslee WR, Versage EM, Wright EJ, et al.** Examination of preventive interventions for families with depression: evidence of change. *Develop Psychopathol.* 1997;9:109–30.

89. **Beardslee WR, Swatling S, Hoke L, et al.** From cognitive information to shared meaning: healing principles in prevention intervention. *Psychiatry.* 1998;61:112–29.

90. **Puskar KR, Lamb J, Tusaie-Mumford K.** Teaching kids to cope: a preventive mental health nursing strategy for adolescents. *J Child Adolesc Psychiatr Nurs.* 1997;10:18–28.

91. **Jaycox LH, Reivich KJ, Gillham J, Seligman MEP.** Prevention of depressive symptoms in school children. *Behav Res Ther.* 1994;32:801–16.

92. **Clarke GN, Hawkins W, Murphy M, et al.** Targeted prevention of unipolar depressive disorder in an at-risk sample of high school adolescents: a randomized trial of a group cognitive intervention. *J Am Acad Child Adolesc Psychiatry.* 1995;34:312–21.

93. **Prien Rf, Kupfer DJ.** Continuation drug therapy for major depressive episodes: how long should it be maintained? *Am J Psychiatry.* 1986;143:18–23.

94. **Kupfer D, Frank E, Perel J, et al.** Five-year outcomes for maintenance therapies in recurrent depression. *Arch Gen Psychiatry.* 1992;49:769–73.

95. **Lin EHB, Katon WJ, Von Korff M, et al.** Relapse of depression in primary care: rate and clinical predictors. *Arch Fam Med.* 1998;7:443–9.

96. **Reimherr FW, Amsterdam JD, Quitkin FM, et al.** Optimal length of continuation therapy in depression: a prospective assessment during long-term fluoxetine treatment. *Am J Psychiatry.* 1998;155:1247–53.

97. **Angst J.** Clinical indications for a prophylactic treatment of depression. *Adv Biol Psychiatry.* 1981;7:218–29.

98. **Schulberg HC, Katon WJ, Simon GE, Rush AJ.** Treating major depression in primary care practice: an update of the Agency for Health Care Policy and Research practice guidelines. *Arch Gen Psychiatry.* 1998;55:1121–7.

99. **Canadian Task Force on the Periodic Health Examination.** *Canadian Guide to Clinical Preventive Health Care.* Ottawa, Canada: Canada Communication Group; 1994:450–5.

100. **Depression Guideline Panel.** *Depression in Primary Care,* vol. 1, no. 5. Rockville, MD: Department of Health and Human Services, Public Health Service, Agency for Health Care and Policy and Research [Pub no. 93-0550].

101. **American Academy of Family Physicians.** *Age Charts for Periodic Health Examination.* Kansas City, MO: American Academy of Family Physicians; 1994.

102. **American Medical Association.** *Guidelines for Adolescent Preventive Services (GAPS): Recommendations and Rationale.* Chicago: American Medical Association; 1992:131–9.

103. **Besseghini VH.** Depression and suicide in children and adolescents. *Ann NY Acad Sci.* 1997;816:94–8.

KEY REFERENCES

Anthony JC, Petronis KR. Suspected risk factors for depression among adults 18–44 years old. *Epidemiology.* 1991;2:123–32.

Katon W, Schulberg H. Epidemiology of depression in primary care. *Gen Hosp Psychiatry.* 1992;14:237–47.

Kessler RC, McGonagle KA, Zhao S, et al. Lifetime and 12-month prevalence of DSM-III-R psychiatric disorders in the United States: results from the National Comorbidity Survey. *Arch Gen Psychiatry.* 1994;51:8–19.

Paykel ES. Contribution of life events to causation of psychiatric illness. *Psychol Med.* 1978;8:245–53.

Reimherr FW, Amsterdam JD, Quitkin FM, et al. Optimal length of continuation therapy in depression: a prospective assessment during long-term fluoxetine treatment. *Am J Psychiatry.* 1998;155:1247–53.

U.S. Preventive Services Task Force. *Guide to Clinical Preventive Services,* 2nd ed. Alexandria, VA: International Medical Publishing; 1996.

Vartiainen E, Puska P, Pekkanen, et al. Serum cholesterol and mortality from accidents, suicide, and other violent causes. *Br Med J.* 1994;309:445–7.

Weissman MM, Leaf PJ, Tischler GL, Blazer DG, et al. Affective disorders in five United States communities. *Psychol Med* 1988;18:141–53.

3

■ ■ ■

Diagnosis

Michael J. Roy, MD, MPH

Kurt Kroenke, MD

"After a frustrated internist received the results of my very normal, very healthy tests, she decided to bail out. In parting, she dismissed me with, 'There's nothing more I can do for you. Why don't you get a job?'"

D epression is common, and it is especially prevalent in people who are seeking medical care. Depressive symptoms that do not meet criteria for major disorders are even more prevalent and are associated with significant impairment in social and occupational functioning. However, for a variety of reasons, depression frequently goes undiagnosed. Although time-consuming, screening methods developed to help diagnose depression often have been impractical to use in the busy primary care setting, more recent studies have shown that a simple question or two are highly sensitive for detecting depression. Confirmation of a depressive diagnosis can then be achieved with a few questions focusing on the DSM-IV criteria (Table 3.1).

Challenges to Diagnosing Depression in Primary Care

At least one in every four patients treated in the primary care setting has a mental disorder (1,2), and there is significant associated morbidity and functional impairment with such conditions (2–6). Although it has been estimated that 88% of individuals who are worried about having a psychological distur-

---

Table 3.1   DSM-IV Criteria for Major Depressive Episode*

---

1. Depressed mood most of the day

2. Markedly decreased interest or pleasure in all or almost all activities most of the day

3. Significant unintended weight change or appetite change

4. Insomnia or hypersomnia

5. Psychomotor agitation or retardation

6. Fatigue or loss of energy

7. Feelings of worthlessness or excessive or inappropriate guilt

8. Diminished ability to think or concentrate

9. Recurrent thoughts of death, suicidal ideation, or a suicide attempt

---

* At least five of the above symptoms must be present nearly every day for a 2-week period. In addition, the symptoms should not be the result of substance abuse, a medication, or a medical condition, and should not be better accounted for by bereavement.
Adapted from American Psychiatric Association. *Diagnostic and Statistical Manual of Mental Disorders*, 4th ed. Washington, DC: American Psychiatric Association; 1994.

bance seek the help of a general medical practitioner first (7), it also has been reported widely that primary care physicians miss the diagnosis of depression at least half of the time (8–10). Some believe that the increased emphasis on recognizing depression during the past decade may be improving case detection, but there remain numerous barriers to diagnosis in the primary care setting. First, primary care providers may not have had extensive training in the diagnosis of mood disorders. Second, patients often present with somatic symptoms that could have many potential causes, and primary care physicians may be more attuned to seeking organic rather than psychological causes. Compounding this problem, patients will often have comorbid medical conditions; Coulehan and coworkers (11) found that primary care physicians had a lower detection rate for major depression in patients who also have more severe medical problems. Unfortunately, patients with depression often do have a greater burden of medical illness than do nondepressed patients (12,13). Third, physicians may not yet know their patients well enough to diagnose depression accurately. A recent study found that family physicians more effectively identified depression in patients with whom they were more familiar and in those who had histories of depression and/or greater distress or vegetative symptoms (14). Additionally, the stigmatization surrounding mental illness may lead patients and physicians striving for greater rapport to avoid directly discussing mood disorders. Ironically, perhaps contrary to many physicians' beliefs, patients seem to derive greater satisfaction from the discussion of psychosocial issues than from biomedical subjects (15). Finally, doctors face progressively more onerous time constraints, trying to squeeze greater numbers of health-screening measures into shorter appointment times. The typical general medical office visit is reported to be 15 minutes or less, compared with 30 minutes or more for mental health specialists (16).

Screening Instruments

Because of the challenges of and obstacles to diagnosing depression in the primary care setting, screening methods need to be brief, easily remembered, and accurate to receive broad acceptance in primary care. The ideal screening instrument should have some additional features as well. Klinkman (17) categorizes competing demands in the patient-physician interaction that will limit the rate of detection of mental disorders. His four domains are 1) physician characteristics, including skills, knowledge, and attitudes about psychosocial issues; 2) patient characteristics; 3) the structure of the health care system; and 4) the public policy environment. An effective diagnostic tool therefore should be able to overcome gaps in physician knowledge and skills as well as in patient concerns and fears of stigmatization. Ideally, it should facilitate the education of both physicians and patients. In addition, it should be compatible with restrictions on time and reimbursement. Although some changes in the medical arena may make diagnosis of depression more difficult, there is one that may be helpful: greater attention to outcomes. Recognition of depression by primary physicians is associated with initiation of treatment and improved outcomes, including social functioning (9,18). Therefore, screening instruments that facilitate diagnosis should appeal to managed care, third-party payers, and physicians.

Schwenk (19) identified four characteristics that a screening test for depression in the primary care setting should have to be useful: 1) the disease (depression) must have sufficient prevalence and morbidity to influence the quality and/or duration of life significantly; 2) the screening test must be safe, accurate, and inexpensive; 3) detection of new cases must result in better outcomes than waiting until the disease becomes clinically apparent without such a screening test; and 4) the outcome of cases detected and treated in primary care should compare favorably with detection and treatment in a mental health setting.

Early Instruments

A variety of instruments have been developed to facilitate identification of affective disorders. Several are broad screens that elicit symptoms of general psychological distress without making specific diagnoses. The General Health Questionnaire (GHQ) and the Hopkins Symptoms Checklist (HSCL) have multiple versions with differing (generally large) numbers of questions that screen predominantly for general psychiatric illness (20). The 21-item Beck Depression Inventory, 20-item Zung Self-Assessment Depression Scale (SDS), and the 20-item Center for Epidemiologic Studies Depression Screen (CES-D) are instruments that have been used widely to screen for depression and to assess the severity of depression and response to therapy (20,21). Another depression-specific screen, the Popoff Index of Depression, has only 15 items but has received less attention in the literature (20). The CES-D looks for mood and vegetative symptoms in the preceding week and has been reported to predict depression more consistently than the SDS or HSCL; however, it has had a significant false-positive rate (identifying patients with other mental disorders or no disorder as being depressed) (21). The Medical Outcomes Study Depression Scale (MOS-D) was an attempt to improve on the CES-D by combining six of its 20 items with two from a widely used, lay-administered instrument, the Diagnostic Interview Schedule (DIS) (21). In addition, rather than weighing the items equally, an attempt is made to improve diagnostic accuracy by applying a logistic regression technique that requires the use of a calculator. A review of each of the above screening instruments found no significant differences between them in regard to sensitivity and specificity (20). However, such tools have been criticized for their ability "to detect hassles, stress, and distress more than they detect specific diagnoses" (19), and time constraints in primary care have continued to limit the use of formal questionnaires.

Simplifying Screening
Recently, several simple approaches have been developed by busy primary care providers to facilitate screening for depression.

THE SDDS AND THE PRIME-MD
Two multidimensional questionnaires use a limited number of questions to screen specifically for depression. Each is designed to make criteria-based diagnoses of DSM-IV disorders and can detect disorders that commonly coexist with depression (e.g., alcoholism, anxiety and somatoform disorders) (DSM-IV disorders are listed in Table 3.2). For depression, the SDDS (Symptom-Driven Diagnostic System-Primary Care) (22) asks five questions, whereas the PRIME-MD (Primary Care Evaluation of Mental Disorders) pares screening down to two questions: During the past month, have you 1) "often been bothered by feeling down, depressed, or hopeless?"; and 2) "had little interest or pleasure in doing things?" (2). Each of these approaches picks up as many cases as the more comprehensive instruments, with similar specificity as well. The initial PRIME-MD validation study found that a positive response to one of the two questions had 86% sensitivity and 75% specificity for depression, which are identical to the 20-item Zung Depression Scale. A more recent study in a population with a higher prevalence of depression yielded 96% sensitivity and 57% specificity, rates comparable with six more cumbersome measures (23). Mulrow and coworkers (20) de-

Table 3.2   DSM-IV Depressive Disorders

• Major depression	• Bereavement*
Mild, moderate, severe	• Depression not otherwise specified
With psychotic features	• Subthreshold and other minor depressions
With melancholia	• Mixed anxiety and depression
Atypical	• Adjustment disorder with depressed mood
Rapid-cycling	
Postpartum	• Premenstrual dysphoric disorder
Seasonal	• Depression due to a general medical condition
• Dysthymic disorder	
• Bipolar disorder (depressed phase)	• Depression due to a medication or substance

* Bereavement has a diagnostic code in DSM-IV and in ICD, but it is not a disorder per se.
Adapted from American Psychiatric Association. *Diagnostic and Statistical Manual of Mental Disorders*, 4th ed. Washington, DC: American Psychiatric Association; 1994.

termined that the use of any of the case-finding instruments would miss approximately 20% of depression cases, a significant improvement, however, over the estimated 50% to 70% that are missed in routine practice. In addition, there is evidence that sensitivity is greater for more severe cases of depression, so cases that are missed are likely to be milder.

The PRIME-MD has been validated in urban primary care and academic centers and in rural medical practices (2,23–24). The PRIME-MD has two phases. The initial phase is a one-page questionnaire (PQ), which includes the previously described two questions to screen for depressive disorders, that is completed by the patient. The second phase is known as the Clinician Evaluation Guide (CEG), and if either of the two screening questions for depression is positive, it will lead the clinician to ask a series of nine questions based on the DSM-IV criteria for depression. Physicians using the CEG were able to identify twice as many mental disorders than they had detected without the tool, with high specificity. A version of the PRIME-MD that uses interactive voice-response technology for computerized telephone interviews also has been validated (25). Another version, known as the Patient Health Questionnaire (PHQ), can be self-administered entirely by patients before seeing their physicians. The PHQ enables physicians to scan patient responses quickly and to discern which DSM-IV diagnostic categories patients meet; it has been found to be as accurate as the original PRIME-MD (25a).

A SINGLE QUESTION
Williams and coworkers (18) found that even a single question, "Have you felt sad or depressed much of the time in the past year?", had similar sensi-

tivity to and only slightly less specificity than more comprehensive questionnaires (85% and 66%, respectively). The characteristics of this "diagnostic test" compare favorably with many of the tests commonly used by primary care providers for cancer or heart disease screening. As the authors note, this question can be answered quickly by patients in a waiting room, or it can be incorporated easily into a review of systems.

The S4 Model

Given the propensity for depressed primary care patients to present with physical complaints, Kroenke and coworkers (26) developed a screening method analogous to the CAGE questionnaire screen for alcoholism. Their S4 model incorporates the following four simple predictors of mood and anxiety disorders (2):

1. An affirmative response to "During the past week have you been under stress?"

2. A score of greater than 5 in response to "Describe how bad your symptom is, from 10 (unbearable) to 0 (none at all)?"

3. Poor or fair answer to "In general, would you say your health is excellent, very good, good, fair, or poor?"

4. Five or more of the 15 somatic symptoms on the PRIME-MD Patient Questionnaire

Physical symptom count in particular can be viewed as a "sed rate" for psychological conditions because, as it increases, the likelihood of a psychological diagnosis rises greatly (26). In fact, on analysis of the Medical Outcomes Study data, Wells and coworkers (27) concluded that symptom count in combination with a simple measure of functional status could be a better predictor of outcome than DSM-IV disorder status. This might be especially relevant in primary care, where patients have a penchant for presenting with complaints about functional status rather than their mood. They further suggested that a classification system based on such factors might meet less resistance from primary care physicians and patients.

Recommendations for Screening

The high prevalence of depressive disorders in primary care, the marked associated morbidity, and the availability of effective interventions should lead to widespread use of a simple question or set of screening questions. Administration can occur by phone before an appointment, by ancillary personnel in the office, or by the physician during the encounter. Therefore, the first two of Schwenk's postulates are satisfied: 1) the disease (depression) must have sufficient prevalence and morbidity to significantly influence the quality and/or duration of life; and 2) the screening test must be safe, accurate, and inexpensive. Some believe that depressive symptomatology seen in the primary care setting is clinically mild and may not warrant treatment. Although the impairment associated with even sub-threshold depressions would refute this "clinically insignificant" argument (4,6,28), the use of screening questionnaires remains controversial. The U.S. Preventive Services Task Force concluded that "there is insufficient evidence to recommend either for or against routine use of standardized screening questionnaires to screen for depression in asymptomatic primary care patients" (29). Simple screening methods coupled with new evidence from the Treatment Effectiveness Project (30) about efficacy of therapy for minor depression may justify wider use of screening.

Confirming the Diagnosis

To confirm a diagnosis in a patient with a positive screen, health care providers can refer directly to DSM-IV criteria (*see* Table 3.1), use an instrument that is based on them, or request evaluation by a mental health specialist. Several confirmatory instruments are based on DSM-IV criteria for depression: the PRIME-MD CEG for primary care providers (2), the DIS for lay interviewers (31), and the Structured Clinical Interview for DSM-III-R (32) for mental health specialists. Two popular mnemonics based on DSM-IV criteria are SIG= E CAPS ("the prescription for depressed patients is energy capsules"), or SPACE DIGS. Both stand for similar symptoms:

- Sleep disturbance
- Psychomotor retardation or agitation
- Appetite disturbance
- Concentration impairment
- Energy level low
- Depressed mood
- Interest in activities lost
- Guilt or worthlessness
- Suicidal ideation

Persistence of at least five of the nine symptoms for more than 2 weeks is sufficient for a diagnosis of major depression. Recently, Brody and coworkers (33) attempted to simplify this process further, while improving the specificity of the PRIME-MD. They identified four depressive symptoms that accounted for most of the functional impairment: sleep disturbance, anhedonia, low self-esteem, and decreased appetite (and coined a catchy mnemonic, SALSA). Patients with a depressive disorder almost always had two or more of the four symptoms, as did another 5% of the study population, who also had significantly impaired function, despite falling short of major depression.

Presentations in the Primary Care Setting

Depressed patients often present to their primary physician or to an urgent care site with complaints of insomnia, fatigue, or weight change, rather than depressed mood. Most depressed patients seen initially in primary care do not spontaneously volunteer emotional distress as a chief complaint (7). In fact, it is common for depressed patients principally to report physical symptoms that are not even diagnostic criteria for depression (e.g., dyspepsia, joint or muscle pain, headaches). In general, depressed patients tend to have more physical symptoms than other primary care patients (10). It is important for the physician to think about depression when patients present with physical complaints and to ask routinely about depressed mood and loss of interest in activities. Depression should be considered up front, rather than as a diagnosis of exclusion made after performing numerous costly and time-consuming diagnostic tests for symptoms that do not have a clear organic basis. Not only does extensive testing delay treatment, incurring the potential for interim morbidity and mortality, but it may undermine satisfaction in patients who want to talk about psychosocial issues (15,34,35). Individuals with depressive disorders commonly report high rates of functional impairment (6) and use medical care heavily (5), but often this may be contributed to by physicians who relentlessly hunt for organic causes. Impairment and service use are elevated even for patients with depressive symptoms or subthreshold diagnoses. Some researchers have found that formal DSM-IV diagnoses often are not made in primary care and that patients are treated without an exact diagnosis. As long as significant variables (e.g., suicidality, psychosis, bipolar features) are ruled out, this may not be necessarily inappropriate (36).

The first episode of major depression may occur at any age, but onset before 30 years of age is most common. The course is variable, with a typical untreated episode lasting from 6 to 24 months, and more than half of patients having a recurrence (37). The diagnosis of depression is outlined in Figure 3.1.

Risk Factors

It also behooves primary care physicians to pay attention to risk factors for depression, enabling them to lower the threshold for screening higher-risk patients. Risk factors are listed in Table 3.3.

Classification of Depressive Disorders

Major Depression

Number of Episodes
Major depressive episodes may be single or recurrent. The number of episodes has implications for choice and duration of treatment and progno-

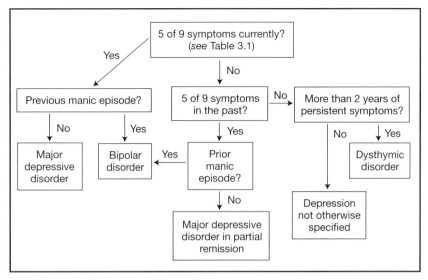

Figure 3.1   Diagnosis of depression. (Adapted from Depression Guideline Panel, U.S. Department of Health and Human Services. Detection and diagnosis. *Depression in Primary Care*, vol. 1. Washington, DC: U.S. Government Printing Office; 1993:20.)

sis. It may be difficult, if not impossible, to determine the number of episodes in a patient with long-standing depression with incomplete remission between period exacerbations.

Severity and Specifiers

The severity and subtype (if present) of major depression also have implications for prognosis and choice of treatment. Major depressive episodes can be classified as mild, moderate, severe without psychotic features, or severe with psychotic features. For diagnosis of a depressive disorder with psychotic features (i.e., delusions or hallucinations), the psychotic features should never be present without mood symptoms. In addition, the psychotic features, if present, are typically depressive in content or are "mood congruent" (e.g., the delusion that one's body is riddled with cancer). Schizoaffective disorder, however, features periods of 2 weeks or more in which delusions and hallucinations occur without mood disturbances. Several other specifiers may be added to characterize the disorder more accurately (38):

- **With melancholic features:** More common in older patients; remarkable for loss of pleasure or lack of reactivity to pleasurable stimuli and worse symptoms in the morning
- **With atypical features:** More common in younger patients, with two subtypes described; the anxious type is characterized by prominent anxiety, reactive mood, insomnia, phobic symptoms, and symptoms of sympathetic arousal; the vegetative form

---

Table 3.3   Risk Factors for Depression

• Previous history of depression	• Female sex
• Previous suicide attempts	• Postpartum condition
• Age <40 years at onset	• Lack of social support
• Comorbid medical illnesses	• Current substance abuse
• Stressful life events	• Low socioeconomic status
• Family history of depression	

Table 3.4   Criteria for Dysthymia

• Symptom-free periods should not exceed 2 months

• Chronic depressed mood present for ≥2 years

• Major depression *not* present for at least 6 months

• At least two of the symptoms below accompany depressed mood:

    Poor appetite

    Overeating

    Insomnia

    Low energy or fatigue

    Low self-esteem

    Poor concentration or difficulty making decisions

    Hopelessness

---

features overeating, weight gain, excessive sleep, symptoms, rejection sensitivity, mood that remains reactive, and leaden paralysis (a sensation of limb heaviness).

• **With rapid cycling:** May apply to bipolar disorders in particular, with more than four episodes per year.

Specifiers often have implications for treatment and prognosis.

Dysthymia

Dysthymia is a mild yet long-term depressed mood present more often than not for at least 2 years (Table 3.4). For diagnosis, at least two of the following symptoms should accompany the depressed mood:

• Poor appetite or overeating

• Insomnia or hypersomnia

- Low energy or fatigue
- Low self-esteem
- Poor concentration or difficulty making decisions
- Feelings of hopelessness

Symptom-free periods should not exceed 2 months, and during the first 2 years of the disturbance, criteria for major depressive episode should not be met. In fact, if the patient has a history of major depression, it should be in full remission for at least 6 months to make a diagnosis of dysthymia (otherwise, the diagnosis of major depression in partial remission should be considered). However, after the initial 2 years, major depression may be superimposed, yielding a diagnosis of "double depression." Comorbidity with other psychiatric conditions occurs frequently enough that the presence of dysthymia should lead physicians to look for associated conditions, including alcohol and substance abuse. The Medical Outcomes Study found an even worse prognosis for patients with dysthymia than for those with major depression, accentuating the importance of identifying such patients (27).

Bipolar Disorder

Bipolar disorder is characterized by the presence of mania (bipolar I) or hypomania (bipolar II) in addition to depression. A manic episode may last 1 week or longer and features an abnormally and persistently elevated, expansive, or irritable mood (Case 3.1). During this period, three or more of the following symptoms should be present:

- Inflated self-esteem or grandiosity
- Decreased need for sleep
- Unusually pressured, rapid, and/or prolonged speech
- Racing thoughts or flights of ideas
- Distractibility; increased goal-directed behavior (e.g., sexual, political, religious)
- Excessive involvement in activities that have the potential for significant adverse consequences (e.g., spending sprees, sexual indiscretions), often characteristic of impaired judgment

Hypomanic episodes may last as little as 4 days and are characterized by a clear change in functioning that falls short of engendering marked impairment, in addition to having three or more of the accompanying manic symptoms. Psychotic features also may occur in bipolar disorders and typically reflect manic mood (e.g., grandiose delusions). Cyclothymic disorder parallels dysthymia, defined by 2 years or more of alternating mild depressive and hypomanic episodes.

CASE 3.1 *Bipolar disorder*

A physician 65 years of age was referred by his partner who noted recent despondence. He cut back on his work schedule 9 months before presentation because of fatigue. He consistently awakens 1 to 2 hours before his usual time and is unable to return to sleep. He skips breakfast and lunch most of the time but is still not hungry for dinner. He no longer is eager to see his patients and does not think that he is able to help them much. Many have aged with him, and it seems as if many have died recently. He wishes that he were dead, too, and has contemplated taking an overdose or using carbon monoxide. He recollects other periods of depression in his life, although never for longer than 6 months. He has never taken psychotropic medicines. He has no history of psychosis, but he does recall periods during which he could go nearly without sleep for several days at a time. He had incredible energy at those times, writing several semi-autobiographical books within 3 or 4 days each. Although he has had no sexual drive in the past 9 months, he remembers having multiple partners during the energetic times. His father has similar periods of minimal sleep requirements: once, building the family home in less than a week, and another time nearly losing it in a trip to Las Vegas.

The diagnosis is bipolar II disorder.

Bereavement

The reaction to the death of a loved one may have several of the features of major depression, including depressed mood, sleep disturbance, and altered appetite. If depressive symptoms fail to improve within 2 months, the diagnosis of major depressive episode should be considered. In addition, the following features should prompt consideration of depression as the most apt diagnosis:

- Guilt about things other than what the individual did or did not do at the time their loved one died
- Excessive preoccupation with worthlessness
- Thoughts of death beyond wishing that they had died with, or instead of, the deceased
- Striking psychomotor retardation
- Prolonged, marked functional impairment
- Hallucinations other than transiently hearing the voice or seeing images of the deceased

In one study of widows and widowers, approximately half had no depressive symptoms 2 months after loss of their spouse, and they tended to remain symptom free (39). Of the 21% with major depression after 2 months, many improved by 13 months: 36% no longer had depressive symptoms, and an equal percentage had subsyndromal depression but 28%

still had major depression. Widows and widowers with subsyndromal depression at 2 months fared significantly better: 63% were asymptomatic at 13 months, 28% stayed the same, and 9% developed major depression.

Depression Not Otherwise Specified

Studies in the primary care setting have found that half or more of patients with clinically significant depressive symptoms do not meet criteria for major depression or dysthymia (1,2,40), suggesting that additional diagnostic categories may be necessary. DSM-IV defines depression not otherwise specified (NOS) as encompassing those disorders with depressive features that fail to meet specific criteria for major depression, dysthymia, or adjustment disorder with either depressed or mixed anxiety and depressed mood (38). In many cases, this represents patients who fall short of either the required number of symptoms or the required duration for major depression and dysthymia. Although efforts have been made to classify milder forms of depression as far back as the 1970s, there has yet to be widespread agreement on the best classification and their significance. The following categories, some of which are incorporated in an appendix to DSM-IV intended to stimulate further research, are worthy of discussion.

Subthreshold Depression

Sherbourne and coworkers (41) define subthreshold depression as symptoms of sufficient severity and duration, but of inadequate number, to qualify for major depression (Case 3.2). They analyzed patients with hypertension in the general medical setting, finding that those with subthreshold depression were more similar to patients with depressive disorder than to those without depression. Medical and psychiatric comorbidity was similar between those with full and subthreshold depression, except that those with subthreshold depression had lower rates of panic and anxiety disorders. A family history of depression was common in patients with subthreshold depression (41%), although not to be as common as in patients with full depressive disorders (59%). One in four patients with subthreshold depression develop major depression within 2 years. A recent study indicates that primary care physicians' diagnostic rates for subthreshold mood and anxiety disorders are even lower than for threshold diagnoses (42). In addition, it has been shown that mental health professionals treat patients for subthreshold depression nearly as often as they treat those with depression, whereas primary care providers are far less likely to treat patients with subthreshold depression (41). This may indicate that primary care providers are more inclined to attribute subthreshold depressive symptoms to co-existing medical disorders, which in some studies have been particularly common in patients with subthreshold diagnoses (43). However, there does seem to be evidence in favor of more liberal treatment, particularly because increased disability has been associated with the condition. Compared with major depression, the lifetime prevalence of clinically significant depressive symptoms is fourfold greater, thereby accounting for greater medical service use and social morbidity on a population basis (28). Subthreshold depression can be divided further into minor depression and subsyndromal symptomatic depression (SSD).

CASE 3.2   *Subthreshold depression disorder*

A man 30 years of age, who previously enjoyed working out at the gym and running 3 to 4 miles daily, complains that he has felt tired for most of the past 2 months. He has to push himself to get out and run, tires easily, and has gained 10 pounds. He denies feelings of depression, worthlessness, or suicidal ideation, but he has had some difficulty concentrating on his work as a computer programmer. He has stopped going out with friends after work so he can go home and nap. His father is an alcoholic, so he always limits himself to one drink when he does go out. His mother committed suicide at 40 years of age. A physical examination, complete blood count, serum glucose, and thyroid stimulating hormone level were all within normal limits.

Although he has neither the number of symptoms needed for a diagnosis of major depression nor does their duration qualify for a diagnosis of dysthymia, he does have several depressive symptoms and evidence of an adverse impact on his social and occupational functioning. His family history places him at high risk for depressive disorders.

He meets the criteria for a subthreshold depressive disorder, and treatment should be strongly considered because of his impairment in functioning and family history.

Minor Depression

Minor depression is defined in the DSM-IV appendix as the presence of a sad or depressed mood, or anhedonia, for at least 2 weeks, accompanied by at least two but less than five of the depressive symptoms listed in Table 3.1. Broadhead and coworkers (4) found that this condition carried a 1.6-fold risk for disability compared with asymptomatic individuals, far less than the 4.8-fold risk for major depression. However, the higher prevalence of minor depression rendered it responsible for 51% more disability than major depression in the community (4). PRIME-MD 1000 Study participants with subthreshold diagnoses (e.g., minor depression) reported significantly worse social functioning, mental health, and health perceptions than those without mental disorders (6).

Subsyndromal Symptomatic Depression

As defined by Judd and coworkers (44), SSD is "any two or more simultaneous symptoms of depression, as defined by the DSM-IV criteria (*see* Table 3.1), present for most or all of the time, at least 2 weeks in duration, associated with evidence of social dysfunction, and occurring in individuals who do not meet criteria for diagnoses of minor depression, major depression, or dysthymia." In essence, they separated SSD from minor depression, with patients reporting significant depressed mood or anhedonia in the latter category and patients without these features comprising the former.

Recurrent Brief Depression

Recurrent brief depression (RBD) is defined by Angst and coworkers (45) as the presence of at least five of the nine symptoms of major depression that last less than 2 weeks but recur at least 12 times over the course of 1 year (i.e., approximately once each month). In other words, this encompasses patients who have sufficient symptoms for a diagnosis of major depression but which lack sufficient duration. The typical length of depressive episodes is 1 to 3 days. Angst and Hochstrasser (46) found that patients with this form of depression are depressed for a total of 5 to 6 weeks in a 1-year span, compared with approximately 10 weeks for those with major depression (46). Although premenstrual dysphoria would seem to fit the definition for RBD perfectly, the female-to-male ratio was 1.1 to 1, compared with 1.5 to 1 for major depression. However, a significant percentage went on to develop major depression, and the ratio was 3.5 to 1 for patients with both disorders. Morbidity was significant, as shown by a suicide attempt rate of 14% by 30 years of age. This rate is similar to that of patients with hypomania and dysthymia: less than the rate of major depression (21%) but greater than the rate for minor depression (3.5%). This did not differ significantly from controls (46).

Mixed Anxiety and Depression

Mixed anxiety and depression (MAD) is best viewed as the presence of mixed symptoms of anxiety and depression that are below diagnostic thresholds for either group of disorders. It also has been included in the *International Classification of Diseases*, tenth revision (ICD-10) (47); however, because of continuing controversy about its existence and significance as a separate entity, it was relegated to the appendix of DSM-IV as an area for potential research. It has garnered significant attention in the medical literature in recent years. There is evidence that MAD is particularly common in primary care (48) and that it is associated with significant levels of functional impairment (49), use of nonpsychiatric medical care (50), somatic and emotional symptoms of long duration (51), and previous and comorbid mental disorders (52). In fact, several studies indicate that MAD is similar to major anxiety or depressive disorders in each of these respects

(47–53). However, others fear that mixed anxiety and depression will become a "wastebasket" category for a heterogeneous group of patients and that it will overlap extensively with adjustment reaction (54–55). Some think that minor depression should be diagnosed in lieu of MAD, whereas others suggest categorizing it under generalized anxiety disorder (GAD). Those favoring MAD as a diagnosis view it as "a stable core of subsyndromal symptoms that do not reach the threshold for the diagnosis of GAD or depression, but which, under stress, will decompensate to an overt anxiety disorder or depression" (56). Some view even major mood and anxiety disorders as part of the same spectrum, buttressed by frequent comorbidity and newer treatments that are efficacious for both (57). Still others postulate that major depression and panic disorders are discrete entities but find dysthymia and general anxiety disorder more difficult to separate (58). At the least, it is important to recognize that anxiety frequently co-exists with depression at both subsyndromal and full disorder levels.

Adjustment Disorders

Symptoms that develop within 3 months after the onset of an identifiable psychosocial stressor and that do not meet criteria for another mood or anxiety disorder may represent an adjustment disorder. To make the diagnosis, the response to the stressor should be greater than what normally would be expected, typically impairing social or occupational functioning to some degree. Symptoms should be expected to resolve within 6 months of the termination of the stressor, although a chronic stressor such as a general medical condition could yield a chronic adjustment disorder. Depending on the predominant symptoms, the adjustment disorder may be characterized as "with depressed mood," "with anxiety," or "with mixed anxiety and depressed mood" (38).

CASE 3.3 *Premenstrual dysphoric disorder*

A woman 29 years of age reports that a coworker suggested she see her doctor about premenstrual syndrome. She relates a long history of cramps and headaches that occur for several days before menses. For several years, these symptoms have interfered with sleep; she attributed heightened irritability and emotional lability to the resulting fatigue and noticed that coworkers often avoid her during this time. She avoids her aerobics class and tends to eat a lot of chocolate "to provide energy" when she feels this way. Within a few days after her menstrual flow starts, she feels "back to normal."

The diagnosis is premenstrual dysphoric disorder.

Affective Disorders Specific to Women

Premenstrual Dysphoric Disorder

This diagnosis should be considered in women with mood symptoms that are temporally related to their menstrual cycle (Case 3.3). As defined by research criteria in the appendix to DSM-IV, symptom onset should be in the week before menses with complete remission within a week after menses. Five or more of the symptoms listed in Table 3.5 (38) should be reported, and the symptoms should interfere markedly with work, school, or usual social activities and relationships; should be confirmed by prospective daily ratings for at least two consecutive cycles; and should not represent merely an exacerbation of another mental disorder. PMDD has been identified in 3% to 5% of menstruating women and, like other disorders, subthreshold symptoms seem to be much more common than the disorder itself (59). There are additional parallels with mood disorders, including evidence of disturbances in serotonin metabolism (60). The diagnosis should be considered in women who develop symptoms of recurring dysphoria, irritability, and tension in association with menstrual periods.

Postpartum Depression

DSM-IV uses a specifier to describe a mood disorder that starts within 4 weeks of delivery. Postpartum blues, characterized by 1 to 4 days of labile mood and tearfulness, is reported to occur in 50% to 80% of women within

---

Table 3.5   Criteria for Premenstrual Dysphoric Disorder*

1. Markedly depressed mood, feelings of hopelessness, or self-deprecating thoughts

2. Marked anxiety, tension, feelings of being "keyed up" or "on edge"

3. Marked affective lability

4. Persistent and marked anger or irritability or increased interpersonal conflicts

5. Decreased interest in usual activities

6. Subjective sense of difficulty concentrating

7. Lethargy, easy fatigability, or marked lack of energy

8. Marked change in appetite, overeating, or specific food craving

9. Hypersomnia or insomnia

10. Feeling overwhelmed or out of control

11. Other physical symptoms (e.g., breast tenderness or swelling, headaches, joint or muscle aches)

---

* Symptom onset should occur the week before menses; complete remission should occur the week after. At least five of the above symptoms should be reported, including one of the first four.

5 days after delivery (37). Postpartum depression has been reported in 10% to 15% of women at 3 to 6 months postpartum, more frequently in those with a psychiatric history. Life stressors related to delivery and child care are also risk factors (61). Psychosis is far less common than depression and may occur with or without depressive symptoms. Typically beginning within 3 days after delivery, psychosis has a good prognosis but often recurs with subsequent pregnancy. As might be expected, the risk of depression after perinatal death has been found to be even higher (RR 2.4) than after a live birth (62). Miscarriage also is associated with depression, with a relative risk of 2.5 compared with women who had not been pregnant in the previous year (63). Factors that particularly raise risk after miscarriage include being childless and having a previous history of major depression.

Perimenopausal Symptoms
Although initial studies indicated an increased prevalence of depression in women at the time of menopause, the studies had methodologic flaws, and at this time a significant increase in risk is not thought to be associated with menopause (64). However, mild mood and anxiety symptoms may be more common perimenopausally, particularly for women with prolonged menopausal physical symptoms (e.g., hot flashes). Some researchers believe that estrogen replacement therapy may be helpful for mild psychological symptoms in such cases. In women who do develop depression at menopause, a previous history of depression, again, seems to be the strongest predictor (65).

Depression in the Elderly

Although the presentation of depression in the elderly does not differ greatly from that in younger patients, there are additional factors to consider. Depression and dementia are both common in geriatric populations; in fact, their co-existence is more common than pseudodementia (depression mimicking dementia). The elderly are more likely to be on multiple nonpsychotropic medications that must be taken into account both as potential causes of depression and in regard to medication interactions if antidepressants are prescribed. Similar concerns are raised by the heightened potential for comorbid medical conditions. Although age alone may not increase the risk of depression, the many conditions that become more common with age do seem to result in a significantly higher prevalence of depressive symptoms in older individuals (66).

Seasonal Affective Disorder

Seasonal affective disorder (SAD) is not recognized by DSM-IV, although there is a specifier, "with seasonal pattern," for major depression. This requires a regular temporal relationship between the onset of the episodes at a particular time of the year, full remissions at a particular time of the year, and at least two major depressive episodes within the past 2 years that demonstrate the temporal seasonal relationship (38). Although most of the population in one study reported at least mild seasonal changes in mood and behavior, SAD is more common in women and has a peak prevalence at 20 to 40 years of age (67). Northern latitudes apparently predispose to SAD, probably because of the decrement in sun exposure that occurs in winter months (68). Typically, depressive symptoms develop in the fall or winter and remit in the spring. However, a "summer SAD," which is exacerbated in sunny summer months and ameliorated in the winter, also has been reported (67). Most patients in the first reported case series of SAD also met criteria for a bipolar disorder (69). A subsyndromal form of SAD seems to be two to three times more common than the full disorder (67). Researchers at the National Institute of Mental Health have published diagnostic criteria and a questionnaire to screen for the disorder. Their Seasonal Pattern Assessment Questionnaire may be administered in person or by phone (70). There is also a 24-item Structured Interview Guide for the Hamilton Depression Rating Scale, Seasonal Affective Disorder Version (71). However, it is probably more practical for primary care physicians to simply consider seasonal patterns in depressed patients because this may affect the choice of therapy in some cases. For patients manifesting consistent significant seasonal variation, more detailed screening with one of these instruments, or referral, is warranted.

Mood Disorders Caused by a General Medical Condition

Most patients with a nonpsychiatric general medical condition do not have a depressive disorder, but the prevalence of clinically significant depressive symptoms has been reported to be 12% to 36% (37). Therefore, screening for mood disorders in patients with other medical conditions is warranted. The co-existence of the mood disorder and medical condition may be co-incidental, or they may be related biologically and/or psychologically. If the patient is on medication for a medical condition, the first consideration is whether the depressive symptoms could be induced by the medication; if so, alternative treatment should be considered. If the medical condition is one known to be a biological cause of depression (e.g., hypothyroidism or Cushing's disease), primary treatment of the underlying medical disorder should be the initial step. However, if the depression seems to be psychologically induced, such as a reaction to the prognosis of a malignancy or HIV infection, treatment of the depression should not be delayed. Likewise, coincident depression that does not seem to be a consequence of the medical condition(s) deserves prompt treatment. In cases in which the relationship between the general medical condition and the mood disorder is not clear, it is prudent to screen for major depression and to treat it when it is identified. Chronic diseases such as diabetes mellitus and coronary artery disease in particular may be associated with greater risk for mood disorders. There is also a strikingly high prevalence of depression in patients with neurological conditions, particularly cerebrovascular accidents, and Parkinson's disease and probably multiple sclerosis, Alzheimer's disease, and traumatic brain injury (72).

When depression is identified, how extensively does a clinician need to investigate for underlying medical conditions? In general, a good history and physical examination is the best place to start and may be all that is necessary. Table 3.6 addresses more specific medical conditions, although it should be noted that evidence of etiology, beyond mere association, is frequently lacking.

Symptom-Based Diagnoses

Symptom-based diagnoses, including chronic fatigue syndrome, fibromyalgia, irritable bowel syndrome, and headache syndromes, are often made in patients who meet criteria for mood and other mental disorders. Symptoms comprising criteria for such diagnoses overlap with the criteria for, or are

Table 3.6   Proposed Evaluation to Rule Out Medical Conditions in Depressed Patients

Condition	Evaluation
Hypothyroidism	Thyroid function tests
Malignancy	Careful history and physical examination; directed testing if abnormalities exist
Sleep apnea	History, sleep study
Connective tissue disease	Sedimentation rate
HIV	Antibody test
Cushing's disease	Dexamethasone-suppression testing
Hyperparathyroidism	Parathyroid hormone level
Parkinson's disease	History and physical examination
Alzheimer's disease	Mini-Mental Status Examination; assess for other causes of dementia
Other chronic diseases (e.g., diabetes mellitus, heart failure)	History and physical examination; glucose, blood urea nitrogen, and creatinine testing

commonly associated with, mood disorders. A Venn diagram of the disorders would demonstrate large areas of overlap, although the relationship between mood disorders and other symptom-based diagnoses remains controversial (73). Moreover, clinical trials have shown that antidepressants may be effective in the treatment of fibromyalgia, irritable bowel syndrome, chronic headache, pain disorders, and other symptom syndromes (74).

Medication-Related Mood Disorders

Mood disorders may be induced by medications as either idiosyncratic reactions or, with a small number of medications, as a biological effect in a predictable percentage of those who take the medicine at a specified dose. Medications that have been well documented to have a biological effect are relatively few. Of several antihypertensives suspected to cause depression, the only convincing relationship has been with reserpine, which is rarely used today (37). Even reserpine seems relatively safe at low doses for patients without personal or family histories of depression. Beta-blockers, particularly propranolol, have been indicted in some studies, reports, and case series. In such uncontrolled studies, the association may be spurious, simply reflecting the co-occurrence of two common conditions in the general population: hypertension and depression. Alternatively, propranolol-related side effects (e.g., fatigue, reduced energy) might suggest depression if clear definitions are not used. Larger, more rigorous studies generally have not shown a relationship between beta-blockers and depression or cognitive impairment (75–78).

Hormonal therapy also has been a source of concern about depression. Again, there is only one class of medication that clearly heightens the risk for mood disorders: glucocorticoids (e.g., prednisone). Mood disorders, with or without psychosis, most often occur shortly after beginning treatment and have been reported to be more common at higher doses in women and in patients being treated for systemic lupus erythematosis. There is no clear evidence of an association between other hormonal therapies and mood disorders (37). Although there have been studies suggesting higher rates of depression in patients taking anabolic steroids or oral contraceptives, the studies have been flawed, unconfirmed, or both. The best advice is to evaluate patients taking such agents for mood disorders, recognizing that the agents may be associated but not necessarily etiologic.

Substance-Induced Mood Disorders

Alcoholism should be considered as a distinct disorder separate from major depression. The prevalence of alcoholism in patients with primary depression is probably no greater than for nondepressed patients, and numerous studies have found that alcoholism is rarely a result of depression (37).

However, the conditions commonly co-exist, and some studies have found evidence of gender differences in their relationship. Women raised by alcoholic fathers seem to have a higher rate of depression (79), and women (as opposed to men) may attempt to self-medicate their depression with alcohol (37). Even when alcoholism is thought to be the primary disorder, diagnosing depression is important because it can modify the course of the alcoholism. Appropriate treatment improves prognosis.

Cocaine and amphetamines can mimic mania, whereas tricyclic antidepressants and selective serotonin-reuptake inhibitors (SSRIs) can precipitate manic or hypomanic episodes in patients with genetic predispositions for bipolar disorders. Use of cocaine or other stimulants should be considered in patients presenting with bipolar symptoms. In addition, patients who abruptly stop taking stimulants often exhibit depressive symptoms.

Psychiatric Comorbidity

Among the disorders that are more common in depressed than non-depressed patients are panic and anxiety disorders, obsessive-compulsive disorder, eating disorders, somatization, and personality disorders. The possibility of some of these should be considered because their presence may influence treatment plans. Likewise, the identification of another psychiatric condition should lead to an inquiry for depressive symptoms.

Somatization deserves special consideration, given that more than half of patients who present in a primary care setting with affective disorders have significant somatic components to their illness. Somatic pain has been present in 60% to 100% of depressed patients in some studies, and chronic pain is particularly nettlesome. In fact, Katon and coworkers (80) note that the presentation of depression with overt emotional symptoms is a relatively recent, Western phenomenon and that patients from non-Western cultures may be even more likely to display a predominance of somatic symptoms. Patients with multiple unexplained symptoms should be carefully evaluated for the presence of mood and anxiety disorders.

Suicidal Ideation

Suicide risk should be assessed in all depressed patients. Suicide is one of the leading causes of death in U.S. citizens under 45 years of age. Thoughts or plans of suicide constitute one of the nine diagnostic criteria for depression, and it has been reported that as many as two thirds of patients who commit suicide have seen a physician in the month before killing themselves (81). Patients are often reluctant to bring up the issue of suicide, but will usually talk about it when physicians ask. In addition to depression, risk factors include unemployment, substance abuse, recent adverse life events, and living alone. To determine the degree of immediate risk, a patient should be queried about specificity of their plans, including method and availability of means.

Recommendations

Physicians should routinely ask patients a question or two about depression as part of their health maintenance/preventive medicine assessment. Although depressed patients often do not volunteer emotional complaints spontaneously, patients in general are comfortable when their doctors inquire about psychosocial concerns (2). When patients have positive responses to screening questions, they should be queried further about depressive symptoms and associated impairment in occupational, social, and familial roles. A significant percentage are likely to have a major depressive disorder, and an even higher number will have depressive symptoms that fall short of major depression but that nevertheless produce significant disability and distress. Advances in treatment have made management of depression by primary care physicians increasingly effective and feasible.

■   ■   ■

Key Points

- Depressed patients in a primary care setting are more likely to present with physical rather than emotional complaints.
- The diagnosis of depression is missed in primary care at least half of the time.
- Screening for depression can handled effectively with as little as one or two questions, such as "Have you felt sad or depressed much of the time in the past year?"
- Subthreshold mood disorders are more common than major depression and dysthymia and as such are responsible for a greater degree of disability on a population basis.
- The high prevalence of depressive disorders, associated morbidity, and availability of simple screening measures make a cogent argument for routinely evaluating primary care patients for depression.

■   ■   ■

REFERENCES

 1. **Barrett JE, Barrett JA, Oxman TE, Gerber PD.** The prevalence of psychiatric disorders in a primary care practice. *Arch Gen Psychiatry.* 1988;45:1100–6.

 2. **Spitzer RL, Williams JBW, Kroenke K, et al.** Utility of a new procedure for diagnosing mental disorders in primary care. *JAMA.* 1994;272:1749–56.

 3. **Wells KB, Stewart A, Hays RD, et al.** The functioning and well-being of depressed patients: results from the Medical Outcomes Study. *JAMA.* 1989;262: 914–19.

 4. **Broadhead WE, Blazer DG, George LK, Tse CK.** Depression, disability days, and days lost from work in a prospective epidemiologic survey. *JAMA.* 1990;264: 2524–28.

 5. **Von Korff M, Ormel J, Katon W, Lin EHB.** Disability and depression among high utilizers of health care: a longitudinal analysis. *Arch Gen Psychiatry.* 1992;49: 91–100.

 6. **Spitzer RL, Kroenke K, Linzer M, et al.** Health-related quality of life in primary care patients with mental disorders: results from the PRIME-MD 1000 study. *JAMA.* 1995;274:1511–17.

 7. **Tollefson G, Hughes E, Derro RA, et al.** Depressive syndromes in a primary care setting: evaluation, classification, and outcome. *Compr Psychiatry.* 1983;24:144–53.

 8. **Linn LS, Yager J.** Recognition of depression and anxiety by primary physicians. *Psychosomatics.* 1984;24:593–600.

 9. **Ormel J, Van der Brink W, Koeter MWJ, et al.** Recognition, management and outcome of psychological disorders in primary care: a naturalistic follow-up study. *Psychol Med.* 1990;20:909–23.

10. **Perez-Stable EJ, Miranda J, Munoz RF, Ying Y.** Depression in medical outpatients: underrecognition and misdiagnosis. *Arch Intern Med.* 1990;150:1083–88.

11. **Coulehan JL, Schulberg HC, Block MR, et al.** Medical comorbidity of major depressive disorder in a primary care medical practice. *Arch Intern Med.* 1990;150: 2363–67.

12. **Covinsky KE, Fortinsky RH, Palmer RM, et al.** Relation between symptoms of depression and health status outcomes in acutely ill hospitalized older persons. *Ann Intern Med.* 1997;126:417–25.

13. **Callahan CM, Kesterson JG, Tierney WM.** Association of symptoms of depression with diagnostic test charges among older adults. *Ann Intern Med.* 1997;126: 426–32.

14. **Klinkman MS, Coyne JC, Gallo S, Schwenk TL.** False positives, false negatives, and the validity of diagnosis of major depression in primary care. *Arch Fam Med.* 1998;7:451–61.

15. **Bertakis KD, Roter DR, Putnam SM.** The relationship of physician medical interview style to patient satisfaction. *J Fam Pract.* 1991;32:175–81.

16. **Kroenke K.** Discovering depression in medical patients: reasonable expectations. *Ann Intern Med.* 1997;126:463–65.

17. **Klinkman MS.** Competing demands in psychosocial care: a model for the identification and treatment of depressive disorders in primary care. *Gen Hosp Psychiatry.* 1997;19:98–111.

18. **Williams JBW, Mulrow CD, Kroenke K, et al.** Case finding for depression in primary care: a randomized trial. *Am J Med.* 1999;106:36–43.

19. **Schwenk TL.** Screening for depression in primary care: a disease in search of a tests. *J Gen Intern Med.* 1996;11:437–39.

20. **Mulrow CD, Williams JW, Gerety MB, et al.** Case-finding instruments for depression in primary care settings. *Ann Intern Med.* 1995;122:913–21.

21. **Burnam MA, Wells KB, Leake B, Landsverk J.** Development of a brief screening instrument for detecting depressive disorders. *Med Care.* 1988;26:775–89.

22. **Leon AC, Olfson M, Weissman M, et al.** Brief screens for mental disorders in primary care: a validation study. *J Gen Intern Med.* 1996;11:424–8.

23. **Whooley MA, Avins AL, Miranda J, Browner WS.** Case-finding instruments for depression: two questions are as good as many. *J Gen Intern Med.* 1997;12:439–45.

24. **Philbrick JT, Connelly JE, Wofford AB.** The prevalence of mental disorders in rural office practice. *J Gen Intern Med.* 1996;11:9–15.

25. **Kobak KA, Taylor LV, Dotti SL, et al.** A computer-administered telephone interview to identify mental disorders. *JAMA.* 1997;278:905–19.

25a. **Spitzer RL, Kroenke K, William JBW, and the Patient Health Questionnaire Primary Care Study Group.** Validation and utility of a self-report version of PRIME-MD: the PHQ Primary Care Study. *JAMA.* 1999;282:1737–44.

26. **Kroenke K, Jackson JL, Chamberlin J.** Depressive and anxiety disorders in patients presenting with physical complaints: clinical predictors and outcome. *Am J Med.* 1997;103:339–47.

27. **Wells KB, Burnam A, Rogers W, et al.** The course of depression in adult outpatients: results from the Medical Outcomes Study. *Arch Gen Psychiatry.* 1992;49: 788–94.

28. **Johnson J, Weissman MM, Klerman GL.** Service utilization and social morbidity associated with depressive symptoms in the community. *JAMA.* 1992;267:1478–83.

29. **U.S. Preventive Services Task Force.** *Guide to Clinical Preventive Services,* 2nd ed. Baltimore: Williams & Wilkins; 1996.

30. **Barrett JE, Katon W, Williams JW.** *Treatment of Minor Depression and Dysthymia in Primary Care: Response to Paroxetine and Problem-Solving Therapy.* Paper presented at Improving Care for Depression in Organized Health Care Systems, Seattle, 1999 Feb 25.

31. **Robins LN, Helzer JE, Croughan C, Ratcliff KS.** National Institute of Mental Health Diagnostic Interview Schedule: its history, characteristics, and validity. *Arch Gen Psychiatry.* 1981;38:381–9.

32. **Spitzer RL, Williams JBW, Gibbon M, et al.** *Structured Clinical Interview for DSM-IIIR, Non-Patient Edition* (SCID-NP, Version 1.0). Washington, DC: American Psychiatric Press; 1990.

33. **Brody DS, Hahn SR, Spitzer RL, et al.** Identifying patients with depression in the primary care setting. *Arch Intern Med.* 1998;158:2469–75.

34. **Good MD, Good BJ, Cleary PD.** Do patient attitudes influence physician recognition of psychosocial problems in primary care? *J Fam Pract.* 1987;25:53–59.

35. **Hall JA, Dornan MC.** What patients like about their medical care and how often they are asked: a meta-analysis of the satisfaction literature. *Soc Sci Med.* 1988;27: 935–39.

36. **Broadhead WE, Clapp-Channing NE, Finch JN, Copeland JA.** Effects of medical illness and somatic symptoms on treatment of depression in a family medicine residency practice. *Gen Hosp Psychiatry.* 1989;11:194–200.

37. **Depression Guideline Panel, U.S. Department of Health and Human Services.** Detection and diagnosis. *Depression in Primary Care,* vol. 1. Washington, DC: U.S. Government Printing Office; 1993.

38. **American Psychiatric Association.** *Diagnostic and Statistical Manual of Mental Disorders,* 4th ed. Washington, DC: American Psychiatric Association; 1994.

39. **Zisook S, Shuchter SR, Sledge PA, et al.** The spectrum of depressive phenomena after spousal bereavement. *J Clin Psychiatry.* 1994;55(Suppl):29–36.

40. **Angst J, Hochstrasser B.** Recurrent brief depression: the Zurich Study. *J Clin Psychiatry.* 1994;55(Suppl):3–9.

41. **Sherbourne CD, Wells KB, Hays RD, et al.** Subthreshold depression and depressive disorder: clinical characteristics of general medical and mental health specialty outpatients. *Am J Psychiatry.* 1994;151:1777–84.

42. **Cass AR, Volk RJ, Nease DE.** Health-related quality of life in primary care patients with recognized and unrecognized mood and anxiety disorders. *Int J Psychiatr Med.* 1999;29:293–309.

43. **Coulehan JL, Block MR, Janosky JE, Arena VC.** Depressive symptomatology and medical co-morbidity in a primary care clinic.

44. **Judd LL, Rapaport MH, Paulus MP, Brown JL.** Subsyndromal symptomatic depression: a new mood disorder? *J Clin Psychiatry.* 1994;55(Suppl):18–28.

45. **Angst J, Merikangas K, Scheidegger P, Wicki W.** Recurrent brief depression: a new subtype of affective disorder. *J Affect Disord.* 1990;19:87–98.

46. **Angst J, Hochstrasser B.** Recurrent brief depression: the Zurich study. *J Clin Psychiatry.* 1994;55(Suppl):3–9.

47. **World Health Organization.** *The International Classification of Diseases,* 10th rev. Geneva, Switzerland: World Health Organization; 1992.

48. **Stein MB, Kirk P, Prabhu V, et al.** Mixed anxiety and depression in a primary care clinic. *J Affect Disord.* 1995;3479–84.

49. **Fawcett J.** The detection and consequences of anxiety in clinical depression. *J Clin Psychiatry.* 1997;58(Suppl 8):35–40.

50. **Roy-Burne PP.** Generalized anxiety and mixed anxiety-depression: association with disability and health care utilization. *J Clin Psychiatry.* 1996(Suppl 7);57:86–91.

51. **Katon W, Roy-Burne PP.** Mixed anxiety and depression. *J Abnorm Psychol.* 1991;100:337–45.

52. **Boulenger JP, Fournier M, Rosales D, Lavallee YJ.** Mixed anxiety and depression: from theory to practice. *J Clin Psychiatry.* 1997;58(Suppl 8):27–34.

53. **Zinbarg RE, Barlow DH, Liebowitz M, et al.** The DSM-IV field trial for mixed anxiety-depression. *Am J Psychiatry.* 1994;151:1153–62.

54. **Preskorn SH, Fast GA.** Beyond signs and symptoms: the case against a mixed anxiety and depression category. *J Clin Psychiatry.* 1993;54(Suppl):24–32.

55. **Liebowitz MR.** Mixed anxiety and depression: should it be included in DSM-IV? *J Clin Psychiatry.* 1993;54(Suppl):4–7,17–20.

56. **Stahl SM.** Mixed anxiety and depression: clinical implications. *J Clin Psychiatry.* 1993;54(Suppl):33–38.

57. **Stahl SM.** Mixed depression and anxiety: serotonin-1A receptors as a common pharmacologic link. *J Clin Psychiatry.* 1997;58(Suppl 8):20–26.

58. **Liebowitz MR, Hollander E, Schneier F, et al.** Anxiety and depression: discrete diagnostic entities? *J Clin Psychopharmacol.* 1990;10:S61-6.

59. **Rivera-Tovar AD, Frank E.** Late luteal phase dysphoric disorder in young women. *Am J Psychiatry.* 1990;147:1634–36.

60. **Rapkin AJ.** The role of serotonin in premenstrual syndrome. *Clin Obstet Gynecol.* 1992;35:629–36.

61. **O'Hara MW, Neunaber DJ, Zekoski EM.** Prospective study of postpartum depression: prevalence, course, and predictive factors. *J Abnorm Psychol.* 1984;93:158–71.

62. **Clarke M, Williams AJ.** Depression in women after perinatal death. *Lancet.* 1979;1:916–7.

63. **Neugebauer RN, Kline J, Shrout P, et al.** Major depressive disorder in the 6 months after miscarriage. *JAMA.* 1997;277:383–88.

64. **Pearlstein T, Rosen K, Stone AB.** Mood disorders and menopause. *Endocrinol Metab Clin North Am.* 1997;26:279–94.

65. **Avis NE, Brambilla D, McKinlay SM, Vass K.** A longitudinal analysis of the association between menopause and depression: results from the Massachusetts Women's Health Study. *Ann Epidemiol.* 1994;4:214–20.

66. **Lebowitz BD, Pearson JL, Schneider LS, et al.** Diagnosis and treatment of depression in late life: consensus statement update. *JAMA.* 1997;278:1186–90.

67. **Kasper S, Wehr TA, Bartko JJ, et al.** Epidemiologic findings of seasonal changes in mood and behavior. *Arch Gen Psychiatry.* 1989;46823–33.

68. **Rosen LN, Targum SD, Terman M, et al.** Prevalence of seasonal affective disorder at four latitudes. *Psychiatry Res.* 1990;31:131–44.

69. **Rosenthal NE, Sack DA, Gillin C, et al.** Seasonal affective disorder. A description of the syndrome and preliminary findings with light therapy. *Arch Gen Psychiatry.* 1984;41:72–80.

70. **Rosenthal NE, Genhart M, Sack DA, et al.** Seasonal affective disorder and its relevance to the understanding and treatment of bulimia. In Hudson JL, Pope HG (eds). *Psychobiology of Bulimia.* Washington, DC: American Psychiatric Press; 1987:203–228.

71. **Williams JBW, Link MJ, Rosenthal NE, et al.** *Structured Interview Guide for the Hamilton Depression Rating Scale,* Seasonal Affective Disorder Version (SIGH-SAD). New York: New York State Psychiatric Institute; 1992.

72. **Sutor B, Rummans TA, Jowsey SG, et al.** Major depression in medically ill patients. *Mayo Clin Proc.* 1998;73:329–37.

73. **Kroenke K.** Unexplained physical symptoms and somatoform disorders. In deGruy FV (ed). *Twenty Common Behavioral Problems in Primary Care.* New York: McGraw-Hill. In press.

74. **O'Malley PG, Jackson JL, Santoro J, et al.** Antidepressant therapy for unexplained symptoms and symptom syndromes. *J Fam Pract.* 1999;48:980–90.

75. **Bartels D, Blasser M, Wang A, Swanson P.** Association between depression and propranolol use in ambulatory patients. *Clin Pharm.* 1988;7:146–50.

76. **Ried LD, McFarland BH, Johnson RE, Brody KK.** Beta-blockers and depression: the more the murkier? *Ann Pharmacother.* 1988;32:699–708.

77. **Palac DM, Cornish RD, McDonald WJ, Middaugh DA, et al.** Cognitive function in hypertensives treated with atenolol or propranolol. *J Gen Intern Med.* 1990;5:310–18.

78. **Skinner MH, Futteman A, Morrissette D, et al.** Atenolol compared with nifedipine: effect on cognitive function and mood in elderly hypertensive patients. *Ann Intern Med.* 1992;116:615–23.

79. **Goodwin DW, Schulsinger F, Knopf J, et al.** Psychopathology in adopted and non-adopted daughters of alcoholics. *Arch Gen Psychiatry.* 1977;34:1005–09.

80. **Katon W, Kleinman A, Rosen G.** Depression and somatization: a review. Part I. *Am J Med.* 1982;72:127–135.

81. **Hirschfeld RMA, Russell JM.** Assessment and treatment of suicidal patients. *N Engl J Med.* 1997;337:910–15.

KEY REFERENCES

Depression Guideline Panel, U.S. Department of Health and Human Services. Detection and diagnosis. *Depression in Primary Care,* vol. 1. Washington, DC: U.S. Government Printing Office; 1993.

A good overview and summary of the findings of an expert panel on depression. Includes algorithms and many references.

Mulrow CD, Williams JW, Gerety MB, et al. Case-finding instruments for depression in primary care settings. *Ann Intern Med.* 1995;122:913–21.

Analyzes 18 studies that used nine methods of screening for depression, finding similar accuracy for each, regardless of their length.

Spitzer RL, Williams JBW, Kroenke K, et al. Utility of a new procedure for diagnosing mental disorders in primary care. *JAMA.* 1994;272:1749–56.

Reviews the use and validation of the PRIME-MD in 1000 ambulatory primary care patients.

Whooley MA, Avins AL, Miranda J, Browner WS. Case-finding instruments for depression: two questions are as good as many. *J Gen Intern Med.* 1997;12:439–45.

Demonstrates that two screening questions for depression taken from the PRIME-MD are as effective as more comprehensive measures.

Williams JW, Mulrow CD, Kroenke K, et al. Case-finding for depression in primary care: a randomized trial. *Am J Med.* 1999;106:36–43.

Compares the CES-D with a single question to screen for depression, finding similar sensitivity and slightly diminished specificity. In addition, demonstrates that screening for depression is associated with improved outcomes.

4

■　■　■

Management

Robert K. Schneider, MD

Robert N. Glenn, PhD

James L. Levenson, MD

"I'm simply not strong enough to fight the depression by myself."

General Considerations
in the Management of Depression

Primary care physicians (PCPs) often carry long-term responsibility for the management of depression. Other professionals may be involved at various times in the course of treatment, but many patients return to their PCPs for treatment of both medical problems and symptoms of depression. In many circumstances, PCPs manage depressed patients without the involvement of mental health professionals.

The management of depression in the primary care setting is a complex and dynamic process requiring the physician's attention to recognition, diagnosis, treatment, and follow-up. Each of these elements is covered in depth elsewhere in this book. This chapter presents an overview, integrating these elements with other aspects of management. For the purposes of this chapter, we will assume that the symptoms of depression have been recognized accurately and diagnosed properly as major depression. Treatment for depression is potentially multimodal. The physician and patient have the task of choosing which treatments are appropriate and acceptable to both.

After the diagnosis is made in the physician's mind, the task of "giving" the diagnosis to the patient is next. At this juncture, the use of the very word "depression" is tricky. Informing the patient that he or she is depressed may create problems in acceptance and compliance. Many patients do no understand what depression really is and may interpret the term in a highly negative or self-critical way. It is important to use the patient's own words in describing depressive symptoms by restating the most troubling symptoms. These symptoms will become the target of treatment and will be tracked by the patient and the physician. The physician also should ask about other symptoms that the patient might not have mentioned, particularly neurovegetative symptoms and thoughts about death or dying (*see* section on Management of the Suicidal Patient below). Efficacy of treatment will be determined by tracking the course of the target symptoms over time—the more specifically described the better. "He's depressed and feels helpless" is much less helpful than, "His sleep is reduced to 4 hours, he has stopped going to church, and his back pain has increased." The latter better enables the patient and physician to track the patient's response to treatment in terms understandable, observable, and specific to the patient.

After the target symptoms are identified, they should be tracked carefully over time. Chapter 12 reviews these terms in more depth as part of the Agency for Health Care Policy and Research's practice guidelines. The terms used to follow the target symptoms over time can be remembered as the five R's and the three phases, which allow the physician and the patient to conceptualize the course of depression longitudinally. The five R's are as follows:

1. **Response:** When symptoms have decreased to the point at which the criteria for major depression are no longer met

2. **Remission:** A period during which either there is an improvement of sufficient magnitude that criteria for major depression are no longer met (partial remission) or the patient becomes asymptomatic (full remission)

3. **Relapse:** The return of symptoms after a prolonged full remission that satisfy full diagnostic criteria before recovery has occurred

4. **Recovery:** A prolonged full remission for at least 6 months during which the patient is asymptomatic

5. **Recurrence:** The appearance of a new episode of depression with symptoms that meet full criteria and, thus, can occur only after recovery

The above terms have been defined precisely for research purposes (1), but they also serve to remind us that depression is often a chronic disease, with many patients suffering multiple episodes and some never achieving complete recovery.

The five R's occur in the context of the three treatment phases of depression:

1. **Acute phase:** Begins when treatment is initiated and ends with full remission

2. **Continuation phase:** Begins with full remission and lasts until either the chances of relapse significantly diminish or a relapse occurs (typically 6–9 months in the first episode of depression); the goal during this phase is to prevent relapse

3. **Maintenance phase:** Follows the continuation phase, with the goal being to prevent recurrence; this phase ends if a new recurrent episode of depression begins

When it comes to intervention, the choice is complex between continued observation, psychotherapy, medication, nonmedication/nonpsychotherapy ("adjunctive") interventions, or some combination of these. The relative efficacy of medication versus psychotherapy versus a combination of both in the treatment of depression remains a topic of active study, without clear consensus from the data. Chapter authors in this book vary in their views about the choice of first-line treatment; however, if one interprets the research to date, treatment should be individualized to each patient. The choice should be directed by two organizing principles: the severity of the depression and the patient's preferences. The principles also relate to each other in that the more severe the depression the more treatment options become circumscribed. When the patient is actively suicidal, psychotic, manic, or rapidly deteriorating, an immediate referral to a mental health specialist is indicated regardless of patient preference; somatic treatments (e.g., medication, electroconvulsive therapy) and usually hospitalization are indicated. Fortunately, these cases are atypical in the primary care setting. Far more common is depression that is subsyndromal, mild, or moderate in severity. In these cases, patient preference should direct treatment choice. The major reason for treatment failure is noncompliance or noncompletion of treatment. Patient preference is paramount in obtaining compliance with the treatment selected (*see also* Chapters 5 and 6).

Table 4.1 summarizes the initial steps in the management of depression.

Management of the Suicidal Patient

Risk Assessment

Assessment of the potential for suicide is an essential component in evaluating and treating depression. An evaluation of the patient's suicidal potential should be performed whenever the diagnosis of depression is

---

Table 4.1   Initial Management Steps for Depression

1. Restate the most troubling symptoms

2. Ask about other symptoms (e.g., lack of pleasure, concentration difficulties, low energy, preoccupation with death or suicide)

3. State the target symptoms of treatment and the expectation of change

4. Establish where the patient is in the longitudinal course of the disease (e.g., relapse vs. recurrence)

5. Determine severity of depression

6. Discuss patient's preferences and expectations

---

considered and especially if an antidepressant is prescribed (1a). Identification of depression and suicidal ideation is particularly important in the medical setting because physicians are likely to have contact with people who commit suicide soon thereafter. Approximately 80% of people who end their lives talk about suicide before taking action (1b). Some evidence indicates that half of people (and 75% of elderly) who kill themselves have seen their physicians within a month before they died (1c). Suicide ranks as the ninth leading cause of death each year, with over 30,000 suicides annually. There are at least 10 suicide attempts for each completed suicide (1d). Physicians have the potential to help prevent morbidity and mortality from suicide. Their skill in identifying, evaluating, and interviewing for suicidal ideation/intent can make a crucial difference. Key risk factors for suicide can be identified in the patient's demographics (Case 4.1) (Table 4.2), history (Table 4.3), and current state (Table 4.4) (1,2).

CASE 4.1   *Assessment of suicide risk during initial evaluation for depression*

Mr. L's wife died of breast cancer 6 months ago. He now comes for his yearly check-up. Although Mr. L denies depression, he has stopped hunting and fishing with his friends, both of which are long-time interests. He is white, 63 years old, recently retired, and has chronic obstructive pulmonary disease (COPD) and rheumatoid arthritis.

Many patients with major depression deny feeling depressed, although they usually admit specific symptoms if asked. Mr. L's withdrawal from pleasurable activities is suggestive. He has many risk factors for suicide (older white man, widowed, not working, chronic illness, chronic pain, and access to guns). His physician should evaluate for depression and directly ask about any alcohol use and suicidal thoughts.

Table 4.2   Demographic Risk Factors for Suicide

Age	The highest risk is in adolescents and the elderly
Gender	Women make 10 times more attempts than men, but men succeed at suicide three times more often because they use more lethal methods
Marital Status	Separated, widowed, or divorced
Race	White men and women account for a disproportionate 90% of all suicides
Sexual identity	Homosexuals are at higher risk
Gun ownership	People who live in homes with firearms are five times more likely to die by suicide than those in gun-free homes
Relationships	Persons are at higher risk when living alone and have no social supports
Employment	Unemployed or have lost status in their jobs

Discussing Suicidal Ideation and Plans with the Patient

Patients' anxiety or shame and physicians' discomfort may lead to skirting the topic of suicide. The best approach is to ask the patient directly. A good, empathetic initial question is "Have you felt so bad that life did not seem worth living?". If answered affirmatively (or not answered), the next question should be "Was it bad enough that you thought of ending your life?".

Further steps include the following:

1. What is the frequency of the thoughts (pervasive, intermittent)?
2. Are the thoughts directly related to a recent or upcoming situation?
3. Does the patient have a suicide plan? If so, how well developed is it?
4. How lethal is the described method of suicide?
5. What is the patient's access to the method? Is there a gun or are there drugs in the home?
6. Does the patient have any thoughts or impulses of hurting someone else? (It is not uncommon for suicidal and homicidal thoughts to occur together, particularly if domestic violence is involved.)

Providing the Patient with Immediate Safety

Prevention of suicide requires specific and immediate interventions. Emergency referral to a mental health practitioner is always indicated with acute

Table 4.3   Patient History Risk Factors for Suicide

- Previous suicide attempts, even if minor
- Family history of completed or attempted suicide
- Suicide of a close friend, particularly if an adolescent
- Psychotic or bipolar depression
- Poor coping ability
- Substance abuse
- Personality disorder
- Anniversary of a loss
- Chronic pain
- Chronic debilitating illness (e.g., AIDS, end-stage renal disease)

Table 4.4   Current State Risk Factors for Suicide

- A direct or indirect expression of intent to harm self
- A suicide plan that is well developed
- Poor judgment or impulse control
- Use of alcohol or other substances
- Giving away possessions
- A significant deterioration in functioning and appearance
- A rapid elevation in mood (the patient may have decided on a plan and feels a sense of relief)
- More energy also may help a patient follow through with a plan
- A fantasy of reuniting with deceased loved one

suicidal thoughts or plans or recent attempts. An inpatient admission also may be needed if the patient's or others' safety cannot be protected. Depending on the severity of the crisis, the physician should consider the actions below in the interim before evaluation, admission, or treatment by a mental health provider. If the patient has expressed suicidal ideation or intent, the physician has to determine the extent to which the patient will cooperate with safety issues (e.g., giving up guns); the availability of friends and family to ensure safety or to follow through with more restrictive options; and the risk to another person if violence is also threatened.

The range of alternatives for the physician will depend on the degree to which the patient's safety can be assured. Assessment will be contingent on the following:

1. The patient's willingness to engage in a plan with the physician to not harm himself/herself. This plan can be verbal or written. It can be as simple as the patient's clear agreement to call the practice if they are feeling unable to control thoughts or impulses to harm themselves (3).

2. The availability of family or friends to provide a "suicide watch" (if needed) for a defined period of time or to help in the removal of lethal items from the home. They also should be familiar with the procedures if more restrictive intervention is required (i.e., psychiatric emergency room, involuntary hospitalization).

3. Increased contact with the physician or medical practice until the patient can see a mental health practitioner.

4. The physician will need to implement more restrictive options for the patient's safety if prevention of self-harm cannot be negotiated. The patient can be given the opportunity for a voluntary admission to a hospital. Refusal to agree to this alternative requires an involuntary process. Procedures vary by state or province.

Although these precautions are usually easy to implement, they are not always effective. Patients who become resolutely and persistently intent on killing themselves may succeed despite others' best efforts.

When To Refer to a Mental Health Specialist

Emergency Referral

The first consideration is whether the patient's safety is at risk. All depressed patients with active psychosis (hallucinations or delusions), acute suicidal risk, or dehydration-malnutrition should be urgently referred to a psychiatrist. An emergency referral can be voluntary or involuntary. In a voluntary emergency referral, the patient agrees to the evaluation and is escorted to the place of evaluation, which is usually a general hospital's emergency room or a psychiatric crisis evaluation service. In the event that the patient does not agree to emergency evaluation, involuntary psychiatric hospitalization should be considered. Criteria for involuntary hospitalization, who can file, and legal procedures vary by state or province. Generally a crisis service or magistrate is contacted and a law enforcement officer is sent if necessary to escort the patient to a facility for emergency evaluation. Although some patients may be initially distressed or angry about being coerced into psychiatric care, most are ultimately grateful, recognizing that their physicians and families acted out of concern for them.

Urgent Non-Emergency Referrals

The urgent non-emergency referral is for the unstable, suicidal patient that needs evaluation in the next 24 to 72 hours. The suicidal patient is considered to be relatively safe and can wait because the patient is cooperative with a plan for safety, there is a good supportive environment to observe the patient, there is no access to means for suicide (e.g., removal of guns), and the patient accepts the need for referral. Non-emergency urgent referral also should be attempted for patients without any acute risk for suicide whose depressive symptoms are severely distressing to them. For both emergency and non-emergency urgent referrals, physicians should have established knowledge of available mental health resources in their community and how to access them.

Routine Referrals

Routine referrals will occur much more frequently than emergency or urgent non-emergency referrals. Referral patterns vary within physician groups. The three major variables affecting routine referral are the physician's comfort and aptitude in handling depression, the system of health care in which the physician practices, and the patient's condition and preferences. In systems in which mental health services are integrated with primary care, referral indications and pathways are much clearer. Because most physicians and mental health professionals in the United States are not currently in such systems, the PCP must take more responsibility for referral. Reasons for referral include a patient who wants or could benefit from psychotherapy (see Chapter 6), patients who have not responded to therapeutic trials of antidepressants, comorbid substance abuse, bipolar illness, and a history of psychotic or severe depression. Some patients are not open to referral to a mental health specialist and openly refuse or accept the referral in the office and break the appointment. These situations are challenging and difficult and can isolate the primary physician. In these circumstances a telephone call to a mental health colleague should be made to discuss options. The one thing all referrals have in common is the forethought of the referring physician: awareness of laws, referral procedures, and one's own skills allow for efficient and timely referrals to mental health professionals and ultimately the best outcomes for our patients.

Ethical and Risk-Management Issues

Boundaries

Maintenance of professional boundaries is appropriate in all doctor-patient relationships, but a physician's wish to aid a distressed, depressed patient may lead to crossing boundaries. Depressed patients are more vulnerable and more likely to be dependent, lonely, and unhappy in their primary relationships. In most cases, physicians should remain neutral in patients' major life decisions (e.g., quitting job, divorce). It is often appropriate to encourage an acutely depressed patient to postpone a major decision until feeling better, but physicians should refrain from urging a particular decision. Although it can be tempting, for example, to tell a depressed patient to leave an unhappy marriage, the physician seldom has sufficient knowledge of the patient's entire situation and the potential consequences of this advice. To take such a position undermines the physician's objectivity and erodes the patient's autonomy and capacity for independence. Excessive self-disclosure by physicians also is to be avoided. Although it is said "misery loves company," depressed patients do not want or benefit from having depressed physicians. Doing special favors for patients (e.g., loaning money, supporting unjustified sick leave) also is ill advised because it fosters increased dependency and unrealistic expectations about the physician. For similar reasons, physicians should not have sessions with depressed patients that are unbilled, unusually long, or outside regular office hours. Hugging and kissing patients is usually inappropriate; a lonely depressed patient is especially likely to misinterpret what the physician intended as an innocent expression of affection and concern. Sexual misconduct by physicians who become involved with patients typically starts with the physician's rationalizing of less serious boundary violations with patients who are depressed and hungry for a benevolent, caring parental figure (4).

Confidentiality

Confidentiality is a vital ethical principle in all of medical care, but it is especially important in the treatment of psychiatric disorders. Although stigma associated with depression has decreased in recent years, many people are still reluctant to accept a diagnosis of and treatment for depression. Others are willing but wish to keep it a secret. Family members, employers, schools, and other third parties may ask the physician for information about a depressed patient, but divulging this information requires the patient's permission. Some employers may discriminate against depressed employees. Concern that a history of depression may interfere with obtaining personal health, disability, or life insurance is not unwarranted. This does not apply to group policies, but many insurers do charge more or decline to insure individuals currently or previously treated for depression. Confidentiality, like other ethical principles, is not an absolute and sometimes must give way to an overriding moral imperative. Physicians may break confidentiality with suicidal patients if the purpose is to prevent self-harm (e.g., asking the spouse to remove firearms from the home). Additionally, physicians are legally mandated to report child abuse or neglect, both of which are more frequent with a seriously depressed parent.

Documentation

Nonpsychiatric physicians frequently treat depression in their patients without explicitly documenting diagnosis or treatment. Although this may be an understandable response to concerns about confidentiality (*see* section above), failure to document is a mistake with potentially serious consequences. Written details permit the physician (or a subsequent physician) to track treatment response accurately, recall side effects or compliance problems, and note any referrals made to mental health professionals. Predictably, as more nonpsychiatric physicians prescribe antidepressants, there are more malpractice suits brought against them after poor depression outcomes (especially suicide). Although sketchy documentation may be frequent, it is difficult to claim that it represents the standard of care. If the physician did not document a diagnosis of depression, an evaluation of suicide risk, and what treatment and referrals were given, the plaintiff's attorney is likely to assert that there is no evidence the physician ever did what he/she claims.

Shared Treatment

Shared-treatment arrangements in which a PCP provides pharmacotherapy and a nonmedical therapist provides psychotherapy have become common, raising a number of potential concerns. It is clearly negligent for a physician to prescribe an antidepressant "recommended" by a psychotherapist, without seeing the patient. The physician should not prescribe any psychiatric drug about which he/she is not knowledgeable. Because psychologists, social workers, and counselors are not licensed to prescribe, the physician will be the one bearing liability risk if there is an adverse outcome related to a prescribed antidepressant medication.

Are physicians in shared-treatment relationships responsible only for the part of treatment they provide (typically, medication), or are they responsible for the overall treatment of the patient? The answer is likely to vary with the specifics of the case, but in general, the courts have regarded physicians as having broad authority and responsibility. Furthermore, plaintiffs' attorneys usually try to cast their nets widely, directing them toward deeper pockets. Better patient care and lower malpractice risk can be achieved by clear communication between the physician and nonmedical psychotherapist, with explicit understanding of their relative responsibilities and expectations. In a shared-treatment arrangement, the psychotherapist and physician must be free to discuss the patient. Neither should agree to a patient's insistence that there be no communication. Certainly psychotherapists must still exercise discretion in whether to withhold sensitive information (e.g., the patient having had an extramarital affair). Failure to communicate may deprive both clinicians of essential information (e.g., substance abuse) and also may undermine allocation of responsibility, consequently leading to failure to intervene when the patient is deteriorating (*see* Cases 4.2 and 4.3). The physician may bear some responsibility even for aspects of treatment outside his or her domain, especially if the collaborating therapist is grossly unethical, incompetent, or impaired, as Case 4.3 illustrates.

CASE 4.2   *Miscommunication between primary care physician and psychotherapist*

A psychologist treating Mr. J advised him to consult his PCP for antidepressant medication after Mr. J's depression had worsened despite 8 weeks of psychotherapy. The PCP prescribed fluoxetine. There was no communication by phone or letter between the psychologist and PCP. On a follow-up visit to the PCP, the patient complained his depression was no better, even worse. After careful questioning, Mr. J acknowledged he had stopped taking fluoxetine after a few days because he did not wish to be on any psychiatric drug. The PCP assumed the psychologist would decide what to do next because without medication there was no need for his involvement. The psychologist assumed the PCP was proceeding with pharmacotherapy, because psychotherapy alone had not worked. Mr. J's condition worsened. His wife became alarmed. She called the offices of both the PCP and psychologist, and each suggested she call the other.

If Mr. J commits suicide, both the PCP and the psychologist may be held liable.

CASE 4.3   *Shared treatment: primary care physician's accountability*

Ms. K told her PCP (who was treating her with an antidepressant) that she "loved" the counselor recommended by the PCP's nurse. At subsequent visits, Ms. K spoke so affectionately about her therapist that the PCP grew uneasy about their relationship (of Ms. K and the therapist). It later emerged that the therapist had become sexually involved with Ms. K, was unlicensed, and had no malpractice insurance. If a lawsuit arises, the search for a way to compensate the patient may focus liability on the PCP.

In shared treatment arrangements, the physician has some accountability for knowing the qualifications and competence of the collaborating psychotherapist (and vice versa). Responsibility for having such knowledge is increased when one has referred the patient to the other, and more so if they regularly collaborate in shared cases.

Disability and Its Evaluation

Depression causes as much or more disability (e.g., missed work, days in bed) than chronic medical conditions like diabetes or arthritis (5). Even minor depressive illness results in days lost from work and, because of its greater prevalence, accounts for more total disability days in the community than major depression (6). Consequently, physicians are frequently asked by patients, employers, or insurers (private or Social Security) to complete disability evaluations for depressed patients. Some physicians reflexively release patients with depression from work and support their receipt of disability regardless of whether they meet disability criteria (which vary by occupation and insurance policy). Although such physicians feel they are acting out of loyalty to their patients, uncritical support for disability promotes invalidism and long-term illness. The employer, insurer, and patient each have their own interests; physicians cannot serve all three simultaneously and equally. The same problems arise in school- and work- release evaluations (7). If the depressed patient's physician decides to play this role, he or she should be truthful and inform the patient that filling out disability forms will breach confidentiality. If the provision of accurate information to employer or insurer will potentially harm the doctor-patient relationship, the physician can decline to perform the disability evaluation and recommend an independent examination. In any case, all patients who are unable to work (or attend school) because of depression should be aggressively treated. Depression should only rarely be a cause of permanent disability, as long as the patient has received adequate treatment.

Adjunctive Interventions

In addition to antidepressants, psychotherapy, or both, there are a number of other interventions that may improve outcomes in depression. Some patients are eager for ways to speed recovery, whereas others require encouragement to take an active role in treatment. Some adjunctive interventions have been demonstrated as being beneficial, whereas others remain unproven but potentially helpful.

Exercise

Depression rates are lower in the physically active (8), and generally depressed patients are more physically inactive as a result of the depression itself. Exercise in almost any form (aerobic and less intense forms) is an effective adjunct in the treatment of depression that improves energy, mood, appetite, sleep, and self-esteem. It has been found to be an effective treatment when compared with no treatment (9). Also, exercise's antidepressant qualities continue after depressive symptoms abate (10), making it valuable as part of long-term management and relapse prevention. In general, exercise is safe and effective in the treatment of mild to moderate depression. Severely depressed patients are usually unable to exercise until partly recovered. Prematurely urging them to exercise adds to their feeling of failure and inadequacy. Prescribing exercise may be contraindicated for depressed bulimic patients, who already may be compulsively over-exercising.

Nutrition and Hydration

Although eating correctly and maintaining adequate hydration may seem obvious, they are frequently overlooked in the management of the depressed patient. Reduction in intake of food and fluids, or over-consumption of "junk" food, are often symptoms of depression. If sustained or if the patient was already in a vulnerable state (e.g., chronically ill, elderly), secondary problems can occur, including alteration of medication metabolism and orthostasis secondary to dehydration. If prolonged, electrolyte derangement and vitamin deficiencies may occur. Some depressed patients may benefit from oral nutritional supplements. B-vitamin supplementation has been studied in treatment-resistant depression with mixed results; a daily multivitamin cannot hurt and may help (11).

Sleep Hygiene

A disrupted sleep cycle is a major symptom of depression, and sleep deprivation is a recognized precipitant of depression. Poor sleep quality or quantity contributes to the higher incidence of depression postpartum, in rotating shift workers, in patients with chronic pain, and in patients with substance abuse problems. Some patients have lifestyles entailing long-term poor sleep habits. A review of the patient's sleep pattern and instruction on proper sleep hygiene is often helpful. Simple information sheets can be provided that include reminders to only be in bed when ready for sleep, to not read or watch television in bed for prolonged periods, to avoid drinking fluids before bed that may cause nocturnal urination, and to avoid stimulating substances in the late afternoon or evening. Although treatment of depression may be necessary to improve sleep quality and quantity, improved sleep also may be necessary for remission of depression. Failure to change poor sleep habits will undermine the effectiveness of therapies for depression and promote relapse (Case 4.4).

CASE 4.4 *Prescribing lifestyle changes*

Ms. Q is a nurse and single mother who complains of persistent depression. She has not responded to an initial trial of an antidepressant. She works the late shift and each day takes "catnaps," smokes 2 packs of cigarettes, and drinks 5 cups of coffee and 3 "cokes" to "keep going." She eats primarily fast food and does not see her friends or attend church anymore because "there's no time left after my job and my children."

Successful treatment for her depressive symptoms requires lifestyle changes. Poor sleep habits, smoking, over-consumption of caffeine, and social isolation are all interfering with recovery.

Hypnotic medication can be a valuable adjunct to treatment when depression includes insomnia. This is especially true in the agitated or anxious depressed patient. Typically a low dose of a short-acting or intermediate-acting benzodiazepine or zolpidem is prescribed during the first weeks of therapy until the normalizing effect of the antidepressant on sleep starts. Long-term use of hypnotic drugs should be avoided because they are central nervous system depressants and may lead to dependency and withdrawal, which makes them particularly risky in patients with current or previous substance abuse. If long-term therapy for insomnia is needed, then trazodone is often used (12).

Reduction of Psychoactive Substances

Some substances interfere with antidepressant treatment, and patients frequently consume such substances, in some cases as a form of self-treatment (13,14).

Caffeine is probably the most widely used psychoactive substance. Many patients with depressive symptoms, particularly fatigue and decreased concentration, may self-medicate with caffeine. In addition to coffee, tea, caffeinated soda, and herbal beverages (e.g., Herba Mate), caffeine may be consumed in over-the-counter (OTC) preparations for weight loss, headache, and staying awake. A few patients are especially sensitive to caffeine and experience side effects even at lower doses (1–2 caffeinated drinks). When taken in regular high quantities (greater than 4 caffeinated drinks per day), caffeine may produce anxiety and interfere with sleep. Additionally, a withdrawal syndrome characterized by irritability, depression, lethargy, headache, and decreased concentration may occur, particularly in the late afternoon. Excessive consumption of caffeine interferes with the normalization of sleep that marks the efficacy of antidepressants. Too much caffeine may aggravate side effects of antidepressants, especially SSRIs and bupropion, such as jitteriness, diarrhea, and insomnia.

The OTC decongestants may on their own account cause side effects such as jitteriness and sleeplessness, or they may interact with antidepressants to cause side effects. Because OTC sympathomimetics are nonspecific adrenergic agonists, tachyphylaxis is common; some patients are addicted and use large quantities (e.g., nasal decongestant spray). Sedating antihistamines may aggravate the mental slowing of depression or the sedation side effect of antidepressants. The preferred treatment for allergic upper respiratory symptoms in depressed patients is nonsedating antihistamines. Presentation during cold or allergy season of new side effects in patients on a previously stable antidepressant regimen suggests a possible OTC drug action or interaction.

A wide variety of herbal preparations contain sympathomimetic compounds, primarily "natural" ephedrine (often identified as ephedra or Ma Huang). Like OTC sympathomimetics, such herbal supplements may cause poor sleep and jitteriness in their own right or by interacting with medications.

There is a strong and complicated relationship between smoking and depression. People who have ever smoked are 50% more likely to have depression, and the incidence of depression in smokers is more than twice that in nonsmokers (15). Patients may be smoking for the antidepressant effects of nicotine or to counteract a particular symptom of depression (lack of concentration, fatigue, constipation, etc.). It also has been observed that depressive symptoms appear during smoking cessation in people with a history of depression (16), and smokers whose withdrawal syndrome includes depressive symptoms are less likely to achieve abstinence. Additionally, smoking may interfere with treatment in some patients by inducing hepatic metabolism of some psychiatric drugs.

Because of the strong association between cigarette smoking and depression, antidepressants have been used to assist in smoking cessation. When accompanied by smoking cessation counseling, bupropion has been demonstrated in controlled trials to double 1-year quit rates compared with placebo (12%–16% vs. 24%–35%) (17). Similar results have been found with nortriptyline (18) and in small studies with doxepin (19). Trials of fluoxetine, sertraline, and other antidepressants have generally been unsuccessful.

Alcohol is the quintessential form of self-treatment. In the short term, for some it causes a feeling of well being, relaxation, and helps initiate sleep. Yet because it is a CNS depressant, it eventuates in worsening depression. It ultimately erodes sleep by disrupting REM sleep, decreases motivation and self-esteem, and contributes to poor nutrition. It is appropriate to urge cessation of all alcohol during the initial phases of treatment of depression. When the symptoms of depression have abated, cautious limited resumption of alcohol can be considered. Advising no more than one drink per day is prudent. Patients should be instructed that their sensitivity to alcohol, especially in their psychomotor skills, has been significantly increased by antidepressant medication, and that alcohol may make them more sensitive to the adverse effects of antidepressants. In some patients even small amounts of alcohol will exacerbate depressive symptoms; in these cases, total abstinence from alcohol should be prescribed to achieve and maintain full remission.

Patients should be asked about any other psychoactive substance use. Long-term daily use of marijuana may be associated with depression, apathy, and decreased ability to concentrate. Even occasional usage should be discouraged in actively depressed patients. Cocaine and amphetamines cause the release of brain catecholamines. Repeated usage leads to a vicious cycle of catecholamine depletion with intense feelings of depression, resulting in increased abuse and then ultimately in a "crash." After cessation of regular use of cocaine or amphetamines, there are often depressive withdrawal symptoms.

Relaxation Techniques

Meditation, yoga, tai chi, and other mind-body therapies may be helpful in managing some of the anxiety symptoms associated with depression, and there are easy-to-learn forms adapted for general-use relaxation techniques. These techniques become particularly important if the patient doesn't wish to or shouldn't be prescribed a benzodiazepine. These practices, although simple, require effort and motivation on the patient's part. Depressed patients often lack energy and motivation, which usually makes relaxation techniques impractical in the moderately to severely depressed patient. However, in the mildly depressed patient with anxiety or in long-term treatment, relaxation techniques can be an important adjunct. Many psychotherapists and physical and occupational therapists are familiar with and can teach relaxation techniques to patients, and there are increasing numbers of nonmedical sources for depressed patients as well.

Religious Involvement

Isolation and disconnection from social support are often seen in depression. Depression occurs less often in people with religious involvement than in those with no religious involvement. Recent studies have shown a decreased likelihood of depression in frequent church attendees (20). It is unclear what provides the protective value. Social support, instillation of hope, a sense of life's meaning, and acceptance of suffering or other spiritual values are some benefits that could explain religion's protective value. It seems that the cognition of an ordered world (faith and trust in God) offers some protective value for the psychological symptoms of depression but less for the somatic symptoms of depression (21). Although a physician cannot "prescribe" religion, a careful review of past religious involvement may uncover a potential avenue for support that could be reinvigorated with the physician's encouragement. Sometimes depression is precipitated by a loss that challenges the patient's faith and/or causes spiritual alienation. Clergy or pastoral counselors can provide meaningful help to depressed patients with these "psychoreligious" conflicts.

Support Groups and Other Social Involvement

Social isolation is a risk factor for, a symptom of, and cause of depression. Steps taken to counter social isolation directly are helpful. This may be as simple as the physician encouraging the depressed patient to have more contact with family, friends, and community. For patients with chronic or recurrent depression, as with other chronic medical illnesses, support groups can be helpful by providing an opportunity to share experiences with others who have the same condition. Physicians should learn what resources are locally available. National sources of information about mental health referral, support groups, and depression in general are listed at the end of this chapter.

Patient Educational Material

Many patients and their families can benefit from educational material, and the organizations listed at the end of this chapter are good sources for printed and Web-based information. For those who wish more in-depth information, there are a number of good books (Table 4.5). Educational materials are useful adjuncts to treatment, but they are primarily effective in reinforcing information provided by the physician, his or her staff, and mental health professionals. Clinical research suggests that if the educational material is not supported by the health care staff, then there is little impact on patient behavior (22). Patient educational material should not replace patient-physician dialogue, which remains one of the most powerful means of behavior change in patients.

Light Therapy

Seasonal affective disorder (SAD) is a mood disorder consisting of recurrent episodes of major depression that occur with a seasonal pattern, most com-

Table 4.5   Recommended Self-Help Books on Depression

- *Feeling Good: The New Mood Therapy* and *The Feeling Good Handbook* by David D. Burns

- *Breaking the Patterns of Depression* by Michael D. Yapko

- *The Pain Behind the Mask: Overcoming Masculine Depression* by John Lynch and Christopher T. Kilmartin

monly with depressive episodes during the fall and winter, with full remission to normal mood (or a switch to hypomania or mania) during the spring and summer. Randomized controlled trials with light therapy have demonstrated short-term improvement in SAD, but little is known about light therapy's long-term benefits (23). A variety of modalities have been tested, including light boxes, light visors, and dawn simulators. The therapeutic effects are mediated via the eyes, not the skin. The spectrum of light seems unimportant, but intensity is probably a requirement to achieve benefits, on the order of 10,000 lux. The ideal timing remains controversial, but most controlled trials have shown morning light to be superior to evening light (24). The optimal dose has not been determined. Side effects include minor visual complaints, headache, insomnia, and over-activation (including, rarely, mania) (25). Most light therapy modalities screen out UV rays, so adverse cutaneous reactions are limited to patients with photosensitivity. There have been no reports of basal cell cancer or cataracts with light therapy. No ocular changes have been detected even after years of treatment, and there are no defined ocular contraindications (26). There is no evidence of similar benefit from tanning salons (eyes are usually covered and high UV light exposure does carry risks). There is no evidence that replacing home or office light bulbs with bulbs of different spectra provides any benefit. There is some evidence of modest acute benefits of light therapy in nonseasonal depression (27), but no evidence that it can be used instead of standard therapies. Even in SAD, light therapy is not adequate as sole treatment if symptoms are severe.

St. John's Wort and Other Alternative Medicine Therapies

St. John's wort, a common flowering plant (*Hypericum perforatum*), is widely sold in the United States as a dietary supplement. The FDA does not evaluate it and does not monitor its purity or safety. St. John's wort is licensed in Germany for the treatment of anxiety, depression, and insomnia. Many Americans now take this preparation for depressive symptoms. Hypericin, a naphthodiathrone, is considered the active ingredient. It is not known if hypericum crosses the blood brain barrier, but *in vitro* it inhibits the uptake of the neurotransmitters serotonin, norepinephrine, and dopamine and binds to GABA receptors. How the body metabolizes and excretes hypericum is unknown at this time (28). Most of the studies (29) using hypericum for the treatment of depression come from Europe and use different definitions for depression, making it difficult to interpret the results. However, it does seem that hypericum is safe and may be effective in the treatment of mild depression. Most experienced physicians consider it ineffective for severe depression. St. John's wort should not be combined with SSRIs because of the risk of serotonin syndrome.

Patients may turn to a wide variety of other herbal or nutritional remedies purported to have antidepressant effects, such as gingko, kava, melatonin, megavitamin doses, DHEA, chromium, inositol, and *S*-adenosyl methionine. Some other herbal agents include ginseng, royal jelly, wild oats, lemon balm, wood betony, and basil (30,31). Physicians should carefully ask patients what they may be taking.

■   ■   ■

Key Points

- An assessment of suicidality should be performed on every patient suspected of having depression

- Although physicians vary in experience and comfort in managing depression, mental health referral should be made if the patient is acutely suicidal, psychotic, severely depressed, or unresponsive to antidepressants.

- Appropriate boundaries in the doctor-patient relationship should be maintained with depressed patients.

- Patient confidentiality may be broken when dealing with a suicidal patient.

- Explicit documentation of symptoms, diagnosis, and treatment is important for clinical and medical-legal reasons.

- Lifestyle interventions (e.g., exercise, nutrition, sleep hygiene, relaxation techniques, religious involvement, social contact, psychoeducation) can play important roles in treatment for minor depression and as adjuncts to treatment in moderate and severe depression.

- Overuse of psychoactive substances such as caffeine, nicotine, over-the-counter medications, herbal remedies, alcohol, and other substances of abuse may aggravate depression and interfere with recovery.

• There is much interest in but fewer data on alternative remedies such as St. John's wort and light therapy.

■   ■   ■

Resources

Depression Awareness, Recognition, and Treatment (D/ART) Program, National Institute of Mental Health: 1-800-421-4211; 301-443-4140.

Depression and Related Affective Disorders Association (DRADA): Meyer 3-181, 600 North Wolfe Street, Baltimore, MD 21287-7381; 955-4647; 202-955-5800 (Washington, DC); drada@jhmi.edu.

Depressives Anonymous: Recovery from Depression: 329 E. 62nd St., New York, NY 10021; 212-689-2600.

National Depressive and Manic-Depressive Association: 730 North Franklin Street, Suite 501, Chicago, IL 60610; 1-800-82-NDMDA6; 312-642-0049; fax: 312-642-7243.

National Foundation for Depressive Illness: P.O. Box 2257, New York, NY 10116; 800-239-1265; 800-248-4344.

National Institute of Mental Health: 5600 Fishers Lane, Rm. 15C05, Rockville, MD 20857; 301-443-4513.

National Mental Health Association: 1021 Prince Street, Alexandria, VA 22314-2971; 703-684-7722; fax 703-684-5968.

Mental Health Information Center: 800-969-NMHA.

TY Line: 800-433-5959; www.nmha.org.

The Mental Health Foundation: www.mentalhealth.org.uk.

American Psychiatric Association: 1400 K St. NW, Washington, DC 20005; 202-682-6220; www.psych.org.

American Psychological Association: 750 1st St. NE, Washington, DC 20002-4242; 202-336-5500; www.apa.org.

■   ■   ■

REFERENCES

1. **Frank E, Prien RF, Jarrett JB, et al.** Conceptualization and rationale for consensus definitions of terms in major depression: remission, recovery, relapse, and recurrence. *Arch Gen Psychiatry.* 1991;48:851–5.

1a. **Harris EC, Barraclough B.** Suicide as an outcome for mental disorders. *Br J Psych.* 1997;170:205–28.

1b. **Barraclough B, Brunch J, Nelson B, et al.** A hundred cases of suicide: clinical aspects. *Br J Psychiatry.* 1974;125:355–73.

1c. **NIH Consensus Development Panel on Depression in Late Life.** Diagnosis and treatment of depression in late life. *JAMA.* 1992;268:1018–24.

1d. **Peters KD, Murphy SL.** Deaths: final data for 1996. In *Natl Vital Stat Rep*, vol. 47, no. 9. Hyattsville, MD: National Center for Health Statistics; 1998 [DHHS Publication No. (PHS)99-1120].

2. **Lish JD, Zimmermann M, Farber NJ, et al.** Suicide screening in a primary care setting at a Veterans Affairs Medical Center. *Psychosomatics.* 1996;37:413–24.

3. **Gliatto MF, Rai AK.** Evaluation and treatment of patients with suicidal ideation. *Am Fam Phys.* 1999; 59:1500–6.

4. **Gabbard GO, Nadelson C.** Professional boundaries in the physician-patient relationship. *JAMA.* 1995;273:1445–9.

5. **Wells KB, et al.** The functioning and well-being of depressed patients: results from the Medical Outcomes Study. *JAMA.* 1989;262:914–9.

6. **Broadhead WE, Blazer DG, George LK, Tse CK.** Depression, disability days, and days lost from work in a prospective epidemiologic study. *JAMA.* 1990;264:2524–8.

7. **Holleman WL, Holleman MC.** School and work release evaluations. *JAMA.* 1988;260:3629–34.

8. **Paffenbarger RS Jr, Lee IM, Leung R.** Physical activity and personal characteristics associated with depresson and suicide in American college men. *Acta Psychiatr Scand Suppl.* 1994;377:16–22.

9. **Martinsen EW.** Physical activity and depression: clinical experience. *Acta Psychiatr Scand Suppl.* 1994;377:23–7.

10. **Martinsen EW.** Benefits of exercise for the treatment of depression. *Sports Med.* 1990;9:380–9.

11. **Fava M, Borus JS, Alpert JE, et al.** Folate, vitamin B12, and homocysteine in major depressive disorder. *Am J Psychiatry.* 1997;154:426–8.

12. **Neylan TC.** Treatment of sleep disturbances in depressed patients. *J Clin Psychiatry.* 1995;56(Suppl 2):56–61.

13. **Leibenluft E, Fiero PL, Bartko JJ, et al.** Depressive symptoms and the self-reported use of alcohol, caffeine, and carbohydrates in normal volunteers and four groups of psychiatric outpatients. *Am J Psychiatry.* 1993;150:294–301.

14. **Worthington J, Fava M, Agustin C, et al.** Consumption of alcohol, nicotine, and caffeine among depressed outpatients. Relationship with response to treatment. *Psychosomatics.* 1996;37:518–22.

15. **Regier DA, Goldberg ID, Taube AC.** The de facto U.S. mental health services system: a public health perspective. *Arch Gen Psychiatry.* 1978;35:685–93.

16. **Covey LS, Glassman AH, Stetner F.** Depression and depressive symptoms in smoking cessation. *Compr Psychiatry.* 1990;31:350–354.

17. **Hurt RD, Sachs DP, Glover ED, et al.** A comparison of sustained-release bupropion and placebo for smoking cessation. *N Engl J Med.* 1997;23:1195–202.

18. **Hall SM, Reus VI, Munoz RF, et al.** Nortriptyline and cognitive-behavioral therapy in the treatment of cigarette smoking. *Arch Gen Psychiatry.* 1998;55:683–90.

19. **Murphy JK, Edwards NB, Downs AD, et al.** Effects of doxepin on withdrawal symptoms in smoking cessation. *Am J Psychiatry.* 1990;147:1353–7.

20. **Koenig HG, Hays JC, George LK, et al.** Modeling the cross-sectional relationships between religion, physical health, social support, and depressive symptoms. *Am J Ger Psychiatry.* 1997;5:131–44.

21. **Koenig HG, Cohen HJ, Blazer DG, et al.** Religious coping and cognitive symptoms of depression in elderly medical patients. *Psychosomatics.* 1995;36:369–75.

22. **Robinson P, Katon W, Von Korff M, et al.** The education of depressed primary care patients: What do patients think of interactive booklets and a video? *J Fam Pract.* 1997;44:562–71.

23. **Eastman CI, Young MA, Fogg LF, et al.** Bright light treatment of winter depression: a placebo-controlled trial. *Arch Gen Psychiatry.* 1998;55:883–9.

24. **Lewy AJ, BauerVK, Cutler NL, et al.** Morning vs. evening light treatment of patients with winter depression. *Arch Gen Psychiatry.* 1998;55:890–6.

25. **Labbate LA, Lafer B, Thibault A, et al.** Side effects induced by bright light treatment for seasonal affective disorder. *J Clin Psychiatry.* 1994;55:189–91.

26. **Gallin PF, Terman M, Reme CE, et al.** Ophthalmologic examination of patients with seasonal affective disorder, before and after bright light therapy. *Am J Ophthalmol.* 1995;119:202–10.

27. **Kripke DF.** Light treatment for nonseasonal depression: speed, efficacy, and combined treatment. *J Affect Disord.* 1998;49:109–17.

28. St. John's wort. *Medical Letter.* 1997;39:1011–6.

29. **Linde K, Ramirez G, Mulrow CD, et al.** St. John's wort for depression: an overview and meta-analysis of randomised clinical trials. *Br Med J.* 1996;313:253.

30. **Edzard E, Rand JI, Stevinson C.** Complementary therapies for depression. *Arch Gen Psychiatry.* 1998;55:1026–32.

31. **Eisenberg DM, Davis RB, Ettner SL, et al.** Trends in alternative medicine use in the United States, 1990–1997: results of a follow-up national survey. *JAMA.* 1998; 280:1569-75.

KEY REFERENCES

Edzard E, Rand JI, Stevinson C. Complementary therapies for depression. *Arch Gen Psychiatry.* 1998;55:1026–32.

The authors offer the most complete review to date on complementary and alternative therapies for depression.

Gabbard GO, Nadelson C. Professional boundaries in the physician-patient relationship. *JAMA.* 1995;273:1445–9.

Gabbard and Nadelson are two of the most respected psychiatrists in the field. Their discussion on boundaries is readable and applicable to all.

Harris EC, Barraclough B. Suicide as an outcome for mental illness. *Br J Psychiatry.* 1997;170:205–28.

A large meta-analysis of 249 reports of suicide risk of all mental disorders that illustrates that an assessment of suicidality should be performed on not only patients with depression but on all patients with a mental illness.

Wells KB, et al. The functioning and well-being of depressed patients: results from the Medical Outcomes Study. *JAMA.* 1989;262:914–9.

The Medical Outcomes Study is the seminal study demonstrating similar functional impairment in medical and psychiatric illnesess.

5

■ ■ ■

Psychopharmacology

Charles DeBattista, MD

David L. Smith, MD

Alan F. Schatzberg, MD

"Medicine helps. That is, most of the time."

In the 1990s, antidepressants emerged as some of the most commonly prescribed drugs (1). Between 1988—the year Prozac was introduced— and 1993, the number of patients on antidepressants in the United States doubled. Since 1993, antidepressant use has redoubled, with sales approaching $6 billion annually. This unprecedented increase is a result of safer, easier-to-use agents that primary care physicians feel comfortable using over the potentially toxic tricyclic antidepressants (TCAs) and monoamine oxidase inhibitors (MAOIs). Currently, more than 80% of all antidepressants are prescribed by nonpsychiatric physicians, especially those in primary care (2,3).

Despite the fact that more people than ever are being treated with antidepressants, many patients who could benefit from treatment are never diagnosed, and those who are diagnosed often receive suboptimal treatment. Several surveys have reported that the diagnosis of major depression is made in fewer than 50% of patients in primary care settings who meet the criteria for diagnosis (4). Even if the diagnosis is made, the chance that a patient will take an antidepressant at therapeutic doses for an adequate duration is small. Most patients do not refill prescriptions and often stop taking the medication at the first sign that they are feeling better.

General Principles of Antidepressant Use

Selecting an Antidepressant

The choice of antidepressant depends on a number of variables that are specific to the drug as well as to the patient (5). Drug-specific variables include efficacy, side-effect profile, safety, and cost. It is difficult to demonstrate that one antidepressant is consistently more effective than another. A given antidepressant is likely to lead to a significant improvement in a depressive episode 50% to 70% of the time (6); however, with each failure of an antidepressant, the chance of responding to a subsequent trial is reduced.

The side-effect profile differs significantly from one class of agents to another because of differing neurotransmitter effects. The TCAs are characterized by anticholinergic, antihistaminic side effects, whereas the selective serotonin-reuptake inhibitors (SSRIs) produce more serotonin-specific side effects, including headache, gastrointestinal upset, and sexual dysfunction. Most of the newer antidepressants, including the SSRIs, venlafaxine, bupropion, nefazodone, and mirtazapine, enjoy a much higher therapeutic index than do the TCAs and MAOIs. The newer antidepressants are rarely life-threatening when taken in overdose alone, whereas overdoses of small amounts of TCAs may be lethal.

The cost of antidepressants is a major concern to patients, clinicians, and third-party payers. Compared with generic TCAs or MAOIs, the formulary cost of newer antidepressants is considerable. A month's supply of fluoxetine may cost $85 or more compared with the $8 or so for generic imipramine (7). However, the formulary costs are only a fraction of the total expense of treating a depressed patient. If imipramine is prescribed, additional factors to be considered include the cost of potential electrocardiograms, periodic serum-level testing, and more frequent office visits than generally are required for a SSRI prescription. Additionally, the heavier side-effect burden of TCAs leads to a higher percentage of incomplete or inadequate treatment trials compared with the newer antidepressants. When these other factors are considered, it seems to be more cost effective to prescribe a SSRI rather than a TCA.

Patient parameters in choosing an antidepressant include medical status, age, gender, patient preference, and history of response. For example, if a patient's depression is characterized by significant psychomotor retardation, an activating antidepressant may be preferred, whereas a patient with an agitated depression or prominent insomnia may better tolerate a more sedating antidepressant. Patients with a history of cardiac disease should avoid TCAs; those with a history of seizure disorder or stroke may be advised to avoid amoxapine, maprotiline, and bupropion because of their higher seizure risk; and patients with obesity probably should not take TCAs or mirtazapine as first-line agents.

Patients taking multiple medications may better tolerate drugs such as citalopram or venlafaxine because these have less potential for drug interaction than other agents. As a rule, older patients tend to tolerate the newer antidepressants better than the TCAs and MAOIs. Nonetheless, some geriatric patients will not be able to tolerate the orthostasis associated with higher doses of trazodone, the hypertensive effects seen with high-dose venlafaxine, or the dizziness that may occur with SSRIs.

Gender differences in antidepressant response are beginning to be appreciated. Women may tolerate and respond to SSRIs better than do men (8). Conversely, men may respond to and tolerate TCAs better than do women. Even so, newer, less dangerous antidepressants should be considered before trying a TCA.

The patient's antidepressant history is often useful in the selection of an antidepressant. A history of response to a particular agent might lead appropriately to a retrial. Likewise, a history of intolerable sexual side effects in a patient might suggest using nefazodone, bupropion, or mirtazapine (Case 5.1). In this information age, patients may have researched antidepressants and have specific requests. However, patients rarely have the advantage of a larger clinical perspective. It is important to consider the rationale behind the patient's request when choosing a specific antidepressant. The patient-related factors that influence the choice of an antidepressant are summarized in Table 5.1.

When all of these patient- and drug-specific characteristics are matched, it is evident that newer antidepressants, including the SSRIs, are first-line agents for most patients. The MAOIs and TCAs, by virtue of their lower therapeutic index, difficulty of use, and greater potential for serious drug interactions, are now second- or third-line agents. However, the TCAs and MAOIs still have an important place in the treatment of depression and should be considered for certain patients.

CASE 5.1 *Selecting an antidepressant and therapeutic dose*

A woman 42 years of age presents with complaints of depressed mood and fatigue. Associated symptoms include insomnia, loss of interest in usual activities, and excessively guilty thinking. She has had one previous similar episode, which responded well to paroxetine (Paxil) 20 mg/d, although she had significant and bothersome decreased libido for the duration of the treatment. She is prescribed nefazodone (Serzone) starting at 100 mg bid, increasing to 150 mg bid after 1 week. This antidepressant is chosen because there is evidence that it is less likely to cause sexual dysfunction than the SSRIs. She does not respond significantly to this dose after 4 weeks, so it is increased in 100 mg/d increments to 250 mg bid. At this dosage, the patient experiences a sustained remission with minimal side-effect burden.

Dose and Duration

When antidepressants are employed by clinicians inexperienced in treating depression, they are often given in inadequate doses for inadequate durations. All available antidepressants require approximately 3 to 8 weeks to achieve maximal benefit. Although some patients may respond in the first weeks, particularly with improvement in sleep and anxiety, trials of less than 4 weeks at therapeutic doses are generally inadequate. The available data, however, would suggest that if the patient does not respond at all to a given dose for 4 weeks, then he or she is unlikely to respond at that dose even if the trial is considerably longer (9). Thus, the dose should be increased as tolerated by the patient or a switch to a different antidepressant should be considered.

What constitutes a therapeutic dose of a given antidepressant is sometimes debatable. It is clear, for example, that 20 mg/d of some SSRIs such as fluoxetine, paroxetine, or citalopram is probably therapeutic for most patients. However, that does not indicate that higher doses might not be more efficacious. If 20 mg/d does not produce at least a partial response at 4 weeks, then a higher dosage seems to be indicated. For other classes of antidepressants, some clinicians have suggested that two thirds of the max-

Table 5.1   Patient-Related Factors in Selecting an Antidepressant

Patient-Related Factors	More-Preferred Agents	Less-Preferred Agents
Agitation, anxiety, or insomnia	Sedating antidepressant	Activating antidepressant
Psychomotor retardation or hypersomnia	Activating antidepressant	Sedating antidepressant
History of heart disease	SSRI or other newer antidepressant	TCA
History of seizure	SSRI or other newer antidepressant (except bupropion)	Amoxapine, maprotiline, bupropion
Obesity	SSRI, bupropion	TCA, mirtazapine
Multiple medications	Venlafaxine, citalopram	Fluoxetine, sertraline, paroxetine, fluvoxamine
Sexual dysfunction	Nefazodone, bupropion, and mirtazapine	SSRI, TCA, MAOI

MAOI = monoamine oxidase inhibitor; SSRI = selective serotonin-reuptake inhibitor; TCA = tricyclic antidepressant.

imum dose was a reasonable target for a therapeutic trial. Therefore, 200 mg imipramine, 60 mg phenelzine, and 300 mg bupropion might be the minimum doses for at least 4 weeks before a higher dose or a different medication would be considered (10).

Nonetheless, not every patient will respond even to an adequate trial of an antidepressant. The overall efficacy of a first trial of an antidepressant is probably in the range of 50% to 70%. The remaining patients usually can be described as either partial responders (decreased but still significant symptoms of depression) or nonresponders (no significant improvement in symptoms). Many strategies have been tried for patients in these groups, including switching to new antidepressants, adding an augmentation agent (e.g., lithium, L-triiodothyronine), combining more than one antidepressant, or other nonmedication treat-

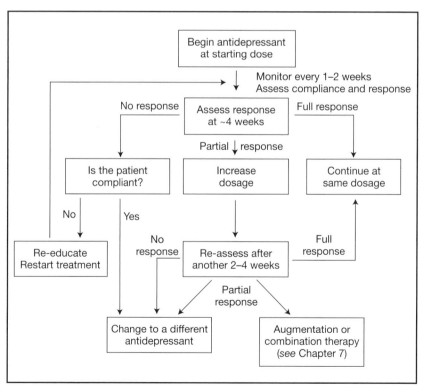

Figure 5.1 Algorithm for selecting dose and duration of treatment with antidepressants.

ments (e.g., electroconvulsive therapy). Unfortunately, there are little empirical data to guide the clinician; our general preference is to try an augmentation or combination strategy with the patient's first agent if there is a partial response and to switch to a new antidepressant of a different class if there is no significant response. Figure 5.1 provides an algorithmic approach to the pharmacologic treatment of depression. The approaches to treatment-refractory depression are reviewed in detail in Chapter 7.

Adverse Effects Common to Most Antidepressants

In general, the different classes of antidepressants vary significantly in their side-effect profiles, which are discussed in each section below. However, every antidepressant has some properties common to the entire group. All antidepressants have the potential to induce a manic episode or to provoke rapid cycling between manic and depressed states. Patients with histories of bipolar disorder are most at risk for developing this effect, but it can occur even in patients with no previous history of mania or hypomania.

Almost all antidepressants have the potential to cause a discontinuation syndrome if they are stopped abruptly. This syndrome is thought not to be caused by classic dependence on the medication, but rather by the abrupt change in monoamine neurotransmission as the medication plasma levels fall. The symptoms of the discontinuation syndrome tend to be similar to the symptoms of beginning an antidepressant and include dizziness, gastrointestinal upset, and jitteriness. Antidepressants with short half-lives (e.g., venlafaxine) seem to be more likely to cause a discontinuation syndrome than those with long half-lives (e.g., fluoxetine). Because of this possible adverse effect, it is prudent to taper most antidepressants gradually.

There have been case reports of the syndrome of inappropriate antidiuretic-hormone release (SIADH) and consequent hyponatremia with many antidepressants. The mechanism of this effect is not known. Although antidepressant-induced SIADH is relatively rare, risk factors seem to be the advanced age of the patient and the use of serotonergic antidepressants.

Selective Serotonin-Reuptake Inhibitors

The SSRIs are now the dominant class of antidepressants and are among the most prescribed medications in the world (11). During 1998, three SSRIs—fluoxetine (Prozac), paroxetine (Paxil), and sertraline (Zoloft)—accounted for more than $5 billion in U.S. sales alone. Another SSRI, citalopram (Celexa)—released in the United States in 1998 and available in

Europe since 1989—is the most popular SSRI in many European countries. Available since 1993, fluvoxamine (Luvox) has been well studied in the treatment of major depression—even though its only FDA-approved indication is for obsessive-compulsive disorder—and seems similar to the other SSRIs.

Indications

The primary indication for the SSRIs is the treatment of major depression. The SSRIs have been better studied in mild to moderate depression in outpatients than they have been in more severely depressed inpatients (12). Some investigators have suggested that the SSRIs may not be as effective as the TCAs or venlafaxine in more seriously depressed patients (13), but this remains to be proven. The SSRIs have proven to be "broad-spectrum antidepressants," meaning that in addition to being effective for depression they have been shown to be useful for the treatment of several anxiety disorders and other psychiatric conditions. Currently, paroxetine and sertraline are FDA approved for the treatment of both panic disorder and obsessive-compulsive disorder (14). In addition, there is some indication that the SSRIs may be effective in the treatment of bulimia nervosa, impulse-control disorders, and negative symptoms of schizophrenia. Nonpsychiatric uses have included migraine prophylaxis, although the SSRIs have not been as popular or as well studied as the TCAs for this purpose. Likewise, the efficacy of the SSRIs is not as well demonstrated as that of the TCAs for the treatment of chronic pain syndromes. The SSRIs have been used in the management of chronic fatigue syndrome, which may represent major depression in some patients. Finally, some clinicians have used SSRIs that induce delayed orgasm to treat premature ejaculation.

Mechanism of Action

As their name implies, the SSRIs inhibit the reuptake of serotonin in the synaptic cleft. However, the SSRIs are not as selective as once thought. For example, paroxetine seems to have both anticholinergic effects and norepinephrine-reuptake–blocking properties (15). Sertraline may block the reuptake of dopamine, at least *in vitro*. Nonetheless, the SSRIs are more selective than previous classes of antidepressants, such as the TCAs and MAOIs (16).

Side Effects

The most common side effects of the SSRIs can be grouped in three major categories: gastrointestinal upset, central nervous system (CNS) activation, and sexual side effects (17). Gastrointestinal upset occurs in up to 30% of patients, and includes symptoms like nausea, vomiting, diarrhea, heartburn, and reflux. These symptoms tend to be present in the first few weeks of treatment, but nausea is no more common than with placebo by the fourth week of treatment. Most patients habituate to the nausea but may have more persistent problems with diarrhea. Instructing the patient to take the drug with food circumvents the nausea in most cases. Anecdotally, the heartburn can be managed with over-the-counter H_2 blockers such as famotidine (Pepcid) 20 mg/d (10). SSRI-induced diarrhea sometimes responds to bulk-forming agents and other antidiarrheals such as lomotil.

Activation in the CNS may include symptoms such as initial insomnia, restlessness, and agitation. Up to 20% of patients experience these side effects, which are associated most commonly with fluoxetine. Anxious, agitated patients sometimes may be exquisitely sensitive to the activating effects of fluoxetine. Fluoxetine is administered in the morning to mitigate problems with insomnia. Occasionally, adjunctive agents such as a benzodiazepine or trazodone are given to manage insomnia or agitation associated with SSRIs.

Sexual side effects occur in 30% to 40% of patients and include decreased libido, delayed orgasm, anorgasmy, and occasionally erectile problems (18). Many adjunctive agents (e.g., bupropion, amantadine, buspirone, cyproheptadine, yohimbine, amphetamines, ginkgo biloba) have been suggested as treatments of SSRI-induced side effects (19). Some strategies seem to work anecdotally in some patients, but no single strategy works in all patients. To date, none of these adjunctive strategies has been subjected to double-blind studies. Other strategies have included withholding the dose of SSRIs with short half-lives (e.g., paroxetine, sertraline) the day before anticipated sexual activity. However, this strategy seems less likely to work with drugs that have longer half-lives (e.g., fluoxetine, citalopram). Another common strategy is to switch to drugs that are less likely to have sexual side effects, including bupropion, mirtazapine, and nefazodone.

Other potential side effects include excessive perspiration, nocturnal myoclonus, headaches, and occasionally extrapyramidal symptoms such as dystonia.

Discontinuation symptoms are sometimes associated with the rapid withdrawal of SSRIs with short half-lives, such as sertraline, paroxetine, and fluvoxamine. Patients may experience headache, nausea, tremulousness, and other symptoms; hence, tapering SSRIs that have short half-lives over the course of several weeks is advised. Prozac generally can be discontinued suddenly without difficulty because its long half-life results in a slow elimination over weeks.

Drug Interactions

The most serious interactions of the SSRIs are those in combination with the MAOIs (20). Less serious but still significant interactions include the tendency of the SSRIs to inhibit competitively certain cytochrome P450 interactions and thus effectively raise the serum level of drugs dependent on those isoenzymes for their metabolism (21). For example, paroxetine and fluoxetine are potent inhibitors of the 2D6 isoenzyme and therefore can raise the serum levels of TCAs if administered concurrently (Case 5.2). The result is enhanced toxicity from the TCAs. Fluvoxamine and nefazodone can inhibit the metabolism of the 3A3/4 isoenzyme (*see* section below), whereas citalopram is a relatively weak inhibitor of the cytochrome P450 system. (*See* Chapter 13 for more information on drug interactions.)

CASE 5.2   *Drug interaction with a selective serotonin-reuptake inhibitor*

A man 50 years of age with a history of diabetic neuropathy, for which he has taken low-dose amitriptyline (50 mg qhs) for several years, presents with signs and symptoms of major depression. He is prescribed fluoxetine (Prozac) 20 mg/d. Three days later he notes significant difficulty with dry mouth, constipation, and blurry vision. These anticholinergic effects are explained by fluoxetine's inhibition of the cytochrome P450 2D6 isoenzyme, which consequently decreased the metabolism of the amitriptyline. Fluoxetine is discontinued, and the patient is changed to a regimen of citalopram (Celexa) 20 mg/d, which does not inhibit the cytochrome P450 2D6 system.

Dosing

For most of the SSRIs, the starting dose is the therapeutic dose. However, there is some evidence that increasing the dose may help some patients who have not responded to a given dose. Overall, a medication such as fluoxetine has a fairly flat dose-response curve, with 60 mg not seeming much more efficacious than 20 mg across all patients with major depression (22). However, a given patient who has not responded at 20 mg may respond at 40 or 60 mg.

The SSRIs are dosed once per day except for fluvoxamine, which is administered one tablet twice daily at dosages above 100 mg/d. Fluoxetine should be given in the morning to reduce the risk of treatment-induced insomnia. The other SSRIs can be given at any time during the day. However, timing of the dose may need to be changed if the patient experiences insomnia or daytime somnolence. Starting and maximum dosages are shown in Table 5.2.

Table 5.2   Dosaging of Selective Serotonin-Reuptake Inhibitors

Drug	Starting Dosage	Maximum Dosage
Fluoxetine (Prozac)	10–20 mg/d	60 mg/d
Sertraline (Zoloft)	50 mg/d	200 mg/d
Paroxetine (Paxil)	10–20 mg/d	60 mg/d
Fluvoxamine (Luvox)	50 mg/d	150 mg bid
Citalopram (Celexa)	10–20 mg/d	60 mg/d

Venlafaxine

Available since 1994, venlafaxine (Effexor) not only blocks the reuptake of serotonin, making it similar to the SSRIs but also blocks the reuptake of norepinephrine, especially at higher doses. Its main indication is for the treatment of major depression, and there has been preliminary evidence that suggests it may have a particular role in the treatment of melancholic depressions (13) and treatment-refractory depressions (23).

The side-effect profile of venlafaxine is also much like that of the SSRIs, with gastrointestinal symptoms (especially nausea), insomnia, somnolence, and sexual dysfunction seen more commonly than with placebo. One side effect that does seem more related to venlafaxine's noradrenergic effects is hypertension, although it tends to be minor and is seen mostly at higher dosages (> 225 mg/d) (24). The short-half life of venlafaxine seems to contribute to its potential for causing a discontinuation syndrome (particularly dizziness) if it is stopped abruptly.

Drug Interactions

Venlafaxine has been implicated in the development of serotonin syndrome, so its co-administration with MAOIs is contraindicated. Venlafaxine's effect on the cytochrome P450 system is weak, and it seems unlikely to inhibit the metabolism of other medications. It is also weakly protein-bound; thus, it is relatively unlikely to displace other tightly bound medications like warfarin and phenytoin. (See Chapter 13 for more information on drug interactions.)

Dosing

With immediate-release venlafaxine, dosing is generally started at 18.75 mg bid and titrated upwards by 18.75 mg every 3 days to reach 37.5 mg bid. If further increases are needed, it can be increased by approximately 75 mg/wk. Venlafaxine also is marketed in a sustained-release formulation (Ef-

Table 5.3   Dosaging of Venlafaxine

Drug	Starting Dosage	Maximum Dosage
Venlafaxine (Effexor)	18.75 mg bid or 37.5 mg/d (XR)	375 mg/d

fexor-XR), which can be taken in a single daily dose. The maximum dosage of venlafaxine is 375 mg/d (Table 5.3).

5HT-2 Antagonists

The 5HT-2 antagonists are nefazodone (Serzone) and trazodone (Desyrel). Trazodone was released in 1981 and for awhile was among the most popular antidepressants because it represented the first safe serotonergic antidepressant released in the U.S. market. Nefazodone became available in 1996 and is chemically related to trazodone; however, nefazodone has a more benign side-effect profile and has been studied more thoroughly in patients with serious depressive episodes than has trazodone.

Indications

The primary indication for nefazodone and trazodone is major depression. However, trazodone is used more commonly as a hypnotic (25). At low doses it can be quite sedating yet does not carry the addictive potential of benzodiazepine hypnotics. Both trazodone and nefazodone seem to be effective in the management of generalized anxiety, and there is preliminary evidence of nefazodone ameliorating the symptoms of panic disorder.

Mechanism of Action

As the name indicates, these agents enhance serotonergic tone by blocking the 5HT-2 receptor (26). However, they have a complex pharmacology. In addition to their 5HT-2 antagonism, the drugs also weakly block the reuptake of serotonin and are alpha-adrenergic antagonists. Trazodone is also a potent antihistamine, which accounts for its sedative effects. It also blocks alpha-2 adrenergic activity, which contributes to a tendency to produce priapism.

Side Effects

Nefazodone and trazodone affect similar neurotransmitters but have different affinities for their receptors (27). For example, trazodone is quite sedating because of its strong antihistaminic effects, but nefazodone is much less sedating because of weak H_1 antagonism. Similarly, trazodone is more likely than nefazodone to induce orthostatic hypotension secondary to its potent alpha-1 adrenergic–blocking properties. However, nefazodone can induce dizziness and orthostatic changes at high doses.

Sexual side effects are uncommon with this class of agents. However, there is a low incidence of priapism (1 in 6000) in men treated with trazodone. No cases of priapism have been reported with nefazodone. Gastrointestinal side effects occur less commonly with the 5HT-2 antagonists than with the SSRIs. If dyspepsia occurs on an empty stomach with nefazodone, patients may be advised to take the medication with meals. Other side effects that are more common than with the SSRIs are asthenia, blurred vision, constipation, dry mouth, and confusion.

Drug Interactions

Nefazodone is a potent inhibitor of the cytochrome P450 isoenzyme 3A3/4 and, as such, can inhibit the metabolism of a variety of agents, including steroids, calcium-channel blockers, and certain benzodiazepines (e.g., alprazolam [Xanax]) (28). More importantly, it can inhibit effectively the metabolism of drugs like cisapride (Propulsid) and astemizole (Hismanal), leading to a cardiotoxicity that may result in ventricular arrhythmias. (*See* Chapter 13 for more information on drug interactions.)

Trazodone rarely has been associated with respiratory arrest when taken in large overdoses in combination with other CNS depressants. In addition, the combination of trazodone with antihypertensive agents may lead to more severe orthostatic hypotension.

Dosing

Both nefazodone and trazodone should be taken in divided doses secondary to their short half-lives (29). The usual starting antidepressant dosage for both drugs is 50 to 100 mg bid (Table 5.4). Dosages this low may be adequate for the treatment of anxiety and agitation. Higher dosages in the range of 300–600 mg/d seem to be required for optimal antidepressant effects.

As a hypnotic, trazodone is prescribed at 50 to 100 mg at night approximately 1 to 2 hours before bedtime. For optimal hypnotic effects, it may be better to advise patients to take the drug on an empty stomach.

Atypical Antidepressants

There are two antidepressants that do not fit neatly into other classes of agents and therefore are sometimes lumped together as being "atypical":

Table 5.4   Dosaging of 5HT-2 Antagonists

Drug	Starting Dosage	Maximum Dosage
Nefazodone (Serzone)	50–100 mg bid	600 mg/d
Trazodone (Desyrel)	50 qhs (hypnotic); 100 mg bid (antidepressant)	600 mg/d

mirtazapine (Remeron; available since 1996) and bupropion (Wellbutrin; available since 1986). Mirtazapine and bupropion are chemically distinct, but they do have similar mechanisms of action.

Mechanism of Action

Bupropion is believed to act primarily as an indirect agonist of norepinephrine, although it also has dopamine-reuptake–blocking properties at high doses. Bupropion is metabolized into a number of amphetamine-like products. Its mechanism of action, however, is not completely understood.

Mirtazapine has a complex pharmacology with presynaptic alpha-2 adrenergic antagonism thought to be among its more important effects. In addition, the drug is a 5HT-2 antagonist and may block the reuptake of serotonin.

Indications

Bupropion and mirtazapine are both primarily indicated for the treatment of major depression. Bupropion also has an FDA indication for smoking cessation under the trade name Zyban. Bupropion has been studied in the treatment of attention-deficit disorder and as an adjunctive agent to standard antidepressants, such as the SSRIs, to augment antidepressant effects and to reverse sexual side effects of serotonergic antidepressants. (See Chapter 13 for more information on drug interactions.)

Adverse Effects

The most serious adverse effects associated with bupropion are seizures. The risk of seizures is approximately 0.4% at dosages below 450 mg/d (approximately the same as most other antidepressants) but climbs to 2.3% at dosages above 450 mg/d. A sustained-release preparation (SR), which is quickly supplanting the immediate-release form, does not seem to be associated with any higher risk of seizures than other antidepressants. Risk factors for seizures with bupropion include a previous history of head trauma, seizures, or eating disorders such as bulimia. Other more common adverse effects of bupropion include CNS activation with insomnia, restlessness, agitation, and tremor. Sexual side effects are uncommon.

Mirtazapine is highly antihistaminic and, as such, is associated with sedation and weight gain. The sedation may be less problematic with dosages greater than 30 mg/d, which may be correlated with increased levels of a stimulating metabolite of mirtazapine, m-chlorophenylpiperazine (mCPP). Other less-problematic side effects include gastrointestinal upset and dry mouth. Although data are limited on the concomitant use of bupropion and other medications, drug interactions with this agent are discussed in Chapter 13. The starting and maximum dosages of bupropion and mirtazapine are shown in Table 5.5.

Tricyclic Antidepressants

The TCAs were discovered by chance, when imipramine was studied as a potential antipsychotic agent in 1958. Although it was ineffective for psychosis, it was noted to have antidepressant effects.

Mechanism of Action

The TCAs all have a similar chemical structure because most of them are based on a three-ring nucleus (hence the term *tricyclic*), although two available TCAs are actually tetracyclic. Except for clomipramine, which strongly inhibits the reuptake of both monoamines, the TCAs are potent blockers of norepinephrine reuptake and relatively weak blockers of serotonin reuptake. The TCAs do not block the reuptake of dopamine. In addition, TCAs are relatively strong antagonists of muscarinic, histaminic, and alpha-adrenergic receptors. TCAs also influence cardiac conduction in the same manner that class 1A antiarrhythmics do.

Table 5.5   Dosaging of Bupropion and Mirtazapine

Drug	Starting Dosage	Maximum Dosage
Bupropion (Wellbutrin SR)	100 mg bid	200 mg bid
Mirtazapine (Remeron)	15 mg qhs	45 mg qhs

Clinical Use

The most common use of TCAs—and the principal FDA indication for all but one of them—is for the treatment of major depression. Clomipramine, with its potent serotonin effects, is FDA indicated for the treatment of obsessive-compulsive disorder but not depression, although European experience indicates that it also is useful as an antidepressant. TCAs also have been used successfully for the treatment of panic, agoraphobia, generalized anxiety, bulimia, childhood enuresis, headaches, and chronic pain.

Because of their relatively heavy side-effect burden and low therapeutic index, the TCAs largely have been supplanted by the SSRIs and other, newer antidepressants for first-line treatment of depression. One potential exception is in the treatment of severe, melancholic depression, in which there is debate about whether the TCAs may actually be more effective than the SSRIs (30).

Because there is significant homogeneity within the group, choosing between TCAs is, to some degree, a matter of physician preference. Based on side-effect profiles, the secondary amines desipramine and nortriptyline are relatively more benign in terms of antihistaminic, anticholinergic, and anti–alpha-adrenergic effects than are tertiary amines such as imipramine and amitriptyline, although their potential for causing these side effects is still much greater than that of the SSRIs.

As with MAOIs, it is generally better to start with low initial doses and to increase the dose gradually into the therapeutic range during several days or weeks. This allows patients time to become accustomed to side effects and to tolerate higher target-dose levels. Starting and maximum dosages are shown in Table 5.6.

Laboratory studies that are important to consider when prescribing a TCA are TCA plasma levels and an electrocardiogram (ECG). A pretreatment ECG is indicated in patients with a personal or family history of heart disease and for elderly patients because some patients have unrecognized conduction deficits that could be exacerbated by the quinidine-like effect of TCAs. A follow-up ECG should then be obtained for these patients when they are on a stable dose of the antidepressant. Trough plasma levels of TCAs (drawn 8–12 hours after the most recent dose) should be considered under the following circumstances: when a patient fails to respond to a TCA in the usual dose range, when a patient has significant side effects at low doses, when there are questions about patient compliance, and after the addition of or change in the dose of another medication that affects TCA metabolism. Clinicians should remember that TCAs have a low therapeutic index and that there is a high degree of individual variability in drug metabolism (~10% of the population are considered "poor metabolizers"). Plasma levels are particularly helpful when using nortriptyline, which is unique among the TCAs in having a well-defined therapeutic window of plasma levels that correspond to clinical response.

Table 5.6   Dosaging of Tricyclic Antidepressants

Drug	Starting Dosage	Maximum Dosage
Amitriptyline (Elavil)	25 mg/d	300 mg/d
Amoxapine (Asendin)	50 mg/d	400 mg/d
Clomipramine (Anafranil)	25 mg/d	250 mg/d
Desipramine (Norpramin)	25 mg/d	300 mg/d
Doxepin (Sinequan)	25 mg/d	300 mg/d
Imipramine (Tofranil)	25 mg/d	300 mg/d
Nortriptyline (Pamelor)	10–25 mg/d	150 mg/d
Protriptyline (Vivactil)	10 mg/d	50 mg/d
Trimipramine (Surmontil)	25 mg/d	300 mg/d

Adverse Effects

Most of the typical TCA side effects correlate with their profile of receptor interactions. Antimuscarinic (anticholinergic) effects include confusion, accommodation difficulties (blurry vision), dry mouth, dry skin, constipation, urinary retention, and erectile dysfunction. Antihistaminic effects include sedation and weight gain. Anti–alpha-adrenergic effects lead to orthostasis and dizziness. Also, enhancement of monoamine activity can lead to symptoms of excessive CNS stimulation, including tremor and insomnia. The above symptoms often are manageable by forewarning patients that some side effects are to be expected and by gradually titrating the dose to allow the patient time to accommodate. It is also important to remember that medically ill and elderly patients are particularly sensitive to the adverse effects of TCAs and require cautious dosing if a TCA is prescribed.

The TCAs exert a quinidine-like effect on cardiac conduction, even at therapeutic doses. In overdose, this effect is dangerous because the drugs can become arrhythmogenic, even for patients without underlying cardiac disease. The potential lethality of TCAs in overdose is in sharp contrast to the safety of SSRIs and other, newer antidepressants and can occur after ingesting as little as 1-week's worth of TCA medication. For this reason, we do not recommend prescribing TCAs to patients who are actively suicidal or who have histories of previous overdoses.

The TCAs may be somewhat more likely than are other antidepressants to provoke a manic episode or to cause rapid cycling between manic and depressed states (31). For this reason, they are undesirable in patients with histories of mania or bipolar disorder.

Drug Interactions

Because most TCAs are metabolized by the hepatic enzyme cytochrome P450 IID6 (CYP2D6), any medication that affects this enzyme can change the plasma level of a TCA significantly, potentially elevating it to toxic levels. These CYP2D6 inhibitors include SSRI antidepressants (especially fluoxetine, paroxetine, and sertraline), phenothiazines, flecainide, quinidine, and cimetidine.

Other drug interactions are the result of additive effects between TCAs and other medications. Examples include cardiac toxicity from the co-administration of TCAs and other agents that have quinidine-like effects, excessive sedation from the combination of TCAs and CNS depressants, additive sympathetic effects with sympathomimetic agents (especially intravenous), additive anticholinergic effects when TCAs are combined with other medications that have anticholinergic properties, and increased risk of orthostasis with the combination of TCAs and antihypertensives. Hypertensive crisis, seizures, and even death may occur when a TCA is added to a MAOI.

The TCAs inhibit the neuronal uptake of guanethidine and consequently block its antihypertensive effect, and they can interfere with the effects of clonidine as a result of increased synaptic levels of norepinephrine. (*See* Chapter 13 for more information on drug interactions.)

Discontinuation of Treatment

The abrupt discontinuation of TCAs has been associated with a "discontinuation syndrome," typically beginning within 1 to 2 days, with symptoms of fatigue, nausea, dizziness, and other flu-like symptoms. Discontinuation symptoms may last up to a week or longer and are more associated with anticholinergic tricyclics, such as amitriptyline. For this reason, and because with a reduced dose it is necessary to monitor for recurrence of the psychiatric symptoms, it is prudent to taper the dose of TCAs gradually. A common strategy is to decrease the dose by 25% every 1 to 2 weeks.

Monoamine Oxidase Inhibitors

The first effective pharmacotherapy for depression was the MAOIs. The discovery that they had antidepressant qualities was serendipitous: the MAOI iproniazid, which is no longer available in the United States because of concerns about hepatic toxicity, was used originally as an antituberculosis agent in the early 1950s and was noted incidentally to elevate the mood of tuberculosis patients.

Although the use of other available MAOIs has declined over time—mostly because of the advent of other classes of antidepressants that are generally easier to use—MAOIs still occupy an important place in the anti-depressant armamentarium, particularly for depression refractory to other antidepressants.

Mechanism of Action

The MAOIs, as their name suggests, inhibit the action of the enzyme monoamine oxidase (MAO), which is found in various organs in the body, including the brain and the gastrointestinal tract. The two principle forms of MAO are MAO-A and MAO-B. MAO-A degrades norepinephrine, serotonin, and tyramine; MAO-B degrades certain other amines like phenylethylamine. Some substrates like dopamine are degraded by both types of MAO. The MAOI antidepressants currently available in the United States—phenelzine, tranylcypromine, and the newly re-introduced isocarboxazid—preferentially inhibit MAO-A in an irreversible manner that requires new protein synthesis to restore enzyme activity.

The MAOIs act within the terminals of monoamine-containing presynaptic neurons, where they block the deamination of serotonin, norepinephrine, and dopamine by MAO-A. This leads to increased neurotransmission in monoamine synapses.

Indications

As previously mentioned, the most common use for MAOIs in contemporary psychiatry is for patients with treatment-refractory depression. MAOIs also have been suggested to have an advantage over TCAs in the treatment of atypical depression (i.e., depression with hypersomnia, increased appetite and weight, and a preservation of mood reactivity) (32), although their use for this indication has diminished because the SSRI antidepressants also seem to treat the atypical subtype. Other demonstrated uses for MAOIs are for the anxiety disorders, social phobia, and panic disorder, but again they largely have been replaced (at least as first-line treatments) by the SSRIs.

The practical use of MAOIs is complicated by two serious potential adverse effects: serotonin syndrome and hypertensive crises. Both are avoidable, but avoidance requires the physician and patient to have a significant knowledge of drug and food interactions, and the patient must adhere carefully to dietary and medication restrictions.

To minimize nuisance side effects, MAOIs generally require titration from a relatively low initial dose to a therapeutic dose over the course of several days to weeks. There is some indication that patients with particularly severe or refractory depressions are more likely to respond to doses at the upper end of the therapeutic range. Therapeutic drug monitoring (checking blood levels of the medication) is not considered useful clinically and is not indicated when prescribing an MAOI. Starting and maximum dosages are shown in Table 5.7.

Serotonin Syndrome and Hypertensive Crises

Serotonin syndrome is a potentially dangerous state related to excessive central serotonergic activity (Case 5.3) (33). Hallmark symptoms are altered mental state, hyperreflexia, myoclonus, autonomic instability, and severe gastrointestinal distress (*see also* Chapter 13). Because MAOIs increase serotonin activity so potently, the addition of any other serotonin agonist generally is contraindicated. Examples of common medications that enhance serotonin tone are serotonergic antidepressants (e.g., SSRIs, venlafaxine, nefazodone, mirtazapine, clomipramine), meperidine (Demerol), dextromethorphan, and sumatriptan (Imitrex).

Table 5.7   Dosaging of Monoamine Oxidase Inhibitors

Drug	*Starting Dosage*	*Maximum Dosage*
Phenelzine (Nardil)	15–30 mg/d	90 mg/d
Tranylcypromine (Parnate)	10 mg/d	40 mg/d

CASE 5.3   *Serotonin syndrome with the use of monoamine oxidase inhibitors*

A woman 58 years of age has a history of migraine headaches, for which she takes Fiorinal (a combination of butalbital, aspirin, and caffeine) on an as-needed basis. She presents to the emergency room with a migraine that does not respond to Fiorinal. She also has a history of recurrent depression that has been treated satisfactorily for the past 10 years with phenelzine (Nardil) 30 mg bid. She has been compliant with her recommended dietary and over-the-counter medication restrictions. In the emergency room she is given an injection of meperidine (Demerol); several hours later she develops confusion; jerky, involuntary muscle movements; diarrhea; and hyperreflexia. The diagnosis is serotonin syndrome as a consequence of meperidine's serotonin agonism acting in combination with the established MAOI therapy. She recovers after 2 days of supportive therapy (intravenous fluids and parenteral benzodiazepines as needed for agitation).

Hypertensive crises are produced via a different mechanism: naturally occurring catecholamines (e.g., tyramine) in food can achieve dangerous concentrations when they are ingested and their metabolism is blocked by MAO. This can lead to an acute hypertensive reaction with violent headaches and an increased risk for stroke. Certain foods like red wines, aged cheeses, dried sausages, and smoked salmon are rich in tyramine and must be strictly avoided by patients on MAOIs because of their potential to cause a hypertensive crisis (the "wine and cheese effect"). Because certain other foods are also rich in tyramine, patients on MAOIs and physicians should be familiar with comprehensive lists of foods to avoid (34). In addition, medications that are sympathomimetic (e.g., stimulants, epinephrine, decongestants such as pseudoephedrine found in many cold and allergy remedies, cough syrups, and nasal sprays) also must be avoided for the same reason. As noted earlier, hypertensive crisis, seizures, and even death may occur when a serotonergic antidepressant is added to a MAOI. (*See* Chapter 13 for more information on drug interactions).

Because newly administered MAOIs must be synthesized to restore enzymatic activity, an MAOI-free period of 2 weeks is required before prescribing another serotonergic or sympathomimetic agent.

Other Adverse Effects

The MAOIs also cause other, usually less-dramatic side effects that nevertheless can cause significant discomfort and complicate treatment. Both MAOIs significantly block alpha-adrenoreceptors and can lead to orthostasis and subsequent dizziness. Patients also may experience either MAOI as being sedating or activating, although phenelzine generally is more likely to be sedating than is tranylcypromine. Other relatively common adverse effects are weight gain and sexual dysfunction, particularly anorgasmia.

Reversible and Selective Inhibitors of MAO-A

A new class of MAOI antidepressants that are not yet available in the United States are termed reversible inhibitors of monoamine oxidase (RIMAs). Examples of this class are moclobemide and brofaromine, which block MAO-A as do traditional MAOIs. However, because they inhibit MAO-A competitively and can be displaced from the enzyme by high concentrations of other substrates, their risk for causing a tyramine-related hypertensive crisis is considerably lower and they require less in the way of dietary vigilance on the part of patients (35). Although RIMAs have an advantage over irreversible MAOIs in terms of dietary restrictions, recent case reports suggest that the risk for serotonin syndrome remains (36).

Selegiline (Eldepryl) is a so-called selective MAOI indicated for the treatment of Parkinson's disease that also has been studied as an antidepressant. At low dosages (5–10 mg/d) it is a selective inhibitor of MAO-B and is much less likely to lead to hypertensive crises. Unfortunately, the dosages that seem to treat depression effectively (20–60 mg/d) (37) also cause selegiline to lose its selectivity for MAO-B.

Stimulants

Stimulants, including amphetamine, methylphenidate, and magnesium pemoline, have been used in medicine since the 1930s for a variety of problems, including attention-deficit–hyperactivity disorder (ADHD) in children, obesity, narcolepsy, and major depression. In recent years, stimulants frequently have been chosen to treat depression in critically or terminally ill patients. It was not until the 1960s that amphetamines (speed, crank) became common drugs of abuse.

There have been a number of trials conducted on stimulants for the treatment of depression (38). In head-to-head comparisons with standard antidepressants, the stimulants have not fared that well. Few trials have suggested superiority of the stimulants over standard antidepressants, and some placebo-controlled trials comparing stimulants to placebo in the treatment of major depression have been negative. Nevertheless, there still is a role for stimulants in the treatment of some major depressive episodes.

Mechanism of Action

Amphetamines immediately flood the cortical synapses with monoamines such as dopamine and norepinephrine (39,40). The result is that users may get intoxicated, especially if the drug is administered intravenously. With continued use of amphetamines, tolerance may develop and the mood-elevating properties of the drug may attenuate; however, other effects of amphetamines, including their ability to produce psychotic symptoms, may increase.

Indications

Stimulants, including methylphenidate, are class II scheduled drugs and in some states require a triplicate DEA (Drug Enforcement Agency) form for their prescription. ADHD is the only disorder for which class II stimulants are approved by the FDA. However, stimulants are used in other disorders in which fatigue is a problem, including chronic fatigue syndrome, AIDS, and depression (41). In major depression, stimulants are most likely to be used as adjunctive agents to augment standard antidepressants. Among the depressed patients who may be candidates for stimulants are those with concurrent ADHD, the depressed medically ill, and those with treatment-resistant geriatric depression. The stimulants have the advantage over standard antidepressants by having an immediate onset of action, and they are useful in mobilizing patients, increasing alertness, and enhancing energy. Their rapid onset of action makes them more attractive than other treatments for depression in the terminally ill.

Adverse Effects

At low doses, stimulants cause few side effects and are well tolerated by most patients. The most common adverse effects of stimulants are those associated with CNS activation. Insomnia, agitation, anxiety, and tremor occur in a dose-dependent fashion. Anorexia is also a common side effect, which may be problematic in cachectic depressed patients. Cardiovascular effects, including tachycardia, arrhythmias, and hypertension, also may occur with higher doses. Hyperpyrexia and seizures may occur in overdose. Benign increases in hepatic enzymes are associated with pemoline use, and there have been some cases of more severe hepatotoxicity with chronic use.

Patients with psychotic depression may experience an exacerbation of psychotic symptoms if they take stimulants. The most common psychotic symptoms with amphetamines include paranoid ideation and delusions. Auditory hallucinations also may occur and persist.

Although addiction is a defined risk of stimulant use, these risks seem to be low for most depressed patients. Candidates for stimulant treatment of depression include patients who have no significant history of substance abuse, those who are reliable, and those who have not responded completely to a standard antidepressant.

Drug Interactions

Stimulants seem to inhibit competitively the metabolism of some CYP2D6-dependent drugs. For example, both methylphenidate and D-amphetamine may raise the levels of TCAs when administered simultaneously.

Pharmacodynamically, the stimulants may lower the seizure threshold further when combined with other agents (e.g., clozapine, bupropion) that lower the seizure threshold.

The use of stimulants with MAOIs generally is contraindicated because of the risk of an ensuing hypertensive crisis. However, in clinical practice,

Table 5.8   Dosaging of Stimulants

Drug	Starting Dosage	Maximum Dosage
D-amphetamine (Dexedrine)	5 mg qd or bid	20 mg bid
Methylphenidate (Ritalin)	5 mg qd or bid	20 mg bid
Pemoline (Cylert)	18.75 mg qd or bid	75 mg bid

stimulants sometimes have been used to combat MAOI-induced sedation and hypotension effectively. (*See* Chapter 13 for more information on drug interactions.)

Dosing

Dosing for the stimulants should start low and be titrated to the lowest dose that achieves the desired effect (Table 5.8). D-amphetamine (Dexedrine) is usually started at 5 mg/d and increased to a maximum of 40 mg/d. Methylphenidate (Ritalin) is typically started at 5 mg bid and also may be increased to 40 mg/d. Pemoline (Cylert) is started at 18.75 mg/d and increased up to a maximum of 112.5 mg/d.

■   ■   ■

Recommendations

The SSRIs and other newer antidepressants should be considered first-line agents for the treatment of depression over the TCAs and MAOIs. Because all antidepressants have approximately equal efficacy, the choice of a specific agent should be influenced by each agent's specific side-effect and safety profiles and the depressed patient's age, gender, medical status, concomitant medications, history of response, and individual preferences.

If a patient's depression does not respond to the usual effective dose of a given antidepressant after 4 to 6 weeks, the dose should be titrated upward toward either to the maximum recommended dose or to the maximum tolerated dose before changing to or adding another agent.

If a patient has no response to the higher dose of a first-choice antidepressant, we recommend changing to a different antidepressant in a different class. If the patient has a partial response, we recommend a combination or an augmentation strategy.

■ ■ ■

Key Points

- Antidepressants are among the most commonly prescribed medications in the United States.

- There are several distinct classes of antidepressants that differ in their mechanisms of action and side-effect profiles.

- Physicians who prescribe antidepressants should be familiar with their side-effect profiles, relative toxicity, and potential drug interactions.

- SSRIs and the other newer generation antidepressants should be considered first-line agents for most patients with major depressive disorder.

- An adequate trial of an initial antidepressant should be pursued for every patient before changing treatments.

■ ■ ■

REFERENCES

1. **Hyalin TR, Buesching DP, Tollefson GD.** Health economic evaluations of antidepressants: a review. *Depression Anxiety.* 1998;7:53–64.

2. **Woster PS, Montgomery PA, Guthrie SK.** Tricyclic antidepressant prescribing by psychiatrists and other physicians. *Am J Hosp Pharm.* 1994;51:381–4.

3. **Olfson M, et al.** Antidepressant prescribing practices of outpatient psychiatrists. *Arch Gen Psychiatry.* 1998;55:310–6.

4. **Brody DS, et al.** Identifying patients with depression in the primary care setting: a more efficient method. *Arch Intern Med.* 1998;158:2469–75.

5. **Huszonek JJ, Dewan MJ, Donnelly MP.** Factors associated with antidepressant choice. *Psychosomatics.* 1995;36:42–7.

6. **DeBattista C.** *Medical Management of Depression,* 2nd ed. Dallas: Essential Medical Information Systems; 1998.

7. **Stewart A.** Choosing an antidepressant: effectiveness based pharmacoeconomics. *J Affect Dis.* 1998;48:125–33.

8. **Kornstein SG.** Gender differences in depression: implications for treatment. *J Clin Psychiatry.* 1997;58(Suppl 15):12–8.

9. **Nierenberg, AA, et al.** Early nonresponse to fluoxetine as a predictor of poor 8-week outcome. *Am J Psychiatry.* 1995;152:1500–3.

10. **Schatzberg, AF.** Dosing strategies for antidepressant agents. *J Clin Psychiatry.* 1991;52(Suppl):14–20.

11. **Schatzberg AF, DeBattista CJ.** *Manual of Clinical Psychopharmacology*, 3rd ed. Washington, DC: APA Press; 1998.

12. **Amsterdam JD.** Selective serotonin-reuptake inhibitor efficacy in severe and melancholic depression. *J Psychopharmacol.* 1998;12(3 Suppl B):S99–111.

13. **Clerc GE, Ruimy P, Verdeau-Palles J.** A double-blind comparison of venlafaxine and fluoxetine in patients hospitalized for major depression and melancholia: the Venlafaxine French Inpatient Study Group. *Int Clin Psychopharmacol.* 1994;9: 139–43.

14. *Physicians' Desk Reference*, 53rd ed. Montvale, NJ: Medical Economics; 1999.

15. **Nemeroff CB.** The clinical pharmacology and use of paroxetine, a new selective serotonin-reuptake inhibitor. *Pharmacotherapy.* 1994;14:127–38.

16. **Goodnick PJ, Goldstein BJ.** Selective serotonin-reuptake inhibitors in affective disorders. Part I: Basic pharmacology. *J Psychopharmacol.* 1998;12(Suppl B):S5–20.

17. **Goldstein BJ, Goodnick PJ.** Selective serotonin-reuptake inhibitors in the treatment of affective disorders. Part III: Tolerability, safety, and pharmacoeconomics. *J Psychopharmacol.* 1998;12(Suppl B):S55–87.

18. **Waldinger MD, Olivier B.** Selective serotonin-reuptake inhibitor–induced sexual dysfunction: clinical and research considerations. *Int Clin Psychopharmacol.* 1998;13(Suppl 6):S27–33.

19. **Woodrum ST, Brown CS.** Management of SSRI-induced sexual dysfunction. *Ann Pharmacother.* 1998;32:1209–15.

20. **Lane R, Baldwin D.** Selective serotonin-reuptake inhibitor–induced serotonin syndrome: review. *J Clin Psychopharmacol.* 1997;17:208- 21.

21. **Baker GB, et al.** Metabolic drug interactions with selective serotonin-reuptake inhibitor (SSRI) antidepressants. *Neurosci Biobehav Rev.* 1998;22:325–33.

22. **Stokes PE.** Ten years of fluoxetine. *Depression Anxiety.* 1998;8(Suppl 1):1–4.

23. **Nierenberg AA, et al.** Venlafaxine for treatment-resistant unipolar depression. *J Clin Psychopharmacol.* 1994;14:419–23.

24. **Thase ME.** Effects of venlafaxine on blood pressure: a meta-analysis of original data from 3744 depressed patients. *J Clin Psychiatry.* 1998;59:502–8.

25. **Cyr M, Brown CS.** Nefazodone: its place among antidepressants. *Ann Pharmacother.* 1996;30:1006–12.

26. **Haria M, Fitton A, McTavish D.** Trazodone: a review of its pharmacology, therapeutic use in depression, and therapeutic potential in other disorders. *Drugs Aging.* 1994;4:331–55.

27. **Greene DS, Barbhaiya RH.** Clinical pharmacokinetics of nefazodone. *Clin Pharmacokin.* 1997;33:260–75.

28. **Davis R, Whittington R, Bryson HM.** Nefazodone: a review of its pharmacology and clinical efficacy in the management of major depression. *Drugs.* 1997;53: 608–36.

29. **Fabre LF.** Trazodone dosing regimen: experience with single daily administration. *J Clin Psychiatry.* 1990;51(Suppl):23–6.

30. **Roose SP, et al.** Comparative efficacy of selective serotonin-reuptake inhibitors and tricyclics in the treatment of melancholia. *Am J Psychiatry.* 1994;151:1735–9.

31. **Wehr TA, Goodwin FK.** Can antidepressants cause mania and worsen the course of affective illness? *Am J Psychiatry.* 1987;144:1403–11.

32. **Quitkin FM, et al.** Atypical depression, panic attacks, and response to imipramine and phenelzine: a replication. *Arch Gen Psychiatry.* 1990;47:935–41.

33. **Sternbach H.** The serotonin syndrome. *Am J Psychiatry* 1991;148:705–13.

34. **Gardner DM, et al.** The making of a user friendly MAOI diet. *J Clin Psychiatry.* 1996;57:99–104.

35. **Cusson JR, Goldenberg E, Larochelle P.** Effect of a novel monoamine oxidase inhibitor, moclobemide, on the sensitivity to intravenous tyramine and norepinephrine in humans. *J Clin Pharmacol.* 1991;31:462- 7.

36. **Neovent PJ, et al.** Five fatal cases of serotonin syndrome after moclobemide-citalopram or moclobemide-clomipramine overdoses (Letter). *Lancet.* 1993;342: 1419.

37. **Sunderland T, et al.** High-dose selegiline in treatment-resistant older depressive patients. *Arch Gen Psychiatry.* 1994;51:607–15.

38. **Satel SL, Nelson JC.** Stimulants in the treatment of depression: a critical overview. *J Clin Psychiatry.* 1989;50:241–9.

39. **Brauer LH, Goudie AJ, de Wit H.** Dopamine ligands and the stimulus effects of amphetamine: animal models versus human laboratory data. *Psychopharmacology.* 1997;130:2–13.

40. **Seiden LS, Sabol KE, Ricaurte GA.** Amphetamine: effects on catecholamine systems and behavior. *Annual Rev Pharmacol Toxicol.* 1993;33:639–77.

41. **Chiarello RJ, Cole JO.** The use of psychostimulants in general psychiatry: a reconsideration. *Arch Gen Psych.* 1987;44:286–95.

KEY REFERENCES

Charney DS, Berman RM, Miller HL. Treatment of depression. In Schatzberg AF and Nemeroff CB (eds). *Textbook of Psychopharmacology,* 2nd ed. Washington, DC: American Psychiatric Press; 1998:705–31.

An excellent review of patient and medication factors that influence the choice of an antidepressant. It includes a detailed discussion of the subtypes of depression and the literature regarding their response to the different classes of antidepressants.

Schatzberg AF, Coles JO, DeBattista C. Antidepressants. In *Manual of Clinical Psychopharmacology,* 3rd ed. Washington, DC: American Psychiatric Press; 1998: 31–112.

A practical overview and guide to the use of antidepressant medications. It includes detailed descriptions of the side-effect profiles of the different antidepressants and strategies for their management.

Thase ME, Rush AJ. Treatment-resistant depression. In Bloom FE, Kupfer DJ (eds). *Psychopharmacology, The Fourth Generation of Progress.* New York: Raven Press; 1995:1081–97.

An excellent review of the literature regarding treatment-resistant depression, including detailed descriptions of treatment adequacy, switching from one antidepressant to another, and the various augmentation/combination strategies.

6

John W. Klocek, PhD

Psychotherapy

"I had always thought of therapy as something other people needed."

When helping a depressed patient decide whether he or she should receive antidepressant treatment, psychotherapy, or a combination of both, it is comforting to know that psychotherapy is an efficacious treatment for major depression (1,2). In controlled randomized clinical trials, psychotherapy has been shown to be superior to placebo and equivalent to other established treatments for mild to moderate clinical depression and an effective treatment for depression as administered by varied clinicians in "real world" clinical settings. Additionally, it has been found that psychotherapy is a valuable addition to the pharmacologic treatment of depression (3) and is effective in reducing relapse (4–6). Given the current status of psychotherapy research and the continuing dominance of managed mental health care, this chapter focuses on those treatments empirically demonstrated to be effective for depression. Additional forms of psychotherapy that may be helpful in addressing a patient's problems are discussed briefly. Subsequently, evidence that psychotherapy significantly reduces the risk of relapse is reviewed. Provided are descriptions of 1) the professionals who perform psychotherapy, 2) recommendations for how (and to whom) to refer for psychotherapy, and 3) techniques the primary care physician may use during office visits to enhance patient care in general.

Definition of Psychotherapy

The term "psychotherapy" means different things to different physicians and often elicits the question, "Just what *is* psychotherapy?" Some erroneously equate psychotherapy with Freudian psychoanalysis. Although psychoanalytically based psychotherapy continues to be practiced, current empirically supported approaches to psychotherapy bear little resemblance to this technique. As with the earlier approaches to psychotherapy, these contemporary approaches emerged from particular theoretical perspectives and emphasize different mechanisms of change. What all psychotherapies have in common is the intent to provide treatment through a careful and empathetic understanding of the individual coupled with the learning of more adaptive behaviors and/or patterns of thinking through systematic interpersonal interaction with a therapist. Similar elements can be used by a primary care physician to enhance the care of patients experiencing depression and other emotional distress.

Severity of Depression and Psychotherapy

How depressed can a patient be and still be referred for psychotherapy? To date, the empirical evidence indicates that psychotherapy is clearly effective with mild and moderate levels of depression (1,2,7). Although mild to moderate depression may be more difficult to detect than the severe depression that requires a psychiatric referral for treatment, it is more common in a primary care setting. Mildly to moderately depressed patients may still have enough motivation to have an interest in actively participating in their treatment for depression, and patients who clearly identify their depression as a result of environmental stressors (e.g., stress, divorce, loss) should be considered even more strongly for psychotherapy, because psychotherapy can provide a remedy specific to the problem.

The efficacy of psychotherapy in independently treating severely depressed patients remains controversial, with recent findings indicating that psychotherapy may indeed be as effective as pharmacotherapy (2,7–9). However, an individual must be capable of actively participating in psychotherapy for it to be a viable treatment option. Thus, although early psychotherapy sessions may serve primarily to enhance medication compliance and instill hope, patients are likely to benefit more fully as they become more able to participate actively. Of course, those patients experiencing particularly severe depressive episodes may benefit initially from pharmacologic management. Other severely depressed patients may benefit initially from both medication *and* psychotherapy (10). The decisions as to which modalities of treatment to pursue must be considered carefully by the physician, fully and clearly discussed with the patient, and subsequently reevaluated for potential modification.

Empirically Supported Psychotherapy

As in the rest of medicine, the age of managed care has brought great changes to the field of mental health care. Perhaps two of the most significant changes are the increasing emphasis on brief treatments and the demand for empirically supported treatments. In an effort to address these questions, mental health practitioners have joined the rest of medicine in bringing an evidenced-based approach to psychotherapy. Accordingly, psychotherapy outcome research has emphasized the careful comparison of a variety of psychotherapeutic techniques with previously established effective treatments for depression. These randomized clinical trials are conducted in a manner similar to randomized clinical trials of newly developed medications. Those psychotherapeutic approaches that are superior to placebo and equivalent to other proficient treatment modalities are deemed to be "empirically supported." Far from a completed task, the search for and evaluation of empirically supported therapies for depression and other clinical disorders continues to be a priority for psychotherapists. To date, three psychotherapeutic approaches can be regarded as being empirically supported for major depressive disorder: behavioral therapy (BT), cognitive-behavioral therapy (CBT), and interpersonal therapy (IPT) (Table 6.1) (2).

Table 6.1   Characteristics of Psychotherapeutic Approaches

Behavioral Therapy

- Is time limited, directive, and goal oriented

- Identifies problematic situations and behaviors

- Helps with social-skills training

- Increases pleasant activities and reduces unpleasant ones

- Is useful for anxiety disorders and depression

Cognitive-Behavioral Therapy

- Is time limited (8–20 weeks) and directive

- Encourages a systematic change in negative thought patterns

- Requires patient monitoring of thoughts and negative thought patterns

- Uses techniques for challenging maladaptive thoughts

Interpersonal Therapy

- Is time limited (12–16 sessions) and directive

- Emphasizes practical, obtainable goals

- Teaches recognition of interpersonal function and dysfunction

- Teaches improvement of coping skills through enhanced interpersonal functioning

To better illustrate the similarities and differences among how these therapeutic approaches conceptualize and treat depression, the case examples illustrating the different therapies use the same hypothetical patient, whom we refer to as "Mary." Basic demographic and referral information and symptomatology for "Mary" are introduced in Case 6.1.

CASE 6.1   *Presenting information*

Mary is a white woman 43 years of age who presents with upset stomach, difficulty sleeping, and fatigue. She has been married for 17 years and has two children, aged 14 and 16 years. She is currently employed at a local advertising firm, which recently was purchased by a large, out-of-town corporation. On further questioning, Mary indicates that she is having trouble producing creative ideas at work because of difficulty concentrating and figuring out what her new boss wants from her. She notes that she has "not been herself" at work or at home and that she has developed a "very short fuse." She reports that she is satisfied with her marriage, although she and her husband don't seem to do as much together as they used to. She reports withdrawing from friends because of fatigue. At this point, Mary becomes quiet and says that she just doesn't seem to enjoy anything anymore. When questioned directly, Mary states that she is not depressed but acknowledges that she often feels "down these days."

Behavioral Therapy

Theories

Behavioral theories of depression primarily focus on observable behaviors and the environmental reinforcers (or lack thereof) that maintain depressive behaviors and cause subjective feelings of sadness. In general, behavioral theorists posit that depression is caused by an aversive experience (e.g., loss of job, death of someone close) and/or significant changes in reinforcers in the environment (11,12), coupled with inaccurate assessment of environmental demands (12), deficiencies in social skills (13), and/or deficiencies in problem-solving skills (14). The feelings of sadness and dysphoria are considered to be the result of too little positive reinforcement from others elicited by the patient (12). Ironically, as the patient begins to engage in depressed behaviors (e.g., withdrawal, sadness, reduced initiative), the sympathetic and concerned responses of others serve to reinforce depressive behaviors (11–14).

Treatment

Behavioral therapy for depression is a time-limited, directive, and goal-oriented therapy (15). The therapist assumes an active role in helping the patient identify problematic situations and behaviors, potential solutions, and coping skills that will address the identified concerns. In addition to requiring patients to monitor mood and activities, BT includes techniques such as social skills training, development of problem-solving skills, and structured programs aimed at increasing pleasant activities and reducing unpleasant events (*see* Table 6.1) (2). For example, a patient may be instructed to engage in behaviors he or she finds enjoyable or relaxing and to use new communication skills to reduce the frequency and impact of interpersonal conflicts at work. Although this approach has been perceived as mechanistic, it should be noted that behavioral therapists do acknowledge the importance of the emotional and subjective experience of depression as a focal point for treatment (16). While maintaining focus on behavioral techniques, the behavioral therapist also addresses the emotional suffering of the individual and provides a caring environment in which change is effected. Case 6.2 illustrates BT in the treatment of depression.

CASE 6.2   *Behavioral therapy*

The behavioral therapist is most interested in the changes in reinforcement that exist in the patient's life (*see* Case 6.1 for the presenting information on the hypothetical patient of this case, whom we call "Mary"). For instance, a significant change in Mary's workplace environment may have removed positive reinforcements that she previously received. Other areas of interest include changes in the positive reinforcement she receives from her husband, children, or both. Removal of any one of these sources may cause Mary to change her behaviors (e.g., to withdraw socially, become more irritable). Ironically, sad and withdrawn behaviors actually may be reinforced by the caring and compassionate response of her husband and friends. These and other changes in behavior—coupled with the dysphoria that Mary would likely feel on removal of sources of positive reinforcement—would be identified as the source of Mary's depressive symptoms.

Efficacy

Numerous well-designed and rigorously controlled studies have demonstrated the efficacy of behavioral treatment of depression. A study published as early as in 1984 demonstrated that BT was as effective as amitriptyline in reducing depression during a 12-week treatment period (17). Furthermore, these effects were maintained above and beyond initial effects with 6 to 8 booster sessions over the course of 6 months. It also has been found that procedures carefully designed to change behaviors thought to maintain depression resulted in significant reductions of depressive symptomatology (18). Most recent studies of behavioral techniques for depression have included the combination of cognitive and behavioral interventions, as reviewed in the section below.

Also, BT has been shown to treat effectively the symptoms of anxiety that so often accompany depression. For example, recent studies have found that BT is effective in treating generalized anxiety disorder, panic disorder (with and without agoraphobia), and social phobia (19). Because symptoms of anxiety and depression are often intertwined and may be mutually exacerbating, BT can provide a way to address both types of symptoms.

Cognitive-Behavioral Therapy

Theory

The cognitivebehavioral theory of depression hypothesizes that systematic patterns of negative and dysfunctional thinking dominate an individual's cognitions and result in the affective, behavioral, motivational, and somatic symptoms of depression (20). Examples of these patterns include the following:

1. **All-or-none thinking:** The tendency to see things in absolute, all-or-none terms

2. **Selective abstraction:** Focusing on negative aspects of a situation to the exclusion of positive aspects

3. **Overgeneralization:** The tendency to draw sweeping conclusions on the basis of a single event or small amount of data

4. **Personalization:** The tendency to relate events to the self—even when there is no evidence to support such personalization

Although these tendencies or patterns of cognitions occasionally may be present in everyone's thinking, in the depressed individual they are considered to comprise a "schema"—a consistent cognitive structure through which most day-to-day events are processed. The continued presence of a negative or maladaptive schema results in a negative view of the self, the world, and the future. As a result of this *negative cognitive triad*, individuals who are depressed view themselves as unworthy, undesirable, deserving of failure, and doomed to such experiences in the future (21). The cycle of negative perceptions and cognitions continues as subsequent events are viewed through a cognitive filter that confirms these expectations (the negative filter might be thought of as the opposite of the proverbial "rose-colored glasses"). Finally, these perceptions and thoughts become "automatic," and internal comments such as "I can't do it," "No one cares," and "I can never change" dominate an individual's thinking (21).

Treatment

Like BT, CBT for depression is a time-limited (8–20 weekly sessions), directive therapy. Because the theory assumes that the negative manner in which one views the self, the world, and the future is the underlying cause of a depressed person's affective and behavioral symptoms, CBT attempts to change the manner in which an individual views himself or herself, the world, and the future. However, it is far more than telling them to "think happy thoughts." CBT asks an individual to systematically and carefully monitor his or her thoughts, assess the presence of negative thinking styles, and use specific techniques to challenge the identified negative patterns (21). Additionally, CBT uses some aspects of the behavioral approach to depression, such as behavioral activation and role-playing in an effort to overcome low levels of motivation and to provide situations in which new cognitive approaches may be practiced and used (see Table 6.1) (21).

A typical course of CBT starts with the description of the cognitive-behavioral approach to depression and the model of therapy (21). Subsequently, the patient is instructed to engage in activities designed to increase his or her activity level and to pursue situations in which thoughts can be self-monitored. As therapy progresses, the patient is taught ways to refine self-monitoring, and he or she also begins to identify the cognitive errors described earlier. As the patient becomes adept at identifying specific types of cognitive errors, the concept of "schema" is introduced by the therapist to provide a framework within which the patient can organize maladaptive thoughts. It is expected that the patient will now begin to challenge the thoughts that comprise his or her negative schema. The therapist assists the patient in challenging these thoughts in a variety of ways.

The final phase of therapy is devoted to practicing these techniques and preparing for the end of therapy by providing strategies to prevent relapse. Behavioral strategies are practiced, more difficult role-playing situations may be used, and the identification and challenging of maladaptive cognitions continue. In addition, the patient and therapist work collaboratively to identify high-risk situations for relapse (e.g., the return of specific distorted cognitions, disrupted sleep patterns). Throughout the treatment, emphasis is placed on teaching the patient to engage in the process of identifying and challenging maladaptive thoughts independent of the therapist (20,21). This focus is intended to ensure the acquisition of skills and awareness that will be of use to the individual if depressive symptomatology recur. Although the patient is informed that returning for "booster sessions" in the future is an option, the strategies and techniques developed during CBT for depression are tools the individual can use independently in the future. Case 6.3 demonstrates how CBT is used in the treatment of depression.

CASE 6.3   *Cognitive-behavioral therapy*

The cognitive-behavioral therapist is interested in the cognitions that accompany the depressive mood and changes in the patient's life (*see* Case 6.1 for the presenting information on the hypothetical patient of this case, whom we call "Mary"). For example, does she attribute her difficulties at work to her one incompetence finally being discovered. The cognitive-behavioral therapist attempts to identify patterns of maladaptive cognitive styles that would account for both changes in behavior and negative affect. Further exploration would seek to identify the degree to which these maladaptive styles are present and in which domains they are most prevalent. The therapist also looks for evidence of negative automatic thoughts. Although some of this can be done through interview, the therapist will likely ask the patient to monitor herself for a week to gather more detailed data. Depressed mood and depressive symptoms are understood to be the result of both maladaptive cognitive styles and the maladaptive behaviors that may result from negative cognitive styles. Additionally, the maladaptive behaviors themselves also may result in depressed symptoms.

Efficacy

Of the empirically validated treatments, CBT has been perhaps the most studied psychotherapeutic treatment for depression. Numerous well-controlled studies have demonstrated the effectiveness of CBT as a treatment for depression (4,8,22,23); careful examination of the studies comparing the efficacy of CBT and pharmacologic interventions indicates that these approaches are nearly equivalent in their efficacy (2,20). Although some studies have found that pharmacologic treatments are superior in reducing symptomatology (7), others have found that CBT is more effective (24). Meta-analytic approaches, which use sophisticated statistical methodology to summarize and analyze data from numerous studies that meet clearly defined scientific standards, also suggest that CBT is at least as effective as pharmacotherapy in treating depression (1,9,25). Although sometimes perceived as a treatment only for mild depressive episodes, it is important to note that CBT has been found to be useful in treating moderate levels of depression as well (1,2).

Interpersonal Therapy

Theory

As its name suggests, interpersonal theory primarily focuses on the interconnections of mood, interpersonal functioning, and personal relationships.

More specifically, interpersonal theory hypothesizes that disturbing events and psychosocial stress may elicit depression, although the presence of close interpersonal relationships may protect one against depression (26,27). After the onset of a depressive episode, interpersonal functioning is further impaired, and the depressed individual further withdraws from others (27). Subsequent impairment of mood, motivation, and cognitive functioning (e.g., indecision) additionally affects an individual's ability to engage in successful and rewarding interpersonal interactions. Clinical depression itself is hypothesized to encompass three component areas (27,28):

1. **Symptom function:** Depressive affect and symptoms

2. **Social and interpersonal relations:** Social role interactions with others

3. **Personality or character problems:** Enduring maladaptive traits influencing reactions to interpersonal events

Interpersonal theory *does not* make etiologic statements about whether impaired social functioning causes depression or vice versa (1,27). Rather, the emphasis is placed on current functioning and strategies to improve future coping and functioning.

Treatment

As with the previously described efficacious treatments, IPT for depression is a time-limited (typically 12–16 sessions), directive psychotherapy (28). Like BT and CBT, the process is collaborative, and the therapist is active in focusing the treatment. Of the three component processes identified above, IPT seeks to intervene only in the first two: symptom function and social and interpersonal processes (27). IPT recognizes that the emphasis on brief treatment precludes expectation of in-depth personality change. Thus, the emphasis is on practical, attainable goals that improve adaptation and function.

Initially, the IPT therapist goes through the DSM-IV diagnostic criteria for depression (*see* Table 3.1) with the patient to demonstrate clearly to the patient that he or she is indeed clinically depressed and in need of treatment. This aspect of the treatment is referred to as "establishing the sick role" and is intended to encourage the patient to acknowledge the importance of devoting energy and resources to getting better (28). Additional goals for the first few sessions include exploration and understanding of interpersonal functioning and dysfunctioning and the development of a treatment plan. The middle phase of therapy continues to focus on current events and functioning. The therapist then selects one of the following four areas as the focus of the IPT treatment:

1. **Grief:** The reaction of the patient to the death of a significant other

2. **Role dispute:** The resolution of an interpersonal dispute that has broadly impacted the patient's life

3. **Role transition:** A significant shift in a patient's interpersonal role (e.g., divorce or marriage, job transitions, being diagnosed with a major medical disease)

4. **Interpersonal deficits:** Long-standing deficits in interpersonal functioning and low levels of interpersonal support

Once selected, the therapist maintains the focus of all future sessions on this particular area. Again, the goal is reduction of depressive symptoms and improved coping through enhanced interpersonal functioning. The final few sessions of IPT are devoted to a review of the therapy and identification of potential future vulnerabilities and indicators of relapse or remission. As with BT and CBT, this is intended to prepare the patient to use the skills learned in therapy if depressive symptoms re-emerge in the future (27,28). Case 6.4 illustrates the use of IPT in a patient with depression.

CASE 6.4 *Interpersonal therapy*

The interpersonal therapist focuses on the interpersonal relationships in the patient's environment (*see* Case 6.1 for the presenting information on the hypothetical patient of this case, whom we call "Mary"). Of particular note are transitions at work, potential transitions at home (e.g., her children are likely striving for greater autonomy and independence, which may greatly change her role as a mother), and potential transitions in her relationships with her friends. The interpersonal therapist discusses with Mary how satisfied she is with interpersonal relationships, talks with her about how she views them, and analyzes with her how she actually goes about interacting with others. The therapist pays particular attention to inaccurate or otherwise problematic perceptions of interpersonal skills. Because interpersonal theory does not make etiologic statements about interpersonal function and depression, the interpersonal therapist is less concerned with which came first; rather, the focus is on how interpersonal deficits maintain or exacerbate depressive symptomatology.

Efficacy

Interpersonal therapy has received a great deal of attention since its introduction. As with BT and CBT, IPT has been found to be an effective treatment for depression (2). Early studies by the developers of IPT indicated its efficacy when compared with amitriptyline. Furthermore, a combination of IPT and amitriptyline was found to be marginally superior to IPT or amitriptyline alone (29). A more recent, well-designed study found that IPT was superior to a control group and equivalent to both imipramine and

CBT for depression (30). The success of IPT as a front-line treatment for depression has been established clearly (2,27).

Other Forms of Psychotherapy

In addition to the previously described methods of psychotherapy, many other approaches to psychotherapy are available. Although some have not been studied systematically, they may still provide a patient with valuable insights and understanding of themselves.

Insight-Oriented Psychotherapies

Insight-oriented (also referred to as psychodynamic) psychotherapies focus on a patient's internal conflicts, psychological defenses, and developmental history. By starting with childhood experiences, the insight-oriented psychotherapist seeks to help the patient identify the determinants of repeating patterns of behavior. For example, insight-oriented therapy may help a woman understand why she has reacted to her husband's reported infidelity with passivity and by becoming depressed. This understanding also may help her to discover what keeps her from becoming angry and standing up for herself. Similarly, a man who becomes depressed when his son departs for college at approximately the same age the man was when his own father died also may be a good candidate for insight-oriented therapy. Such a therapeutic approach may be appropriate particularly when existential questions seem to be inciting a depressive episode. Insight-oriented therapies can be brief, open-ended, or lengthy, and they are often less structured than BT, CBT and IPT. Accordingly, insight-oriented therapies may be able to address a broader range of issues facing a patient. However, as with all psychotherapeutic approaches, access can be a problem, depending on the availability and affordability of skilled therapists and managed care approval (when applicable).

Marital Psychotherapy

Marital psychotherapy should be considered for those patients who are experiencing both depression and marital distress. Such a referral is particularly appropriate for a patient who describes a troubled marriage (or other long-term relationship) preceding or coinciding with the onset of depression. Regardless of which came first—the depression or the relationship problems—a purely pharmacologic approach is unlikely to resolve the relationship difficulties. In making a referral for marital or couples therapy, care should be taken not to place blame on either marital partner because therapeutic success depends on joint participation and shared responsibility for relationship problems.

Group Psychotherapy

Group psychotherapy can be a valuable component of a treatment plan for depression. Group psychotherapy is a term that encompasses a wide variety of approaches, including behavioral, cognitive-behavioral, interpersonal, and insight-oriented techniques. The theoretical orientation of the group will shape the specific techniques used to treat clinical depression in the group; however, the goal is the same: to help patients develop new skills and resources and obtain a better understanding of their depression. Depressed patients who share similar traumatic experiences (e.g., divorce, childhood abuse) may find group therapy particularly helpful. Groups that focus on one topic (e.g., depression) are often designed to last a particular number of sessions, and no new patients may join once the group has started. Thus, it is important to keep in mind that a patient may have to wait several weeks for a new group to begin. Research evaluating the efficacy of group psychotherapy for depression generally has been positive (31).

Combined Pharmacologic and Psychotherapeutic Treatments

Additional research has addressed the question of whether a combination of pharmacotherapy and psychotherapy is superior to each treatment individually during the acute phase of a depressive episode. Although some studies have found that combined treatments are superior to either treatment alone (29,32–34), numerous other studies indicate that combined treatments are not clearly superior to pharmacotherapy alone (7,8,14,24,35) nor to psychotherapy alone (7,8,24,36). However, a recent study (6; reviewed below) suggests that a combination of psychotherapy and pharmacotherapy is a superior *maintenance* treatment for chronic or recurrent depression. The finding that psychotherapy alone, pharmacotherapy alone, and combined protocols are generally equivalent in their demonstrated efficacy for mild to moderate depression provides the physician with a great deal of freedom and confidence in tailoring a treatment regimen to the needs and preferences of the patient.

Relapse Prevention and Psychotherapy

Depression is a disorder known to have a high likelihood of relapse. Thus, after treatment of the acute phase of the depressive episode, maintenance treatment is often necessary. Again, there are considerable data to indicate that psychotherapy and medications are equally effective as maintenance therapies for prevention of relapse. As with psychotherapy for the acute phase of depression, maintenance protocols are intended to provide patients with skills and resources they can use independently. The research described below suggests that patients are able to use these resources to avoid future occurrences of depression.

In one 2-year study of patients who had experienced three or more depressive episodes, it was found that 25% of patients receiving CBT as maintenance therapy relapsed, whereas 80% of those receiving clinical management (i.e., monitoring of medication taper, regular review of clinical status, and provision of advice and recommendations when appropriate) relapsed (5). In another 2-year follow-up study, it was found that CBT was as effective as medication in acute treatment of depression and in long-term maintenance therapy (37), and a recent study found that both IPT and nortriptyline were superior to placebo for the prevention of relapse of depression that had been treated successfully in adults aged 59 years and older. Notably, the combination of IPT and nortriptyline was superior to either treatment alone (6).

Given these and other studies demonstrating the efficacy of psychotherapy in significantly reducing the risk of relapse, psychotherapy should be strongly considered as a component of any treatment program for recurrent depression. In addition to the empirical support for psychotherapy, it makes intuitive sense that the development of new skills, more adaptive coping resources, and the ability to monitor one's own emotional state are likely to help sustain remission. At the very least, it offers physicians another efficacious, front-line treatment option for patients who struggle with chronic or recurrent depression.

Making a Referral for Psychotherapy

Not everyone who seems depressed needs psychotherapy, and psychotherapy is not for everyone. However, psychotherapy should be considered a primary treatment resource rather than a treatment of last resort. Psychotherapy is an effective front-line treatment for mild to moderate clinical depression, and it also may be helpful for individuals who are struggling through difficult periods in their lives but who do not fit neatly into a diagnostic category. It is also helpful as an adjunct to medication in severe depression.

However, some misconceptions about psychotherapy may make some clinicians less willing to make a referral for it. Many health care professionals believe psychotherapy is ineffective in patients who are older, less educated, or from minority cultures. None of these beliefs is accurate. A large amount of research has failed to find any relationship between intelligence, sex, and age on the outcome of psychotherapy—either positive or negative (38). Older patients accept and follow through on mental health referrals at approximately the same rate as their younger counterparts (39). Poor and minority populations underuse psychotherapy because of difficulty in accessing services. Misconceptions and biases about who benefits from psychotherapy can affect who is actually referred, thus depriving some individuals of a valuable treatment option.

Patients, too, may have mistaken ideas about psychotherapy. Common misconceptions include the idea that a referral for psychotherapy means that their physician thinks they are crazy or that psychotherapy occurs on a couch and lasts for years. Such misconceptions are unfortunate because they can deprive patients of a chance to grow and develop in ways that could engender long-term self-care skills, so referring physicians should reassure their patients that contemporary psychotherapy is goal-oriented, effective, time efficient, and bears little resemblance to most media portrayals.

Nevertheless, the stigma and stereotypes of psychotherapy and psychotherapists persist, and making a referral can be difficult, particularly when the patient has sought out the primary care physician because of *physical* symptoms and is not especially receptive to a referral for psychotherapy—even when the physical symptoms indicate possible depression. Drawing extensively on the work of DeGood (40), recommendations for how to facilitate a referral for psychotherapy follow (*see also* Chapter 4).

First, a word of caution. As with any treatment, psychotherapy is not a panacea. In addition, there are individuals who simply are not interested in psychotherapy. The physician should ascertain whether such reluctance is a function of misperceptions that can be dispelled or the result of entrenched attitudes that are unlikely to change, thus negating the possible benefits of psychotherapy. In addition, psychotherapy is not a viable option for patients with significant cognitive impairment. Patients with comorbid depression and active substance abuse present a particular difficulty in referral because 1) both problems must be addressed by a well-trained psychotherapist, and 2) other community and medical resources must be engaged frequently (41). Although the following recommendations may involve a little of the physician's time, some are more a matter of style. A modest investment of time and effort in the referral process is likely to enhance adherence and increases the likelihood of a positive outcome.

Suggestions for Presenting a Referral

Exhibit confidence in the treatment: Perhaps most importantly, a referral to psychotherapy should be presented with the same confidence and certainty that a prescription for an antidepressant medication would be given. As noted earlier, psychotherapeutic approaches have demonstrated empirically an efficacy equivalent to the antidepressants for mild to moderate levels of depression. By presenting it as a front-line treatment option that works, the patient will likely be more receptive.

Reduce the stigma and misunderstanding: Some patients may perceive the referral for psychotherapy as an indication that they are "crazy" or that the depression is their fault. Because many patients are hesitant to express these feelings, it is helpful to ask patients why they are reluctant. For those who fear being labeled "crazy," a discussion of how commonly depression occurs—including in physicians—may help. For those who blame themselves, the physician should explain that guilt and self-blame are often symptoms of depression and that clinical depression is not a result of a weak character or a lack of will power. Neurobiological and pharmacologic research have had the unintended effect of creating the perception that only a drug can cure depression. Simplistic explanations of depression as a "chemical imbalance" or a "serotonin deficiency" may seem appealing as a way to reduce stigma, but they are misleading and ultimately counterproductive. Sometimes physicians use medical analogies to explain the depression. A patient may be told that depression is "just like diabetes." If the message is given that each is cured by a drug (e.g., insulin, antidepressant) that addresses a deficiency, a disservice has been done, for neither condition is so simply eradicated. However, if the physician explains that neither diabetes nor depression is the patient's fault, that both call for counseling and behavior change, and that both conditions can benefit from medication, then the analogy can be helpful.

Discuss rather than challenge: To a patient who already may be feeling defensive about a referral for psychotherapy, a direct challenge to his or her beliefs is not likely to be helpful. Rather, a brief discussion clarifying why the patient feels or thinks the way he or she does potentially will open the door to consideration. Addressing misconceptions (e.g., "only crazy people go to psychotherapists," "you think it's my fault") may further that discussion. Subsequently, presenting the evidence that psychotherapy is an active, efficacious treatment with long-term benefits may help. Because opinions and attitudes sometimes take time to change, do not be surprised if the patient continues to refuse the referral in the office but calls back a day or two later requesting those phone numbers.

Discuss reasonable expectations: As with antidepressant medication, the impact of psychotherapy is not immediate. Clear discussion about duration of treatment (e.g., 8–20 weeks), the potential for "ups and downs" in therapy, and the importance of active participation will go a long way toward preparing the patient for a course of psychotherapy. As noted earlier, many people think of psychotherapy as being an expensive process requiring years on a couch. Even worse, they may have drawn their impressions of psy-

chotherapy and psychotherapists from television or the movies. Researchers have found that, in general, patients prefer shorter-term
therapies and are more likely to follow through with therapy if they
have accurate perceptions of the nature and length of the therapy
(38). Frank discussion of the patient's perceptions and expectations
will facilitate the referral greatly.

Make it the patient's decision: Finally, the decision to participate
in psychotherapy belongs to the patient. Although others (e.g., the
physician, family, friends, an employer, clergy) may be pushing the
patient toward psychotherapy, the decision to pursue psychotherapy must be one with which the patient is comfortable. Noncompliance renders all medical treatments ineffective, but psychotherapy,
like diabetic management, requires active investment in and involvement of the patient.

Who Practices Psychotherapy?

A number of professionals practice psychotherapy, including psychiatrists,
psychologists, and social workers. In addition, listings for "counselors" and
"psychotherapists" can be found in the telephone book. The differences
between these practitioners, their training, and their scope of practice are
important to understand for appropriate referrals. Accordingly, the following descriptions provide a brief summary of the training each type of professional receives, a short description of common approaches to mental
health treatment, and a brief discussion of the scope of practice. Note that
these descriptions are based on generalities and it should be remembered
that there is a great deal of variability among professionals within any disci-
pline. It is also important to note that each state and province has its own
laws on licensure and legally sanctioned scope of practice for each of the
practitioners described below. Finally, it is essential to obtain an understanding of how individual practitioners practice psychotherapy.

Psychiatrists

Psychiatrists attend medical school and then pursue a residency in psychiatry typically lasting 4 years. During their residency, psychiatrists receive intensive training in the diagnosis and treatment of mental disorders. A
significant portion of the training is devoted to psychiatric hospitalization,
neurobiology, somatic therapies (e.g., psychotropic medications, electroconvulsive therapy), and psychiatric illness in the medically ill. Some psychiatrists obtain additional advanced training in child and adolescent or
geriatric psychiatry. Psychiatrists obtain board certification from the Ameri-

can Board of Psychiatry and Neurology. As physicians, psychiatrists are licensed to prescribe medications and can hospitalize patients. On average, the depressed patients treated by psychiatrists are more ill than those treated by other mental health professionals or by primary care physicians.

Although some believe that psychiatrists do nothing but prescribe medications, many psychiatrists do practice psychotherapy. However, it is important to obtain information about their style of practice when making a referral for psychotherapy. Specifically, it is important to determine if "psychotherapy" consists of 15-minute medication evaluations on a monthly basis or weekly 1-hour sessions focused on the previously described approaches to psychotherapy.

Psychologists

Psychologists receive 4 to 5 years of graduate academic education and clinical training in the diagnosis and treatment of mental disorders. Subsequently, they pursue a 1-year clinical internship at a medical center or mental health setting devoted to clinical training. On successful completion of the internship, they are awarded a PhD or PsyD but must be licensed by their state or province first before they are able to call themselves psychologists (in many states and provinces, the term "psychologist" is a legally protected term). In addition to PhD or PsyD, the letters "ABPP" may be listed. This indicates that the clinician has been board certified by the American Board of Professional Psychologists. With a few exceptions (e.g., Guam), psychologists are not licensed to prescribe medications and cannot hospitalize patients in the United States and its territories. Accordingly, individual and group psychotherapies are the primary methods of treatment used by psychologists. Psychologists also have expertise in using and interpreting psychological tests and can be helpful particularly in clarifying difficult diagnostic cases. Psychologists can obtain additional advanced training in behavioral medicine, which emphasizes working collaboratively with multidisciplinary teams to treat mental illnesses in medical patients.

Social Workers

After college, social workers receive 2 years of academic and clinical training. In addition to training in the treatment of mental illness, social workers receive training in case management and in accessing and using social services and resources available in the community. Social workers receive a master's degree in social work (MSW) and may specialize in a variety of areas. However, not all social workers receive training in psychotherapy or choose to practice psychotherapy. Those who do typically must be licensed by their state or province before practicing. States vary in the terminology used in the licensing of social workers. Common terms include

Licensed Clinical Social Worker (LCSW) and Certified Clinical Social Worker (CCSW). Social workers are not licensed to prescribe medications and cannot hospitalize patients.

Counselors and Psychotherapists

In addition to psychiatrists, psychologists, and social workers, numerous other disciplines may be licensed to practice psychotherapy. However, it is also important to note that the terms "psychotherapist" or "counselor" may not be legally protected terms everywhere, so the use of these titles does not necessarily imply professional training, licensing, or regulation.

Furthermore, most states and provinces allow for the licensing of counselors under the term Licensed Professional Counselor (LPC). Again, this title does not imply a particular form of training and may be obtained by individuals with a broad variety of educational and training backgrounds. This license does imply that the individual has met the standards set by the state and is subject to the laws governing their practice. Individuals who obtain an LPC license include those who have a master's degree in clinical or counseling psychology, social workers (in states that do not have licensing for social workers), and psychiatric nurses. Psychiatric nurses who have obtained nurse practitioner training and certification are able to prescribe medications from a limited formulary. Clearly, the broad variety of training and professional experiences encompassed by the titles "psychotherapist" and "counselor" suggests that a careful assessment of training and scope of practice is important when making a referral.

Useful Techniques for the Primary Care Physician

Although this chapter has addressed only briefly the actual techniques used in the empirically supported psychotherapies, primary care physicians may use aspects of these approaches to enhance their own patient care. Note that the use of these techniques does not constitute the use of an empirically supported psychotherapy—to do so would suggest that the physician has 50 minutes per week (or more) to spend with the patient. However, these techniques may enhance care significantly without adding substantially to the primary care physician's already overloaded schedule. Because these techniques are primarily verbal in nature, they may be loosely considered to be psychotherapeutic.

An excellent review of techniques that can be used in a primary care setting is presented in *The Fifteen-Minute Hour: Applied Psychotherapy for the Primary Care Physician* (42). Some of these techniques are discussed below and may be useful with many distressed patients, in addition to those who are depressed.

Listening: Perhaps the most basic and useful technique is listening. A patient will feel that the physician is listening only if the physician sits down, makes eye contact, and pays full attention to what the patient is saying. This may require a few extra minutes, but good listening improves patient satisfaction and, in the long run, actually may save the physician time.

Responding: One of the primary functions of a physician is to attempt to "fix" what is wrong. At times it may be better simply to respond in a way that communicates interest and concern. Rather than providing advice based on what the patient has said, a brief summary and distillation of what the patient has described can be helpful. For example, after a patient's particularly vitriolic description of his inept boss and the problems in working with him, a response along the lines of "So things have been tough at work lately" may be beneficial. It communicates an understanding of the situation and opens dialogue about the impact of those stressors.

Empathy: Another type of response that demonstrates not only interest but empathy is one that addresses the emotional impact of the situations encountered by the patient. Although much lampooned, the question "How do you feel about that?" may deepen the dialogue with a patient. If the patient does have difficulty labeling feelings, an attempt to clarify his or her feelings may help (e.g., "Are you feeling discouraged about this?"). If the patient is clear about his or her feelings, briefly summarizing what he or she has said will again demonstrate that you are listening (e.g., "So you are feeling pretty down about this").

Return control to the patient: Many times, people feel out of control when they encounter emotional or interpersonal difficulties. Rather than giving in to the temptation to dispense advice and reassurance, the physician might attempt to return control (or perceived control) of the situation to the patient. A question along the lines of "What would you like to do about that?" communicates both an understanding that the situation the patient has described is significant and implicitly sends the message that the patient may indeed have the resources necessary to manage the situation.

Given their broad applicability, these techniques can be useful in working with many patients. Although such approaches combined with pharmacotherapy may be sufficient for some patients, these techniques may only begin to illuminate the struggles of others. When it becomes clear that the brief interventions provided by the primary care physician are insufficient, a referral for psychotherapy should be considered.

Conclusion

Psychotherapy has been found to be an effective front-line treatment for clinical depression. Although psychotherapy and its practice can be construed broadly, three specific techniques have been demonstrated empirically to be effective treatments for clinical depression. Given the potential long-term benefits of psychotherapy, a referral for BT, CBT, or IPT should be considered independently or in conjunction with pharmacotherapy for the mildly or moderately depressed patient. Psychotherapy may be the treatment of choice when dealing with problems or difficulties that have a significant psychosocial component (e.g., sadness caused by marital distress), and it can be considered a valuable adjunct to medication for severely depressed patients (although a referral may not be appropriate until the patient is able to participate actively in psychotherapy). Finally, many of the principles and techniques of psychotherapy can be used to enhance medical care. Although these techniques may take practice and adjustment, it is likely that systematic use of psychotherapeutic approaches will enhance patient care as well as patient and physician satisfaction.

■ ■ ■

Key Points

- Psychotherapy is an effective treatment for mild to moderate clinical depression.
- Contemporary psychotherapeutic approaches are goal-oriented, directive, and often time limited.
- Dispelling patient (and physician) misconceptions about psychotherapy can facilitate a referral and offer a patient an additional treatment option.
- Physician use of basic therapeutic techniques can enhance the care of patients who are emotionally distressed.

■ ■ ■

REFERENCES

1. **Antonuccio DO, Danton WG, DeNelsky GY.** Psychotherapy versus medication for depression: challenging the conventional wisdom with data. *Prof Psychol Res Pract.* 1995;26:574–85.
2. **Craighead WE, Craighead LW, Ilardi SS.** Psychosocial treatments for major depressive disorder. In Nathan PE, Gorman JM (eds). *A Guide to Treatments That Work.* New York: Oxford University Press; 1998:226–39.

3. **Weissman MM, Prusoff BA, DiMascio A, et al.** The efficacy of drugs and psychotherapy in the treatment of acute depressive episodes. *Am J Psychiatry.* 1979; 136:555–58.

4. **Evans MD, Hollon SD, DeRubeis RJ, et al.** Differential relapse following cognitive therapy and pharmacotherapy for depression. *Arch Gen Psychiatry.* 1992; 49:802–8.

5. **Fava GA, Rafanelli C, Grandi S, et al.** Prevention of recurrent depression with cognitive-behavioral therapy. *Arch Gen Psychiatry.* 1998;55:816–20.

6. **Reynolds CF, Frank E, Perel JM, et al.** Nortriptyline and interpersonal psychotherapy as maintenance therapies for recurrent major depression: a randomized controlled trial in patients older than 59 years. *JAMA.* 1999;281:39–45.

7. **Elkin I, Shea MT, Watkins JT, et al.** National Institute of Mental Health Treatment of Depression Collaborative Research Program: general effectiveness of treatments. *Arch Gen Psychiarty.* 1989;46:971–82.

8. **Hollon SD, DeRubeis RJ, Evans MD, et al.** Cognitive therapy and pharmacotherapy for depression: singly and in competition. *Arch Gen Psychiatry.* 1992;49: 774–81.

9. **DeRubis RJ, Gelfand LA, Tang TZ, Simons AD.** Medications versus cognitive-behavior therapy for severely depressed outpatients: meta-analysis of four randomized comparisons. *Am J Psychiatry.* 1999;156:1007–13.

10. **Thase ME, Greenhouse JB, Reynolds CF, et al.** Treatment of major depression with psychotherapy or psychotherapy-pharmacotherapy combinations. *Arch Gen Psychiatry.* 1997;54:1009–15.

11. **Skinner BF.** *Science and Human Behavior.* New York: Free Press; 1953.

12. **Lewinsohn PM.** A behavioral approach to depression. In Friedman RJ, Katz MM (eds). *The Psychology of Depression: Contemporary Theory and Research.* New York: Wiley; 1974:157–85.

13. **Coyne JC.** Toward an interactional description of depression. *Psychiatry.* 1976;39: 28–40.

14. **Nezu AM.** A problem-solving formulation of depression: a literature review and proposal of a pluralistic model. *Clin Psychol Rev.* 1987;7:121–44.

15. **Lewinsohn PM, Gotlib IH.** Behavioral theory and treatment of depression. In Beckham EE, Leber WR (eds). *Handbook of Depression.* New York: Guilford Press; 1995:352–75.

16. **Goldfried MR, Davison GC.** *Clinical Behavior Therapy*, exp. ed. New York: Wiley & Sons; 1994.

17. **Hersen H, Bellack AS, Himmelhoch JM, Thase ME.** Effects of social skill training, amitriptyline, and psychotherapy in unipolar depressed women. *Behav Ther.* 1984;15:21–40.

18. **Jacobson NS, Dobson KS, Truax PA, et al.** A component analysis of cognitive-behavioral treatment for depression. *J Consult Clin Psychology.* 1996;64:295–304.

19. **Barlow DH, Esler JL, Vitali AE.** Psychosocial treatments for panic disorders, phobias, and generalized anxiety disorder. In Nathan PE, Gorman JM (eds). *A Guide to Treatments That Work.* New York: Oxford University Press; 1998:288–318.

20. **Sacco WP, Beck AT.** Cognitive theory and therapy. In Beckham EE & Leber WR (eds). *Handbook of Depression.* New York: Guilford Press; 1995:329–52.

21. **Beck AT.** *Cognitive Theory and the Emotional Disorders.* New York: International Universities Press; 1976.

22. **Rush AJ, Beck AT, Kovacs M, Hollon SD.** Comparative efficacy of cognitive therapy in the treatment of depressed outpatients. *Cognitive Ther Res.* 1977;1:17–36.

23. **Simons AD, Murphy GE, Levine JL, Wetzel RD.** Cognitive therapy and pharmacotherapy for depression. *Arch Gen Psychiatry.* 1986;43:43–8.

24. **Murphy GE, Simons AD, Wetzel RD, Lustman PJ.** Cognitive therapy and pharmacotherapy: singly and together in the treatment of depression. *Arch Gen Psychiatry.* 1984;41:33–41.

25. **Hollon SD, Shelton RC, Loosen PT.** Cognitive therapy and pharmacotherapy for depression. *J Consult Clin Psychol.* 1991;54:88–99.

26. **Brown GW, Harris T, Copeland JR.** Depression and loss. *Br J Psychiatry.* 1978; 133:1–18.

27. **Markowitz JC, Weissman MM.** Interpersonal psychotherapy. In Beckham EE, Leber WR (eds). *Handbook of Depression.* New York: Guilford Press; 1995:376–90.

28. **Klerman GL, Weissman MM, Rounsaville BJ, Chevron E.** *Interpersonal Psychotherapy of Depression.* New York: Basic Books; 1984.

29. **Weissman MM, Prusoff BA, DiMascio A, et al.** The efficacy of drugs and psychotherapy in the treatment of acute depressive episodes. *Am J Psychiatry.* 1979; 136:555–58.

30. **Elkin I, Gibbons RD, Shea MT, et al.** Initial severity and differential treatment outcome in the National Institute of Mental Health Treatment of Depression Collaborative Research Program. *J Consult Clin Psychol.* 1995;59:841–47.

31. **Hoberman HM, Lewinsohn PM, Tilson M.** Group treatment of depression: individual predictors of outcome. *J Consult Clin Psychol.* 1988;56:393–98.

32. **Blackburn IM, Bishop S, Glen AIM, et al.** The efficacy of cognitive therapy in depression: a treatment using cognitive therapy and pharmacotherapy, each alone and in combination. *Br J Psychiatry.* 1981;139:181–9.

33. **DiMascio A, Weissman MM, Prusoff BA, et al.** Differential symptom reduction by drugs and psychotherapy in acute depression. *Arch Gen Psychiatry.* 1979;36: 1450–6.

34. **Weissman MM, Klerman GL, Prusoff BA, et al.** Depressed outpatients: results 1 year after treatment with drugs and/or interpersonal psychotherapy. *Arch Gen Psychiatry.* 1981;38:51–5.

35. **Beutler LE, Scogin F, Kirkish P, et al.** Group cognitive therapy and alprazolam in the treatment of depression in older adults. *J Consult Clin Psychol.* 1987;55:550–6.

36. **Blackburn IM, Bishop S.** Changes in cognition with pharmacotherapy and cognitive therapy. *Br J Psychiatry.* 1983;143:609–17.

37. **Blackburn IM, Moore RG.** Controlled acute and follow-up trial of cognitive therapy and pharmacotherapy in outpatients with recurrent depression. *Br J Psychiatry.* 1997;171:328–34.

38. **Garfield SL.** Research on client variables in psychotherapy. In Bergin AE, Garfield SL (eds). *Handbook of Psychotherapy and Behavior Change.* New York: John Wiley & Sons; 1994:192–228.

39. **Sorkin BA, Rudy TE, Hanlon RB, et al.** Chronic pain in old and young patients: differences appear less important than similarities. *J Gerontol.* 1990;45:64–8.

40. **DeGood DE.** Reducing medical patients' reluctance to participate in psychological therapies: the initial session. *Prof Psychol Res Pract.* 1983;14:570–9.

41. **Miller WR, Brown SA.** Why psychologists should treat alcohol and drug problems. *Am Psychol.* 1997;52:1269–79.

42. **Stuart MR, Lieberman JA.** *The Fifteen-Minute Hour: Applied Psychotherapy for the Primary Care Physician,* 2nd ed. Westport, CT: Praeger Publishers/Greenwood Publishing Group; 1993.

KEY REFERENCES

Blackburn IM, Moore RG. Controlled acute and follow-up trial of cognitive therapy and pharmacotherapy in outpatients with recurrent depression. *Br J Psychiatry.* 1997;171:328–34.

A carefully designed and conducted study demonstrating the efficacy of cognitive therapy as a treatment for depression in both the acute and follow-up phases of treatment. The authors note that psychotherapy and medications had the same efficacy.

Craighead WE, Craighead LW, Ilardi SS. Psychosocial treatments for major depressive disorder. In Nathan PE, Gorman JM (eds). *A Guide to Treatments That Work.* New York: Oxford University Press; 1998:226–39.

A clear, concise review of the empirical literature investigating the efficacy of psychosocial interventions for depression. The authors hold to strict standards in identifying which therapies are qualified as empirically supported.

DeGood DE. Reducing medical patients' reluctance to participate in psychological therapies: the initial session. *Prof Psychol Res Pract.* 1983;14:570–79.

Because many patients come to their physician for physical ailments, they may be reluctant to see a psychotherapist. Although written primarily for psychologists in medical settings, this article provides solid recommendations for the physician to help patients understand why they would benefit from a psychotherapeutic intervention.

Stuart MR, Lieberman JA. *The Fifteen-Minute Hour: Applied Psychotherapy for the Primary Care Physician,* 2nd ed. Westport, CT: Praeger Publishers/Greenwood Publishing Group; 1993.

The authors present a clear description of the rationale, the benefits, and the "how to" of the inclusion of basic psychotherapeutic techniques by primary care physicians in their daily practice. Literature on the impact these techniques may have is reviewed.

7

■ ■ ■

Treatment-Resistant Depression

Yvonne M. Greene, MD

William M. McDonald, MD

"But I've since had first-hand experience with another great depression, the kind that takes up residence in the mind like a glum squatter, unwilling to yield and move on."

The modern therapeutic armamentarium available to treat major depression has revolutionized the clinical course of patients with mood disorders. However, clinicians are increasingly aware of the substantial minority of depressed patients who fail to get well despite aggressive treatment. Treatment-resistant depression (TRD) is an important clinical problem. Up to 40% of patients are not responsive to an initial course of antidepressant treatment, and between 10% and 15% of patients remain chronically depressed with significant psychosocial morbidity and high rates of suicide (1–3).

This chapter will define TRD and the clinical variables associated with nonresponse, including adequacy of the antidepressant trial and comorbid medical and psychiatric diagnoses. Strategies for managing TRD (e.g., substitution of an antidepressant with a different mechanism of action, augmentation, combination therapy, psychotherapy, electroconvulsive therapy, transcranial magnetic stimulation) also are reviewed. This discussion focuses on young adults. TRD in the elderly may require different considerations about medication choices (*see* Chapter 8 for a discussion of this topic).

Definition of Treatment-Resistant Depression

TRD is defined as a failure to respond completely to an antidepressant medication (4). Some researchers define absolute treatment resistance as a failure to respond to an adequate treatment trial, i.e., a trial of adequate dose and duration (5). The first step then in determining if a patient has TRD is to evaluate whether the patient has had an antidepressant trial of adequate dose and duration.

What Constitutes an Adequate Trial of Antidepressant Medication?

Clinicians may conclude falsely that a patient has TRD when in fact the patient has not had an adequate dose or duration of antidepressant therapy. A review of pharmacy records in a managed care setting revealed that only 11% of patients requiring antidepressant therapy received an adequate dose or duration of antidepressant (6). Similarly, a case series of patients referred to mental health clinics demonstrated that 15% to 21% of patients had previously received inadequate antidepressant therapy (7).

Duration

Antidepressants are effective because they cause receptor changes within the limbic system. Antidepressants exert their therapeutic effect through different mechanisms (reuptake blockade, agonists, antagonists) at different receptor sites (dopamine, serotonin, norepinephrine). The final common pathway for all antidepressant treatments, including electroconvulsive therapy (ECT), is the down-regulation of beta-adrenergic receptors; this down-regulation takes time, occurring when the central nervous system receptors turn over and are resynthesized. In some patients, an antidepressant effect may take place more quickly, but in most patients the antidepressant response will occur in 4 to 6 weeks (paralleling receptor turnover and resynthesis); therefore, an adequate duration for an antidepressant trial is 4 to 6 weeks (8). For a patient demonstrating a partial response within that time, an additional 4 to 6 weeks (i.e., 10 to 12 weeks total) may improve the response.

One study confirms that the response to an antidepressant is not "all or nothing" but gradual (9). The chance of a patient having a full response to antidepressant therapy after 6 weeks increases if they show an early partial response. In other words, patients who show a partial response at week 1 have a greater than 50% chance of attaining a full antidepressant response at week 6, whereas patients who do not demonstrate at least a partial response until week 3 will have only a one in three chance of having a complete response at week 6. Patients who have no response at week 4 will have a negligible response at week 6 (9); therefore, patients who have a partial response by week 4 should be continued on antidepressants at incremental doses for at least 4 to 6 weeks. Patients who show no response to an antidepressant trial by week 4 should be switched to another medication.

Dose

Basic pharmacologic principles dictate that a drug must be given at a sufficient dose to exert maximal effect. There is a 30-fold range of drug metabolism among individuals taking antidepressants. In addition, numerous reports have discovered that only 16% to 55% of depressed patients are prescribed at least a moderate dose (7,10). For some antidepressants, a plasma-level clinical-response relationship has been defined; medication efficacy may correspond to the presence of adequate antidepressant levels (11). We recommend maximizing antidepressant dose and/or optimizing antidepressant blood levels when patients do not respond to lower doses (Table 7.1).

The clinician must balance his or her judgment regarding the adequacy of the dose and duration of treatment when attempting to provide effective antidepressant therapy. It is usually more effective to provide a longer trial at a higher dose before switching treatment strategies (12) and also to achieve the maximally tolerated therapeutic dose before augmenting an ineffective antidepressant trial (13).

Fixed-dose studies of fluoxetine (14), sertraline (15), and paroxetine (16) indicate that no advantage to the practice of starting patients at higher doses of selective serotonin-reuptake inhibitors (SSRIs). However, this is not true for all new antidepressants. Venlafaxine demonstrates a dosage-dependent response between 75–375 mg/d (17).

When is it time to optimize the antidepressant trial versus switching or augmenting? In patients with a partial response, one study noted that by 8 weeks of therapy with fluoxetine at a dosage of 20 mg/d, increasing the dosage to 40 or 60 mg/d was more effective than adding low dosages of lithium or desipramine (18). In contrast, for patients who lacked any symptomatic response following 4 weeks of fluoxetine treatment, a switch of antidepressants was necessary (13).

Causes of Underdosing

Medication Intolerance

Medication intolerance is an important cause of underdosing (19,20). Discontinuation rates due to inability to tolerate antidepressant medication

Table 7.1   Adequate Dosing Regimens

Antidepressant	Dose (mg)	Plasma level (ng/mL)
Imipramine	200–300	>180
Desipramine	≥300	>150
Nortriptyline	≥100	50–150
Amitriptyline	≥300	>180
Doxepin	300	>180
Protriptyline	≥40	
Clomipramine	≥250	
Trimipramine	≥200	
Maprotiline	≥250	
Phenelzine	≥60	
Tranylcypromine	90	
Trazodone	≥450	
Fluoxetine	80	
Sertraline	≥200	
Paroxetine	50	
Citalopram	80	
Fluvoxamine	300	
Venlafaxine	375	
Bupropion	450	
Mirtazapine	45	

range from 6% to 25% (19,21). The clinician should bear in mind that many antidepressant side effects resolve within days to weeks; if not, patients may tolerate side effects better, especially following signs of clinical improvement. This is particularly true if the side effects are gastrointestinal (e.g., dyspepsia, nausea), which are common in the early weeks of an SSRI trial. Additionally, intolerance to one medication does not predict intolerance to another antidepressant, even one of the same class (22); hence, there may be benefit to changing medications within a class (e.g., SSRIs) if the patient is intolerant of the medication in the first weeks of therapy.

Noncompliance

One study conducted in a managed care setting revealed 28% of patients prescribed their first antidepressant stopped taking it during the first month of therapy, and 44% of patients ceased taking the antidepressant by the third month (21). During the first month of therapy, five educational messages given to the patients were associated with compliance:

1. The patient should take the medication daily.
2. The antidepressants must be taken for 2 to 4 weeks for a noticeable effect.
3. The patient should continue to take the medicine even if feeling better.
4. The patient should not stop taking the antidepressant without checking with the physician.
5. The patient should be given specific instructions as to resolving questions about their antidepressant.

Additionally, inquiring about previous experiences with antidepressants also was correlated with early compliance (21); hence, taking time for medication counseling and using newer antidepressants with more benign side-effect profiles increases patient compliance and diminishes treatment failures (6,21).

Differential Diagnosis

Comorbid Medical Illness

If the patient has received an antidepressant trial of adequate dose and duration, the next step in the approach to evaluating a patient with suspected TRD is to reconsider the differential diagnosis. Unrecognized medical conditions or medication side effects may cause or contribute to the development of a major depression in 35% to 50% of patients (7,23–26). Depression commonly occurs with hypothyroidism, hyperthyroidism, Cushing's syndrome, and stroke (Case 7.1). Subclinical forms of hypothyroidism have been found in 52% of patients with suspected TRD in reports from six clinical studies (25). (*See* Chapter 1 for an in-depth discussion of depression in the medically ill.) Optimal treatment of the medical illness associated with major depression may not lead to a resolution of the depression; continued, aggressive antidepressant therapy may need to be prescribed in conjunction with the medical treatment.

CASE 7.1   *Treatment-resistant depression in a patient with unrecognized hyperthyroidism*

A woman 52 years of age was referred for evaluation of major depression resistant to imipramine (300 mg/d) and sertraline (200 mg/d). She described very low mood for the past 6 months and noted insomnia, anxiety, low energy, diminished concentration, and suicidal ideation.

She had no family history of depression. Review of systems and physical examination revealed mild heat intolerance, a pulse of 88 bpm, and a normal neurological examination. Laboratory studies were remarkable for a thyroid-stimulating hormone level of 0.16. Referral to an endocrinologist revealed mild hyperthyroidism.

Following treatment with radioactive iodine, her depressive symptoms rapidly resolved.

Patients with hyperthyroidism may meet criteria for major depression and present without obvious physical signs of hyperthyroidism (26).

Comorbid Psychiatric Illness

Psychiatric comorbidity, such as anxiety and substance abuse, also can complicate the assessment of depressed patients. The U.S. National Comorbidity Survey has reported that patients diagnosed with major depression also met criteria for panic disorder (10%), generalized anxiety disorder (17%), obsessive-compulsive disorder (60%), and substance abuse (40%) (27). Co-occurrence of major depression and one of the anxiety disorders has been associated with a poorer outcome and increased risk of suicide (28).

Comorbid substance use or abuse is common in depression and is a significant contributor to what might be diagnosed falsely as TRD. As the clinician is reassessing the diagnosis, the investigation also must include the identification of prescribed medications (e.g., antihypertensives, hormones, diuretics; *see also* Chapter 1) that may be contributing to depressive symptoms (29). Alcohol affects anxiety and mood by several mechanisms. In addition to perturbing the balance of central nervous system neurotransmitters, alcohol modifies the clearance and disposition of antidepressant metabolites and interferes with their clinical efficacy (30–32). If depression has been resistant to treatment, it is appropriate to recommend abstinence from alcohol, even in those who do not meet criteria for alcohol abuse.

A complex relationship between depression and personality disorders exists. The clinician must exercise caution when diagnosing a personality disorder in the setting of clinical depression, because depression contributes to personality pathology (33). In patients with co-existing personality disorder and depression, studies report these patients take longer to respond to antidepressants and are less responsive to medications overall (34). Concomitant psychotherapy has been demonstrated to be of assistance (35).

Comorbid Social Pathology

The failure of depression to respond to pharmacotherapy may be due to significant psychosocial problems such as lack of social support, isolation, domestic violence, financial difficulties, marital or other relationship discord, hostile work environment or unstable employment, and religious difficulties (e.g., disconnection from one's faith community). A stressful life event—whether internal or external, acute or chronic—generates challenges to which the patient may not be able to respond. The severity of the stressor is not always predictive of the severity of the depression. Stressor severity is a function of degree, quantity, duration, reversibility, environment, and personal context. To understand the contribution of the stressor to the patient's depression, several factors must be understood: the nature of the stressor, the meaning of the stressor to the patient, and the patient's pre-existing vulnerability. Additionally, actual or perceived support from important relationships may affect the patient's behavioral and emotional responses to the stressor. If depression is not responding to treatment, the physician should identify underlying social problems or stressors. Some of these issues can be addressed in psychotherapy (*see* section on Strategies for Management below and Chapter 6), whereas others may need to be addressed through different modalities such as support groups (*see* Chapter 4).

Depression Subtypes

Psychotic Depression
Major depression accompanied by hallucinations or delusions has been associated with a poor response to antidepressants alone (Case 7.2) (36,37). Response rates with antipsychotics alone are similarly poor (37). When an antidepressant-antipsychotic combination or ECT is used, response rates improve and approach those of non–psychotically depressed patients (37). The psychosis in depression may be subtle with suspicious themes or overt with a patient responding to hallucinations or acting on delusions. The clinician should explore tactfully for these symptoms.

CASE 7.2   *Psychotic depression in a middle-aged man*

A man 49 years of age presented for evaluation of persistent depression, having failed 12-week trials of fluoxetine (40 mg/d) followed by bupropion (450 mg/d). He described a distant history of alcohol abuse, but he had completed an Alcoholics Anonymous program successfully and now completely abstains from drinking. He had a positive family history of depression (his father). He was having great difficulty maintaining his law practice given his anergy, hypersomnia, and desire to be isolated. Additionally, he related intermittent, passive suicidal thoughts and persistent thoughts that his neighbors were deliberately harassing him. He was unable to shake these thoughts and felt they were watching him through his windows. He denied auditory or visual hallucinations or other delusions, including grandiose delusions. He denied periods of mania or hypomania.

Physical examination, review of systems and laboratory studies were notable only for obesity. Risperidone at 0.5 mg twice daily was added to the current bupropion and improved his depressive symptoms. The risperidone was increased to 1.0 mg twice daily and resolved his paranoia.

Atypical Depression

This subtype of major depression is characterized by mood reactivity, increased appetite or weight gain, hypersomnia, leaden paralysis, and a chronic pattern of rejection sensitivity. Patients with atypical depression have been demonstrated to have a greater response to monoamine oxidase inhibitors (MAOIs), than to tricyclic antidepressants (TCAs) or placebo (38–40). One study has shown equal efficacy between fluoxetine and phenelzine in patients with atypical depression suggesting that SSRIs also may be preferable to TCAs in this population (41).

Seasonal Depression

Seasonal depression is defined as a temporal pattern of depressive symptoms that typically begins in autumn or winter, abates in the spring, and occurs over successive years. Numerous studies support the efficacy of light therapy for this population of patients (42–45). These studies also suggest that hypersomnia and carbohydrate cravings may predict responsiveness to phototherapy.

Strategies for Management

Once the clinician has explored the possible conditions that would lead to misdiagnosing a patient with TRD (e.g., an inadequate antidepressant trial, a medical or psychiatric comorbid diagnosis, a subtype of depression), the patient meets the definition for TRD (Fig. 7.1). If the patient has had no response within 4 weeks of the antidepressant trial, an alternative antidepressant should be initiated. If the patient has had a partial response by week 4, the dose

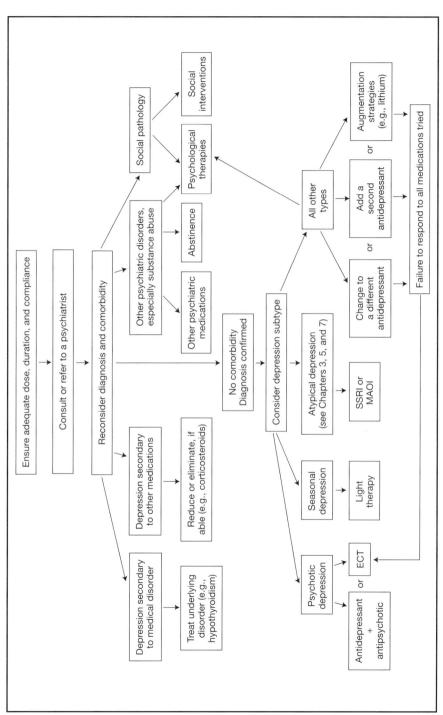

Figure 7.1   Algorithm for treatment-resistant depression. ECT = electroconvulsive therapy; MAOI = monoamine oxidase inhibitor; SSRI = selective serotonin-reuptake inhibitor.

should be increased; if the patient responds, the medication should be continued. If the patient continues to have only a partial response by the 6th to 8th weeks, the antidepressant should be augmented with another agent.

Switching to Another Antidepressant

Alternative monotherapy with a different mechanism of action may be associated with a greater response than switching to a different agent of the same class. Changing antidepressants from an ineffective class to a different class is a rational approach and seems to increase response rates to as high as the more well-studied augmentation strategies (2). As mentioned previously, an alternative antidepressant should be started if the patient has had no response to the initial antidepressant treatment by week 4 of the trial. After withdrawal of the ineffective initial antidepressant, the alternative monotherapy has potential advantages of simplicity, decreased risk of drug interactions, and fewer side effects.

Switching After Treatment Failure with a Selective Serotonin-Reuptake Inhibitor

Currently, most patients begin treatment with a SSRI. Four studies to date have examined switching from one SSRI to another and reported response rates of 26% to 74% (46–49); however, 51% of patients responded to a second SSRI in the one study that examined patients who were all resistant to (rather than intolerant of) the initial SSRI (50). Thus, although there are no controlled data to support the value of switching one SSRI for another, this strategy may be useful for some patients. Alternatively, patients switched from a SSRI to a TCA have been shown to have a response rate of 73% in one study (50). Other antidepressants (e.g., bupropion, nefazodone, mirtazapine) have not been well studied in treatment refractory patients; however, they may be effective because they have different mechanisms of action and are reasonably well tolerated (Case 7.3).

CASE 7.3   A successful switch from a selective serotonin-reuptake inhibitor in a young woman

A woman 26 years of age with a 2-year history of depression presented when her treatment provider was moving away. Her symptoms included diminished appetite, decreased concentration, absent libido, frequent tearfulness, and diminished interest. Her first antidepressant trial was with paroxetine at 20 mg/d for approximately 3 months. She stated she had persistent, daily, mild to moderate headaches with this regimen. Her previous physician then switched her to sertraline, which was of mild benefit at 100 mg/d. She was unable to tolerate a dosage greater than 200 mg/d due to a return of the headaches.

> The patient was tapered off the sertraline and begun on a bupropion-sustained release at 150 mg/d for 5 days, followed by an increase to 150 mg twice daily. She was educated as to the possible side effects, and she complied with the treatment despite daily headaches. She began to note improvement in her sleep and cessation of her headaches in the second week. By the fifth week, she described complete resolution of her depressive symptoms.

Switching After a Treatment Failure with a Tricyclic Antidepressant

Several studies have documented the MAOIs to be 50% to 75% effective in patients failing treatment with a TCA (51–54). The SSRIs also have been studied in TCA-resistant patients, with a review noting response in 43% to 51% of patients who switched to either fluoxetine or paroxetine (55). Switching from one TCA to another is less effective, with response rates ranging from 10% to 30% (2).

Venlafaxine

Several studies have suggested that venlafaxine may be useful in TRD (56,57). One study evaluated venlafaxine in patients who had failed to respond to at least three trials of antidepressants from at least two different classes or ECT and to at least one attempt at augmentation. Approximately one third of the 84 patients responded. Venlafaxine may be effective for a significant minority of patients with strictly defined "triple-resistant" depression (58).

Augmentation Strategies

If the patient continues to have only a partial response to a maximal dose of an antidepressant by the 6th to 8th week of treatment, augmentation should be considered. Although monotherapy simplifies the treatment regimen, assists with compliance, and minimizes side effects, augmentation may be rapid, occurring within 48 hours. Additionally, there is little time lost when the second agent is added to the first, and augmentation avoids the symptomatic exacerbation that results from discontinuation of the initial antidepressant when a second antidepressant is started. Depending on the agent, side effects and cost of augmentation strategies may or may not be advantageous (55). A number of augmentation strategies are available, including lithium, thyroid hormone, buspirone, pindolol, and stimulants.

Lithium Augmentation

Lithium has been the best studied and most commonly used augmentation strategy (58,59). A quantitative analysis of four controlled clinical trials in patients with TRD revealed a 40% response rate (60). A double-blind, placebo-controlled trial of lithium augmentation of fluoxetine or lofepramine (a TCA not available in the United States) revealed a 52% response rate (61). Lithium can lead to a significant and clinically sustained reduction in depressive symptoms within approximately 7 days (62). Many patients will respond to as little as 300–600 mg/d; however, to optimize efficacy, lithium should be administered in a dose significant enough to achieve steady-state plasma concentrations of at least 0.7 mEq/L (63). A 3- to 4-week trial is reasonable to determine response (12). Lithium augmentation of a TCA or SSRI is typically well tolerated, although lithium side effects are more severe in the elderly. Note that patients with bipolar depression respond more frequently than do patients with severe unipolar depression. A lack of response is associated with an overall poor prognosis, with subsequent increases in attempted or completed suicide and hospitalization for depression in lithium nonresponders (64).

Thyroid Hormone Augmentation

The efficacy of thyroid hormone augmentation has been established in many open and several placebo-controlled studies. The form of thyroid hormone impacts efficacy, with T_3 being more effective than T_4 (53% vs. 19%) (65). T_3 has been used successfully to augment SSRIs (66), MAOIs (67), and TCAs (2), with response rates approaching 60%. Cytomel (tri-iodothyronine) at a dosage of 25–50 µg/d typically is used. Generally, Cytomel is well tolerated, with close monitoring recommended for signs of thyrotoxicosis, especially in the elderly. There is some long-term risk of osteoporosis with chronic administration of thyroid hormone at supraphysiologic doses. T_3 augmentation also has been successful in hypothyroid patients receiving therapeutic doses of T_4 (68).

Buspirone Augmentation

Buspirone is an anti-anxiety drug that has been studied in open trials as an augmenting agent (69–71). In these studies with patient populations ranging from 3 to 30 patients, buspirone was used to augment mainly SSRIs and, in some cases, imipramine. The response rates ranged from 36% to exceeding 50%. The typical dosage was 30 mg/d with dosages as high as 50 mg/d. A response was usually noted within a 3-week period, and side effects were negligible to minimal (69–71).

Pindolol Augmentation

Pindolol is a beta-blocker typically used as an antihypertensive agent. It has a high affinity for serotonin receptors. Two early studies touted its use for both rapidity of response and treatment of refractory patients (72,73). Three of four controlled trials of pindolol augmentation, with samples ranging from 40 to 111 patients, reported positive results (74–77). However, the results of these studies were based on speed of response, not on use of pindolol in treatment-resistant patients. A double-blind, placebo-controlled study of 10 refractory patients did not find pindolol more effective than placebo for treatment of refractory depression (78). The dosage used in all of the studies was 2.5 mg thrice daily. At this time, the use of pindolol in treatment-resistant patients remains questionable and requires further study with larger populations.

Stimulant Augmentation

Methylphenidate, amphetamines, and pemoline all have been used as augmenting agents. Open studies suggest they are effective as augmentation agents in the treatment of TRD when used with TCAs and SSRIs (79). However, augmentation efficacy of stimulants has not been verified by controlled trials. Additionally, psychostimulants have the potential of being abused, and patients require close monitoring during treatment. A review of uncontrolled and controlled trials of stimulants in primary depression revealed that although the uncontrolled studies were generally positive, all but one of the 10 controlled studies indicated little advantage of stimulant over placebo (80). Stimulants may be of value in special cases, including the medically ill. When used for augmentation, the typical dosages are dextroamphetamine 5 mg twice daily and methylphenidate 10 mg twice daily (56).

Combination Therapy

Selective Serotonin-Reuptake Inhibitors and Tricyclic Antidepressants

There is unlikely to be any value in combining two similar antidepressants, such as two SSRIs or two TCAs. Combined TCA-SSRI therapy has been studied in several open series of 8 to 30 patients with effectiveness approaching 86% (81–83). Note that several of the patients in one series also had failed ECT (82). The rationale behind this combination is that a noradrenergic tricyclic coupled with a serotonergic SSRI might enhance response. Plasma levels of TCAs should be monitored during TCA-SSRI combination therapy as SSRIs can inhibit the hepatic metabolism of TCAs and increase their concentrations three- to fourfold (84). (*See* Chapter 13 for a more in-depth discussion.)

Selective Serotonin-Reuptake Inhibitors and Bupropion

The combination of SSRIs and bupropion has been described in two open studies of 23 and 27 patients (85,86). Both studies recruited patients who had failed treatment with either a SSRI or bupropion alone and then added the second medication. Efficacy ranged from 35% (85) to 70% (86). Adverse reactions were highly variable between the two studies. To date, there are no controlled trials of this combination strategy. Additionally, there is little information about interactions between these medications.

Psychotherapy

Psychotherapy in conjunction with antidepressants has been shown to be a valuable intervention for TRD. As mentioned earlier, it is indicated particularly in patients with comorbid psychiatric illness or social disorders. Psychotherapy in patients with TRD is unlikely to result in a rapid, dramatic recovery; rather, improvement will be measured by degrees over a period of weeks to months. Effective therapy involves the combination of 1) setting achievable, short-term goals; 2) educating patients about coping strategies; and 3) assisting patients to strengthen areas of weakness (87).

Cognitive-behavioral therapy is a short-term therapy that helps the patient to identify and alter negative cognitive distortions that maintain their depressive symptoms. An open trial of cognitive-behavioral treatment to depressed patients who had failed at least two adequate trials of antidepressants documented that 16 of 19 patients improved significantly (88). Sixty-three percent of patients were determined to be in remission at the conclusion of the trial. Although these preliminary results were exciting, they were obtained at the hands of highly trained cognitive therapists. These data suggest that a trial of cognitive-behavioral therapy performed by an experienced therapist seems to be a reasonable option for patients with TRD. Forms of psychotherapy other than cognitive behavioral therapy are discussed in detail in Chapter 6.

Adjunctive Interventions

Additional interventions, although not sufficiently potent enough to be used in isolation to treat TRD, may be effective in conjunction with other modalities. Strategies such as exercise, sleep hygiene, nutrition, support groups, spiritual assistance, and caffeine reduction are useful in certain patients. These interventions are discussed in detail in Chapter 4.

Electroconvulsive Therapy

ECT should be considered as a treatment for patients who have failed antidepressant medication trials, have not tolerated medications, have severe or psychotic symptoms, remain acutely suicidal or homicidal despite other interventions, or have marked symptoms of agitation, catatonia, or stupor. At present, failure to respond to adequate antidepressant trials is the most common indication for ECT. A randomized trial of right unilateral ECT versus paroxetine in patients who had failed at least two antidepressant trials demonstrated that 71% of ECT patients compared with 28% of paroxetine patients responded (89). Response to ECT can be rapid, occurring within 6 to 12 treatments (i.e., 2 to 4 weeks); thus, ECT remains an essential treatment option in TRD.

Transcranial Magnetic Stimulation

Repetitive transcranial magnetic stimulation (rTMS) is a noninvasive technique for directly stimulating cortical neurons; it stimulates the cerebral cortex with magnetic fields generated by rapidly changing currents passing through a wire coil on the scalp (90). Anesthesia and premedication are not required, and there is no cognitive impairment following treatments. In a 5-month, double-blind, placebo-controlled, cross-over design with five different treatment conditions, 11 of 17 patients under 60 years of age who had been diagnosed with psychotic or TRD responded to left prefrontal rTMS (91). An open trial of left prefrontal rTMS in treatment-refractory patients under 64 years of age demonstrated statistically significant improvement in 16 of 28 patients (92). Similarly, our group recently demonstrated significant improvement in 7 of 14 treatment-refractory patients aged 33 to 76 years following 10 daily left prefrontal rTMS treatments (Unpublished data). This is a promising treatment that soon may become available as an option for TRD.

■   ■   ■

Recommendations

In analyzing a patient's medication trials, consider antidepressants as falling into four separate classes: SSRIs, TCAs, MAOIs, and the newer antidepressants (e.g., atypical antidepressants [e.g., bupropion, mirtazapine], 5HT-2 antagonists [e.g., trazadone, nefazadone], venlafaxine).

- Review the treatment trial parameters to ensure adequate dose and duration.

- Reassess the diagnosis and search for possible unrecognized medical illness or comorbid psychiatric illness.

- Optimize the initial trial to include maximal dose and longer duration for partial responders.

- When a patient fails one class of antidepressants, switch to a different class.

- When a patient has a partial response at a maximal dose at weeks 6 to 8, consider augmentation with lithium, T_3, or another antidepressant.

- Following a failure with augmentation or combination therapy, consider ECT.

■   ■   ■

Key Points

- Between 30% and 40% of depressed patients are resistant to antidepressant treatment.

- Patients who have a partial response by week 4 should be continued on antidepressants at incremental doses for at least 4 to 6 weeks. Patients who show no response to an antidepressant trial by week 4 should be switched to another medication.

- Medication education significantly enhances compliance with treatment.

- 35% to 50% of patients with TRD have unrecognized medical conditions. Comorbid psychiatric illness and social problems also should be considered.

- Alternative monotherapy simplifies the medication regimen and reduces the risk of side effects.

- Augmentation strategies and ECT may provide rapid relief but may carry a greater risk of side effects.

■   ■   ■

REFERENCES

1. **Keller MB, Lavori PW, Mueller TI.** Time to recovery, chronicity, and levels of psychopathology in major depression: a five-year prospective follow-up. *Arch Gen Psych.* 1992;49:809–16.

2. **Thase ME, Rush AJ.** In Bloom SE, Kipfer DJ (eds). *Psychopharmacology: The Fourth Generation of Progress.* New York: Raven Press; 1995:1081–97.

3. **Thase ME, Rush AJ, Kasper S, Nemeroff CB.** Tricyclics and newer antidepressant mediations: treatment options for treatment-resistant depression. *Depression.* 1995;2:152–68.

4. **O'Reardon JP, Amsterdam JD.** Treatment-resistant depression: progress and limitations. *Psychiatr Ann.* 1998;28:633–40.

5. **Nierenberg A, Keck PJ, Samsom J.** Methodological considerations for the study of treatment-resistant depression. In Amsterdam J (ed). *Advances in Neuropsychiatry and Psychopharmacology,* vol. 2. New York: Raven Press; 1991.

6. **Katon W, Von Korff M, Lin E, Bush T, Ormel J.** Adequacy and duration of antidepressant treatment in primary care. *Med Care.* 1992;30:67–76.

7. **Nelsen MR, Dunner DL.** Clinical and differential diagnostic aspects of treatment-resistant depression. *J Psychiatr Res.* 1995;29:43–50.

8. **Depression Guideline Panel.** *Depression in Primary Care, Volume 2: Treatment of Major Depression. Clinical Practice Guideline, Number 5.* Rockville, MD: U.S. Department of Health and Human Services, Public Health Service, Agency for Health Care Policy and Research [AHCPR Pub. no. 93-0551]; April 1993.

9. **Quitkin FM, McGrath PJ, Stewart JW.** Chronological milestones to guide drug changes: When should clinicians switch antidepressants? *Arch Gen Psychiatry.* 1996;53:785–92.

10. **Mueller J, Keller M, Leon A, et al.** Recovery after five years of unremitting major depressive disorder. *Arch Gen Psychiatry.* 1996;53:794–9.

11. **Amsterdam JD, Brunsuick DJ, Mendels J.** The clinical application of tricyclic antidepressant pharmacokinetics and plasma levels. *Am J Psychiatry.* 1980;137:653–62.

12. **Nemeroff C.** Augmentation strategies in patients with refractory depression. *Depression Anxiety.* 1996–7;4:169-81.

13. **Thase ME, Rush AJ.** When at first you don't succeed: sequential strategies for antidepressant nonresponders. *J Clin Psychiatry.* 1997;58:23–9.

14. **Altamura A, Montgomery S, Wernicke J.** The evidence for 20 mg a day of fluoxetine as the optimal in treatment of depression. *Br J Psychiatry.* 1988;153:109–12.

15. **Fabre LF, Abuzzahab FS, Amin M.** Sertraline safety and efficacy in major depression: a double-blind, fixed-dose, comparison with placebo. *Biol Psychiatry.* 1995; 38:592–602.

16. **Dunner DL, Dunbar GC.** Optimal dose regimen for paroxetine. *J Clin Psychiatry.* 1992;53:21–6.

17. **Entsuah AR, Rudolph R, Chitra R.** Effectiveness of venlafaxine treatment in a broad spectrum of depressed patients: a meta-analysis. *Psychopharmacol Bull.* 1995;31:759–66.

18. **Fava M, Rosenbaum JF, Grossbard SJ.** Lithium and tricyclic augmentation of fluoxetine treatment for resistant major depression: a double-blind, controlled study. *Am J Psychiatry.* 1994;151:1372–4.

19. **Quitkin F.** The importance of dosing in prescribing antidepressants. *Br J Psychiatry.* 1985;147:593–7.

20. **Henry JA, Hale AS.** Selective serotonin-reuptake inhibitors: unsuccessful treatment may be related to nonresponse or noncompliance. *Br Med J.* 1994;309:1083.

21. **Lin EHB, Von Korff M, Katon W, et al.** The role of the primary care physician in patients' adherence to antidepressant therapy. *Med Care.* 1995;33:67–74.

22. **Berman RM, Narasimhan M, Charney DS.** Treatment-refractory depression: definitions and characteristics. *Depression Anxiety.* 1997;5:154–64.

23. **Kaplan R.** Obstructive sleep apnea and depression: diagnostic and treatment implications. *Aust N Z J Psychiatry.* 1992;26:586–91.

24. **Green AI, Austin CP.** Psychopathology of pancreatic cancer: a psychobiologic probe. *Psychosomatics.* 1993;34:208–11.

25. **Howland RH.** Thyroid dysfunction in refractory depression: implications for pathophysiology and treatment. *J Clin Psychiatry.* 1993;54:47–54.

26. **Gadde KM, Ranga K, Krishnan R.** Endocrine factors in depression. *Psychiatr Ann.* 1994;10:521–4.

27. **Kessler RC, Nelson CB, McGonagle KA.** Comorbidity of DSM-III-R major depressive disorder in the general population: results from the U.S. National Comorbidity Survey. *Br J Psychiatry.* 1996;30:17–30.

28. **Coryell W, Endicott J, Andreasen N, et al.** Depression and panic attacks: the significance of overlap as reflected in follow-up and family study data. *Am J Psychiatry.* 1988;145:293–300.

29. **Charney D, Miller H, Licinio J, Salomon R.** Treatment of depression. In Nemeroff C (ed). *Textbook of Psychopharmacology.* Washington, DC: APA Press; 1994:575–602.

30. **Castaneda R, Sussman N, Westreich L, et al.** A review of the effects of moderate alcohol intake on the treatment of anxiety and mood disorders. *J Clin Psychiatry.* 1996;57:207–12.

31. **Ciravolo DA, Barnhill JG, Jaffe JH.** Clinical pharmacokinetics of imipramine and desipramine in alcoholics and normal volunteers. *Clin Pharmacol Ther.* 1998;43: 535–8.

32. **Mason BJ, Kocsis MD.** Desipramine treatment of alcoholism. *Psychopharmacol Bull.* 1991;27:155–61.

33. **Fava M, Bouffides E, Pava J.** Personality disorder comorbidity with major depression and response to fluoxetine treatment. *Psychother Psychosom.* 1994;62:160–7.

34. **Ilardi S, Craighead W.** Personality pathology and response to somatic treatments for major depression: a critical review. *Depression.* 1994/5;2:200–17.

35. **Nelsen MR, Dunner DL.** Treatment resistance in unipolar depression and other disorders: diagnostic concerns and treatment possibilities. *Psychiatr Clin North Am.* 1993;16:541–66.

36. **Janicak P, Pandey G, Davis J.** Response of psychiatric and nonpsychiatric depression to phenelzine. *Am J Psychiatry.* 1988;145:93–5.

37. **Spiker D, Weiss J, Dealy R.** The pharmacologic treatment of psychotic depression. *Am J Psychiatry.* 1985;142:430–36.

38. **Quitkin F.** Response to phenelzine and imipramine in placebo nonresponders with atypical depression. *Arch Gen Psychiatry.* 1991;48:319–23.

39. **McGrath P, Stewart J, Harrison W.** Predictive value of symptoms of atypical depression for differential drug treatment outcome. *J Clin Psychopharmacol.* 1992;12: 197–202.

40. **Quitkin FM, Stewart JW, McGrath PJ.** A subgroup of depressives with better response to MAOI than to tricyclic antidepressants or placebo. *Br J Psychiatry.* 1993;163:30–4.

41. **Pande AC, Birkett M, Fechner-Bates S.** Fluoxetine versus phenelzine in atypical depression. *Biol Psychiatry.* 1996;40:1017–20.

42. **Kravchi K, Wirz-Justice W, Graw P.** High intake of sweets late in the day predicts a rapid and persistent response to light therapy in winter depression. *Psychiatry Res.* 1993;46:107–17.

43. **Lam R.** Morning light therapy for winter depression: predictors of response. *Acta Psychiatr Scand.* 1994;89:97–101.

44. **Oren D, Jacobsen F, Wehr T.** Predictors of response to phototherapy in seasonal affective disorder. *Compr Psychiatry.* 1992;33:111–4.

45. **Terman M, Amira L, Terman J.** Predictors of response and nonresponse to light treatment for winter depression. *Am J Psychiatry.* 1996;153:1423–29.

46. **Bronn WA, Harrison W.** Are patients who are intolerant to one SSRI intolerant to another? *Psychopharmacol Bull.* 1992;28:253–6.

47. **Zarate CA, Kando JC, Tohen M, et al.** Does intolerance or lack of response with fluoxetine predict the same will happen with sertraline? *J Clin Psychiatry.* 1996; 57:71.

48. **Apter JT, Thase ME, Birkett M.** *Fluoxetine Treatment in Depressed Patients Who Failed Treatment with Sertraline.* Montego Bay, Jamaica: American Society of Clinical Psychopharmacology Presidents' Day Educational Program; Feb 1986 .

49. **Joffe RT, Levitt AJU, Sokolov STH.** Response to an open trail of a second SSRI in major depression. *J Clin Psychiatry.* 1996;57:114–5.

50. **Peslow ED, Fillippi AM, Goodnick P.** The short- and long-term efficacy of paroxetine HCl: data from a double-blind crossover and from a year long trial vs. imipramine and placebo. *Psychopharmacol Bull.* 1989;25:272–6.

51. **Nolen WA, van de Putte JJ, Dijken WA, et al.** Treatment strategy in depression II: MAO inhibitors in depression resistant to cyclic antidepressants. *Acta Psychiatr Scand.* 1988;78:676–83.

52. **McGrath PJ, Stewart JW, Harrison W, Quitkin FM.** Treatment of tricyclic refractory depression with a monoamine oxidase inhibitor antidepressant. *Psychopharmacol Bull.* 1987;23:169–72.

53. **Thase ME, Melinger AG, McKnight D.** Treatment of imipramine-resistant recurrent depression. Part IV: A double-blind crossover study of tranylcypromine for anergic bipolar depression. *Am J Psychiatry.* 1992;149:195–8.

54. **Nolen WA, Haffmans PMJ, Bonvy PF, Duivenvoorden HJ.** Monoamine oxidase inhibitors in resistant major depression: a double-blind comparison of brofaromine and tranylcypromine in patients resistant to tricyclic antidepressants. *J Affect Disord.* 1993;28:189–97.

55. **Nelson JC.** Overcoming resistance in depression. *J Clin Psychiatry.* 1998;59:13–9.

56. **Nirenberg AA, Feighner JP, Rudolph R, et al.** Venlafaxine for treatment-resistant unipolar depression. *J Clin Psychopharmacol.* 1994;14:419–23.

57. **De Montigny C, Debonnel G, Bergerm R.** *Venlafaxine in Treatment-Resistant Depression: A de Gen-label Multicenter Study.* San Juan, Puerto Rico: 34th annual meeting of the American College of Neuropharmacology; Dec 11, 1995.

58. **Nierenberg AA.** Treatment choice after one antidepressant fails: a survey of Northeastern psychiatrists. *J Clin Psychiatry.* 1991;52:383–5. .

59. **de Montigny C.** Lithium addition in treatment-resistant depression. *Int Clin Psychopharmacol.* 1994;9:31–5.

60. **Austin MPV, Sinza FGM, Goodwin GM.** Lithium augmentation in antidepressant-resistant patients: a quantitative analysis. *Br J Psychiatry.* 1991;159:510–4.

61. **Katona CLE, Abou-Saleh MT, Harrison DA, et al.** Placebo-controlled trial of lithium augmentation of fluoxetine and lofepramine. *Br J Psychiatry.* 1995;165:80–6.

62. **Dinan TG.** Lithium augmentation in sertraline-resistant depression: a preliminary dose-response study. *Acta Psychiatr Scand.* 1993;88:300–1.

63. **Stein G, Bernadt M.** Lithium augmentation therapy in tricyclic-resistant depression: a controlled trail using lithium in low and normal doses. *Br J Psychiatry.* 1993;162:634–40.

64. **Nierenberg AA, Price LH, Charney DS, Hemhger GR.** After lithium augmentation: a retrospective follow-up of patients with antidepressant-refractory depression. *J Affect Disord.* 1990;18:167–75.

65. **Joffe RT, Singer W, Levitt AJ, MacDonald C.** A placebo-controlled comparison of lithium and triiodothyronine augmentation of tricyclic antidepressants in unipolar refractory depression. *Arch Gen Psychiatry.* 1993;50:387–93.

66. **Joffe RT.** Triiodothyronine potentiation of fluoxetine in depressed patients. *Psychoneuroendocrinology.* 1992;17:215–21.

67. **Joffe RT.** Tri-iodothyronine potentiation of the antidepressant effect of phenelzine. *J Clin Psychiatry.* 1988;49:409–10.

68. **Cooke RG, Joffe RT, Levitt AJ.** T_3 augmentation of antidepressant treatment in T_4-replaced thyroid patients. *J Clin Psychiatry.* 1992;53:16–8.

69. **Jacobsen FM.** Possible augmentation of antidepressant response by buspirone. *J Clin Psychiatry.* 1991;52:217–20.

70. **Bakish D.** Fluoxenine potentiation by buspirone: three case histories. *Can J Psychiatry.* 1991;36:749–50.

71. **Joffe RT, Schwller DR.** An open study of buspirone augmentation of serotonin reuptake inhibitors in refractory depression. *J Clin Psychiatry.* 1993;54:269–71.

72. **Artigas F, Perez V, Alvarez E.** Pindolol induces a rapid improvement of depressed patients treated with serotonin-reuptake inhibitors. *Arch Gen Psychiatry.* 1994;51:248–51.

73. **Blier P, Bereron R.** Effectiveness of pindolol with selected antidepressant drugs in the treatment of major depression. *J Clin Psychopharmacology.* 1995;15:217–22.

74. **Berman RM, Darnell AM, Miller HL, et al.** Effect of pindolol in hastening response to fluoxetine in the treatment of major depression: a double-blind, placebo-controlled trial. *Am J Psychiatry.* 1997;154:37–43.

75. **Tome MB, Isaac MT, Harte R, Holland C.** Paroxetine and pindolol: a randomized trial of serotonergic autoreceptor blockade in the reduction of antidepressant latency. *Int Clin Psychopharmacol.* 1997;12:81–9.

76. **Perez V, Gilberte I, Faries D, et al.** Randomized, double-blind, placebo-controlled trial of pindolol in combination with fluoxetine antidepressant treatment. *Lancet.* 1997;349:1594–7.

77. **Zanardi R, Artigas F, Franchini L.** How long should pindolol be associated with paroxetine to improve the antidepressant response? *J Clin Psychopharmacol.* 1997;17:446–50.

78. **Moreno FA, Gilenberg AJ, Bachar K.** Pindolol augmentation of treatment-resistant depressed patients. *J Clin Psychiatry.* 1997;58:437–9.

79. **Stoll AL, Srinivasan SP, Diamond L, et al.** Methylphenidate augmentation of serotonin selective reuptake inhibitors: a case series. *J Clin Psychiatry.* 1996;57:72–6.

80. **Satel SL, Nelson JC.** Stimulants in the treatment of depression: a critical interview. *J Clin Psychiatry.* 1989;50:241–9.

81. **Nelson JC, Mazure CM, Boners MB, Jatlon PI.** A preliminary, open study of the combination of fluoxetine and desipramine for rapid treatment of major depression. *Arch Gen Psychiatry.* 1991;48:303–7.

82. **Seth R, Jennings AL, Bindman J, et al.** Combination treatment with noradrenalin and serotonin-reuptake inhibitors in resistant depression. *Br J Psychiatry.* 1992;161:562–5.

83. **Weiburg JB, Rosenbaum JF, Biederman J.** Fluoxetine added to non-MAOI antidepresssants converts nonresponders to responders: a preliminary report. *J Clin Pstchiatry.* 1989;50:447–9.

84. **Nemeroff CB, DeVance CL, Pollock BG.** Newer antidepressants and the cytochrome P450 system. *Am J Psychiatry.* 1996:153:311–20.

85. **Bodkin JA, Lasser RA, Wines JD, et al.** Combining serotonin-reuptake inhibitors and buproprion in partial responders to antidepressant monotherapy. *J Clin Psychiatry.* 1997;58:137-45.

86. **Boyer WF, Feighner JP.** *The Combined Use of Fluoxetine and Buproprion.* San Francisco: 146th annual meeting of the American Psychiatric Association; May 27, 1993.

87. **Thase ME.** Psychotherapy of refractory depressions. *Depression Anxiety.* 1997;5: 190–201.

88. **Fava GA, Savron G, Grandi S, Rafanelli C.** Cognitive-behavioral management of drug-resistant major depressive disorder. *J Clin Psychiatry.* 1997;58:278–82.

89. **Folkerts HW, Michael N, Jolle R, et al.** Electroconvulsive therapy vs. paroxetine in treatment-resistant depression: a randomized study. *Acta Psychiatr Scand.* 1997; 96:334–42.

90. **George MS, Wassermann EM, Post RM.** Transcranial magnetic stimulation: a neuropsychiatric tool for the 21st century. *J Neuropsychiatr Clin Neurosci.* 1996;8: 373–82.

91. **Pascual-Leone A, Rubio B, Pallardo F, Catala MD.** Rapid-rate transcranial magnetic stimulation of left dorsolateral prefrontal cortex in drug-resistant depression. *Lancet.* 1996;348:233–7.

92. **Epstein CM, Figiel GS, McDonald WM, et al.** Rapid-rate transcranial magnetics stimulation in young and middle-aged refractorally depressed patients. *Psychiatr Ann.* 1998;28:36–9.

KEY REFERENCES

Berman RM, Narasimhan M, Charney DS. Treatment-refractory depression: definitions and characteristics. *Depression Anxiety.* 1997;5:154–64.

The authors review the definition and characteristics of treatment-resistant depression. They describe a methodical approach to evaluating such patients.

O'Reardon JP, Amsterdam JD. Treatment-resistant depression: progress and limitations. *Psychiatr Ann.* 1998;28:633–40.

The authors define treatment-resistant depression versus pseudo–treatment-resistant depression. In addition, they touch on approaches for optimizing treatment and minimizing resistance.

8

∎ ∎ ∎

Late-Life Depression

Christopher C. Colenda, MD, MPH

Lon S. Schneider, MD

Ira R. Katz, MD, PhD

George S. Alexopoulos, MD

Charles F. Reynolds III, MD

onsiderable progress has been made in understanding the diagnosis and treatment of late-life depression. The National Institutes of Health (NIH) held the Consensus Development Conference on Late-Life Depression in 1991 (1). The Consensus Update Conference on the Diagnosis and Treatment of Late-Life Depression was convened by the American Association for Geriatric Psychiatry in 1996 (2). Both conferences summarized the scientific and therapeutic advances for late-life depression that have occurred over the last two decades, underscoring the public health importance of depression late in life.

Late-life depression is a serious illness that is widespread, affecting nearly five million of the 31 million U.S. citizens over 65 years of age, one million of whom suffer from major depression (3). Late-life depression is not part of normal aging, has a chronic and recurrent clinical course, and most importantly is strongly associated with medical comorbidity (3). Failure to recognize depression can lead to serious consequences, such as increased risk of suicide, worsening physical health and cognitive performance, poor compliance with medical treatment, increased use of health care, and diminished quality of life. Despite these consequences, late-life depression remains underdiagnosed in general medical settings, and, when detected, treatments are often not optimal (4).

169

Successful treatment of late-life depression has favorable outcomes for patients and their families and creates significant personal and professional satisfaction. This chapter provides current information about the diagnosis and management of late-life depression.

Clinical and Epidemiologic Overview

Depressive disorders late in life are not a normal reaction to life's uncertainties and troublesome events. They are illnesses that represent a significant and persistent change in an older person's mood that impacts function and quality of life. From a practicing clinician's viewpoint, late-life depression has two primary expressions: major depression and clinically significant minor depression (1,5). Although it is the most serious of the depressive disorders, major depression is the least frequent of the clinically significant late-life depressions. In its fullest form, major depression is a recurrent and life-threatening illness.

The symptoms of clinically significant minor depression (e.g., dysthymia, adjustment disorders) are less severe; nevertheless, they are associated with functional deterioration, excess disability, and increased risk for major depression. Minor late-life depressive disorders are more prevalent, especially in ambulatory settings, and are often accompanied by anxiety symptoms.

Left untreated, late-life depressive disorders have a number of adverse outcomes. Depression in geriatric patients increases disability, functional impairment, and quality of life (6,7). Geriatric patients with minor depression have increased service use and health care costs, have a higher likelihood of developing major depression, and experience greater disability with or without medical comorbidity (5,8). Older adults with late-life depression have increased mortality from both suicide and medical illness. In fact, men over 65 years of age are much more likely to commit suicide than their female counterparts, and elderly white men have the highest suicide rate among all elders (43.7 deaths per 100,000 population) (9). Increased mortality rates also have been found in depressed myocardial infarction patients and among nursing home residents (10,11).

The measured rates of late-life depression depend on the definitions used to classify depression, the populations studied, and the settings in which rates are measured. Figure 8.1 summarizes the prevalence rate data by setting and illness severity (major and minor depressions). Generally speaking, community-based studies consistently find between 15% to 20% of the elderly have symptoms of depression with rates of major depression usually less than 4% (12). Both prevalence and incidence rates of depression are higher in women than in men, particularly for the minor depressions. Epidemiologic studies have failed to resolve the question of whether the incidence of depression increases with age (13).

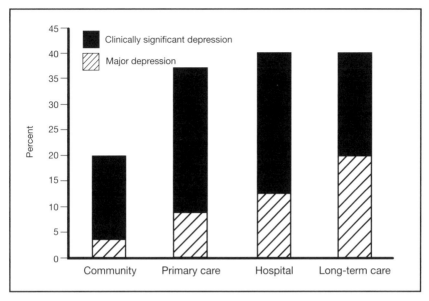

Figure 8.1   Prevalence of late-life depression.

Depression is more common in clinical settings. The prevalence of clinical depression in geriatric primary care practices ranges between 14% and 37%, a higher proportion of which are minor depressions (13). In one recent study, the prevalence of major depression in geriatric primary care settings was approximately 9% (14). In nursing homes and other residential living facilities, major depression has been found in approximately 20% of cognitively intact residents, and clinically significant depression has been observed in over 40% of residents (15). Hospitalized geriatric patients have considerable rates of depression, ranging between 11% and 59% depending on the methodology and instruments used to ascertain cases (16–19). More recent studies in hospitalized medically ill elderly that used more stringent criteria have shown a rate of depression at approximately 35% to 40%, with a ratio of major to minor depression of approximately 1 to 2 (18,19).

Diagnostic Strategies in Late-Life Depression: Problems and Prospects

Recognition of late-life depression by physicians can be challenging for the following reasons:

1. Older patients may not express verbally their depressed ideation, and many of the typical symptoms of depression (e.g., anhedo-

nia, fatigue, somatization, appetite disturbances) could be attributed reasonably to comorbid medical syndromes (20).

2. Psychiatric comorbidity (e.g., anxiety disorders) or dementia syndromes (e.g., Alzheimer's disease, vascular dementia) may have overlapping signs and symptoms that can confound the diagnosis (21).

3. The temporal course of a patient's signs and symptoms for depression become an important criterion when making a diagnosis of depression in late life. Transient symptoms of depression can occur in response to psychosocial stressors, such as a move to a new environment, but remit quickly after the individual adjusts to the new environment. Thus, depending on when the patient was evaluated, false-positive (or in some cases, false-negative) diagnoses could be given to older patients. Although it is important to recognize the risk of "medicalizing" normal reactions to real-life problems, the greater risk may be in failing to recognize and treat clinically significant depressions because they occur in difficult life contexts.

4. The search for biological markers for depression has failed to find any that are sufficiently practical, sensitive, or specific (20). This approach is not as applicable to late-life depression as most nonpsychiatric medical conditions, because physicians tend to use deductive reasoning that connects signs and symptoms with biological markers to arrive at a diagnosis.

Inclusive and Exclusive Diagnostic Approaches

In general, physicians can improve their diagnostic accuracy by actively trying to distinguish those symptoms that could be attributable to general medical conditions from those that could be ascribed to a mood disorder. In ambiguous cases, an "inclusive" approach—in which symptoms are counted toward the diagnosis without consideration of medical causes—increases the sensitivity of making a diagnosis. Conversely, an "exclusive" approach—in which potentially ambiguous symptoms are not considered—can optimize specificity and minimize false-positives in diagnoses. This approach leads to a greater degree of unrecognized depression. The diagnostic strategy that is most appropriate will vary with the clinical context of the patient's presentation. For example, in the research setting, it is important to use the exclusive approach, which maximizes specificity; in the clinical setting, it is more important to err on the side of providing a diagnosis and treatment. Case 8.1 illustrates the differences between an exclusive and an inclusive approach to making a depression diagnosis in a geriatric patient.

CASE 8.1 *Approaches to diagnosis of depression in a hospitalized elderly patient*

A woman 79 years of age who was recently transferred from orthopedic surgery to rehabilitation medicine has not progressed after hip fracture repair as expected. She continually complains of "excruciating" pain at her surgical site, refuses to participate in physical therapy, and has been demanding with the nursing staff. Nurses report that they are able to change her dressing, perform passive range of motion of her leg, and assist her to the toilet without complaint. The patient has several medical conditions, including chronic obstructive pulmonary disease, hypertension, chronic anxiety, and osteoporosis. A psychiatric consultation was requested after the patient overturned her dinner tray, threw milk at the nurse, and became increasingly tachypneic.

On examination, the patient was lying in bed, staring out the window, and in no obvious respiratory distress. When she became aware of the examiner, her respiration rate increased precipitously. Conversation was difficult to initiate, and there was marked poverty of speech. The patient seemed withdrawn and sullen. She expressed distrust and dislike of her rehabilitation treatment team. The patient reported relatively normal appetite but was not sleeping well in the hospital. She admitted feeling restless but denied feeling depressed, "blue," or hopeless. She stated that she felt helpless because she could not walk. She denied feelings of guilt or suicidal ideation but asserted that she was indifferent about the future and looked forward to "seeing her mother again." She reported her mood as being angry. She denied problems with her memory or concentration, and a cognitive screening examination was normal. Her daughter reported that she has been "difficult to deal with as she has gotten older." The daughter reported few signs of depression in her mother before hospitalization 4 weeks ago.

Using the inclusive approach to classify her signs and symptoms, the likelihood of classifying the patient as depressed increases. The excessive pain complaints, angry mood, insomnia, helplessness, irritability, and withdrawal all may be manifestations of depression. A more exclusive approach to the patient's presentation—underscoring the lack of some classic signs and symptoms of depression (e.g., sadness, guilt, hopelessness, appetite disturbance, suicidal ideation) and emphasizing long-standing difficulties—might decrease the likelihood of classifying the patient as depressed. In primary care settings, an inclusive approach is recommended, because failing to detect and treat depression may lead to poor patient outcomes.

Clinical Signs and Symptoms

The clinical signs and symptoms that suggest a diagnosis of depression in geriatric patients are summarized in Table 8.1. Because there is a strong relationship between late-life depression and medical comorbidity, many of these signs and symptoms are similar to those found in depressed medically ill patients, regardless of age. It is important to remember, however, that any combination of signs and symptoms should obligate the clinician to investigate further.

A key symptom of late-life depression is memory complaint. (The association between depression and memory disorders in geriatrics is discussed in more detail later in this chapter.) Because between 18% and 57% of depressed elderly patients present with cognitive impairment that improves with treatment (21,22), it is strongly recommended that any geriatric patient who presents with memory complaints should be evaluated for depression.

Interviewing Strategies

Physicians may wish to frame their inquiry about depression differently with geriatric patients. Elderly depressed patients may not express verbally the typical feelings of sadness or dysphoria. Thus, physicians must be sensitive to atypical presentations of late-life depression in which the predominant symptom may be self-neglect, social withdrawal, anhedonia, pain, cognitive impairment, increased somatization, or hopelessness (23). The persistence of negative emotional responses after an adverse life event is an important signal for physicians to inquire about depression.

Physicians also should be aware of how their personal attitudes and expectations toward aging can influence their ability to detect late-life depression. For example, the prevalence of comorbid medical illness with late-life depression may provide legitimacy to many of the symptoms that are found in depression. This relationship contributes to the false assumption that the geriatric patient has a "good reason" for the depressive symptoms. This can lead to misjudgments about the diagnosis and worthiness of treatment. Additionally, geriatric patients in primary care practices are time consuming, and physicians may not feel they have adequate time to assess and treat elderly patients with depression. Physicians may not be oriented toward or confident in providing the psychosocially based care that is required for the successful treatment of late-life depression (24). These types of concerns have increased under the practice-management pressures generated by managed care, e.g., evaluating more patients in less time. Making a diagnosis of depression in a geriatric patient takes time and patience.

Screening Instruments

Depression screening instruments in geriatric patient populations are strongly recommended. Screening instruments are best used in those patients with specific risk factors for depression (e.g., recent losses, medical illnesses) or to help determine whether patients with unclear clinical signs or symptoms have clinically significant depression.

Table 8.1   Clinical Signs and Symptoms That Should Increase Index of Suspicion for Late-Life Depression

Category	Symptoms
Constitutional symptoms	Vague somatic complaints
	Diffuse pain or focal pain out of proportion to underlying diseases
	Disability out of proportion to severity of underlying diseases
Cognitive symptoms	Memory complaints with impairment of the following cognitive tasks:
	Attention
	Free recall
	Spontaneous elaboration of detail
	Word fluency and syntactic complexity
Health service use	High use of scheduled and unscheduled medical care
	Frequent calls
	Poor compliance with medical treatments
	Refusal of treatments
Psychiatric and behavioral signs	Hopelessness
	Helplessness (especially out of proportion to physical disability)
	Suicidal ideation
	Prolonged grief
	New-onset delusional symptoms
	Anxiety
Clues for residents in long-term care facilities	"Failure to thrive" (apathy, withdrawal, isolation)
	Agitation
	Prolonged rehabilitation
	Unexplained weight loss or malnutrition

Two screening instruments have established performance for late-life depression: the Geriatric Depression Scale (GDS) (25) and the Center for

Epidemiological Studies Depression Scale (CES-D) (26–28). The original CES-D consists of 20 items with five-point responses, and the GDS consists of 30 yes-or-no questions. Both were designed initially as paper-and-pencil, self-report scales, but they are also valid when verbally administered to older patients. Both scales have been validated for use in those with mild to moderate degrees of cognitive impairment, and the GDS remains valid when administered over the telephone (29).

Because of the ease of administration of the GDS (yes-or-no format), the psychometric performance of shorter versions has been explored recently (30,31). In one study, the GDS-10 item scale had a sensitivity of 88% and specificity of 75% for major depression; whereas the GDS-4 item scale (Table 8.2) had a sensitivity of 72%, a specificity of 90%, and a positive predictive value of 86% (30). In this same study, a positive response to the question "Do you often feel helpless?" had a sensitivity of 76% and specificity of 75%.

Therapeutic Approaches

The treatment of depression in elderly patients should be differentiated into acute, continuation, and maintenance phases. Treatment goals vary for each phase. In the acute treatment phase, the primary goal is to achieve symptom remission. Once the patient has improved symptomatically, treatment in the continuation phase attempts to prevent early relapse. The goals of maintenance treatment involve sustaining recovery, preventing recurrences, optimizing quality of life, enhancing functional capacity, and improving general medical health status.

Table 8.2   Four-Item Geriatric Depression Rating Scale (GDS-4)

Question	Response	Interpretation of Response
Are you basically satisfied with your life?	Yes/No	If answer is no, score 1 point
Do you feel that your life is empty?	Yes/No	If answer is yes, score 1 point
Are you afraid that something bad is going to happen to you?	Yes/No	If answer is yes, score 1 point
Do you feel happy most of the time?	Yes/No	If answer is no, score 1 point

Republished with permission from Shah A, Herbert R, Lewis S, et al. Screening for depression among acutely ill geriatric inpatients with a short geriatric depression scale. *Age Ageing.* 1997;26:217–21.

Antidepressant Use: Special Considerations

Research generally confirms that antidepressants with proven efficacy in younger populations are likely to be successful when extended to the elderly. The following factors increase the complexity of choosing antidepressants for the elderly and exert greater influences than age itself on antidepressant treatments in elderly patients.

Polypharmacy

The foremost issue in antidepressant treatment for late-life depression is polypharmacy. Elderly patients use more medications than younger patients, with further increases with increasing age (32). The average individual over 65 years of age uses between two and six prescribed medications and between one and three nonprescribed medications (32). Nursing home residents are prescribed an average of 7 to 8 medications, at least one of which is a psychotropic medication (33,34).

The consequences of polypharmacy are numerous. Drug interactions that lead to adverse reactions are frequent in older patients (35). Polypharmacy also leads to higher noncompliance rates, doubling for patients over 65 years of age when more than three drugs are prescribed (a statistic not found in patients under 65) (36). Polypharmacy leads to high total medication costs that can influence how patients purchase and comply with their medication schedule, especially for those on fixed incomes (37,38). Because newer antidepressants are relatively more expensive, patients may not follow directions, may try to "stretch out" the prescription, or, worse, may not fill the prescription at all. This could lead to suboptimal treatment response and the misperception that the patient is a nonresponder or treatment resistant.

To reduce polypharmacy in the elderly, clinicians are recommended to review an older patient's medication profile (prescribed and over-the-counter) continually. When an antidepressant is required, physicians should use simple dosing strategies and choose dose timing that minimizes medication side effects (39). For more information on drug interactions, *see* Chapter 13.

Age and Antidepressant Pharmacokinetics

In the absence of gastrointestinal pathology, there is no evidence of any clinically significant changes in absorption of antidepressants with normal aging (40). However, gastrointestinal disease or drugs (e.g., antacids, anticholinergic drugs) may alter the absorption of antidepressants through changes in gastric pH levels, intestinal motility, intestinal surface area, or blood flow. Once a medication is absorbed, first-pass metabolism is slowed because hepatic blood flow decreases with age (35).

The liver constitutes the principal site for metabolic transformation of all psychotropic medications, except lithium. Phase I oxidative metabolic pathways, hydrolysis, oxidation, and reduction are part of the cytochrome P450 enzyme system (CP450) (41). Because antidepressants are substrates and inhibitors of the CP450 enzyme systems, potential drug interactions can occur, examples of which are discussed below (42). Phase II metabolism consists of conjugation, which produces inactive water soluble forms (glucuronides) that are generally cleared through the kidney (41).

Age may slow Phase I pathways, thus increasing the plasma concentration of antidepressants, particularly tricyclic antidepressants (TCAs) (35,40). Drug interactions involving Phase I pathways, detailed in Chapter 13, may be especially important in older patients, but there has been little research examining the extent of the possible differences with age (43,44). Phase II metabolism is less affected by age but can be slowed by disease states such as liver failure or severe heart failure, thus effectively changing the clearance rate of antidepressant medications (35,40). The increased proportion of body fat to water with age increases the volume distribution of lipid-soluble medications in the elderly (40). The increased volume of distribution can prolong the half-lives of lipid-soluble medications, such as antidepressants.

Age and/or disease may affect TCA blood levels. TCAs are bound primarily in plasma to the acute phase reactant protein alpha-1-acid glycoprotein (α1-AGP). Although increasing age tends to decrease serum albumin levels, age alone has had inconsistent effects on αl-AGP (increased in some studies and decreased in others) (45,46). Many acute and chronic diseases (e.g., sepsis, cancer, myocardial infarction, arthritis) can increase α1-AGP levels, whereas malnutrition decreases the concentration of α1-AGP (46,47). Changes in concentration of α1-AGP will influence TCA blood levels, which measure the total of free and protein-bound drug.

Excretion of antidepressants, mainly in their hydrophilic forms, can be altered by changes in renal glomerular filtration rate (GFR). Advancing age, medications, and common diseases such as hypertension or diabetes affect GFR. Thus, accumulation of hydrophilic metabolites may occur in some elderly patients, which may be problematic for the water-soluble metabolites of TCAs that affect cardiac conduction (e.g., the 11-hydroxy-nortriptyline metabolite of nortriptyline) (40).

Pharmacodynamic Characteristics of Antidepressants Given in Late Life
Pharmacodynamic actions of antidepressants given in late life have not been well studied. Few studies have examined the question of whether the elderly have a narrower range between therapeutic and toxic concentrations of antidepressants. There is evidence about efficacy: older patients respond to plasma concentrations that are comparable with younger adults for the secondary amine TCAs nortriptyline and desipramine (46–48).

The major concern about pharmacodynamic actions of antidepressants in the elderly is their vulnerability to side effects secondary to changes in the central nervous system, drug interactions, and the impact of comorbid medical illnesses on drug action (35,40,41). Most of the concern has focused on the TCAs, but SSRIs and other antidepressants are not without problems. For purposes of this review, we confine our discussion to three important pharmacodynamic concerns in geriatric patients.

ANTICHOLINERGIC AND ANTIHISTAMINIC EFFECTS

The anticholinergic and antihistaminic effects of TCAs have pharmacodynamic actions that are more pronounced in geriatric patients (35). Because there are fewer neurons in the cerebral cortex, locus ceruleus, and the hippocampus, the elderly may be more susceptible to antihistaminic sedative side effects of TCAs. Reduced cholinergic activity in the central nervous system may increase the risk of confusion and cognitive slowing in older patients receiving TCAs, especially those with pre-existing memory impairment (35,40). Because of changes in peripheral cholinergic activity, older patients are more sensitive to the peripheral anticholinergic side effects of TCAs. This can lead to constipation, ileus, urinary retention, and dry mouth (which can cause serious dental problems in older patients) (51). Prescription of a TCA may acutely worsen symptoms of prostatism.

CARDIOVASCULAR EFFECTS

The TCAs have numerous cardiovascular side effects (most significantly type I anti-arrhythmic properties), may exacerbate pre-existing conduction disease, and have α-1-adrenergic activity (which can cause orthostatic hypotension) (52,53). Plasma concentrations of TCAs and their hydroxylated metabolites are associated positively with cardiac side effects (57,58). In those elderly patients with pre-existing cardiac disease, these effects must be considered when choosing a TCA. Baseline and follow-up ECGs are recommended for elderly patients when TCAs are started. TCAs are considered contraindicated after myocardial infarction. Conversely, the SSRIs as a class are well tolerated by older cardiac patients. They have not shown sustained effects on heart rate or rhythm and have little direct effect on blood pressure (resting or postural) and on cardiac conduction (52,53).

FALLS

The relationship between falls and TCAs has been recognized for many years. Older adults have reduced sensitivity of their carotid baroreceptors and reduced numbers of α-1-adrenergic receptors, making them more vulnerable to the direct hypotensive effects of antidepressants, particularly the older TCAs (35). Many older patients also receive medications for hypertension, and the risk for falls is greatly increased for patients receiving both medication classes (35). This was not considered to be a problem with the SSRIs, but a recent study implicated SSRIs as a risk factor for falls among nursing home residents (54). The study found a positive correlation between increased fall rates and daily doses of either TCAs or SSRIs. Patients who received antidepressants for behavioral symptoms of dementia were also at greater risk for falls compared with patients receiving antidepressants for depression. In summary, to guard against falls in depressed geriatric patients, physicians must monitor the following risk factors: pharmacologic (number and class of medications), physiological (blood pressure, pulse, gait, vision, and cognition), and environmental (physical layout of the patient's environment, shoes, etc.) (55).

Antidepressant Efficacy

There are few randomized clinical trials (RCTs) establishing the efficacy of antidepressant medications in the elderly, particularly the frail elderly or patients over 80 years of age (56). Typical outpatient "geriatric" studies enroll subjects with an average age of only approximately 65 years and allow patients who are as young as 60 to be enrolled. Furthermore, elderly patients who do enter research studies are not typical of the geriatric patient populations seen in primary care. The former are healthier and without significant medical comorbidity, which makes it difficult to generalize findings to patients typically encountered in primary care. Consequently, clinical recommendations are modified largely from experience with young or middle-aged adults (57,58).

Tricyclic Antidepressants and Selective Serotonin-Reuptake Inhibitors
The available evidence indicates that all antidepressants are more effective than placebo in the treatment of acute depression in community-dwelling elderly and that no antidepressant class has superior efficacy over another (59). Approximately 60% of patients show clinical improvement, although many patients have significant residual symptomatology (60–74).

Table 8.3 summarizes starting dosages and final therapeutic dosages for selected antidepressants. Generally, both starting and final therapeutic dosages are lower for elderly patients compared with younger adults. Titration schedules are slower and are governed by side effects. The emergence of anticholinergic, antihistaminic, and α-adrenergic side effects is especially problematic for the tertiary-amine TCAs such as amitriptyline, imipramine, or doxepin. These three medications generally are not recommended for the elderly and are not included in Table 8.3 (51,69). For the secondary-amine TCAs nortriptyline and desipramine, baseline and follow-up ECGs are recommended to monitor geriatric patients for potential cardiac conduction problems. Monitoring blood levels of these two medications also is recommended to achieve a dosage that has been shown to be therapeutic (59).

As a class, SSRIs are better tolerated and have little or no impact on cardiovascular and cognitive functioning in older adults (51,52). Common complaints in the elderly are similar to those in young adults and include

Table 8.3   Dose Recommendations and Special Considerations for Selected Antidepressant Medications in the Elderly

Class	Starting Dosage	Therapeutic Dosage Range	Special Considerations or Comments
Cyclic antidepressants			Baseline ECG recommended for TCAs; monitor orthostatic blood pressure and anticholingeric side effects
Nortriptyline (Pamelor)	10 mg/d	10–75 mg/d	Therapeutic blood level: 50–150 ng/mL; blood level and side-effect tolerance should guide final therapeutic dosage
Desipramine (Norpramin, Pertofrane)	10 mg/d	25–100 mg/d	Therapeutic blood level >125 ng/mL
Selective serotonin-reuptake inhibitors			Controversy exists about whether to pick a fixed dosage versus titration for the SSRIs; it is thought that titration to a final therapeutic dosage helps minimize side effects; final therapeutic dosages are meant to be guides, not hard and fast rules
Fluoxetine (Prozac)	10 mg/d	10–40 mg/d	Prolonged half-life, especially for its active metabolite norfluoxetine; inhibitor of CP450-2D6; the 10-mg starting dosage is recommended for frail elderly patients because of fluoxetine's long-acting metabolite
Sertraline (Zoloft)	25 mg/d	50–200 mg/d	Inhibitor of CP450-2D6
Paroxetine (Paxil)	5–10 mg/d	20–40 mg/d	Inhibitor of CP450-3A3/4 and 1A2
Citalopram (Celexa)	20 mg/d	20–40 mg/d	Weak inhibitor of CP450 system
Other new antidepressants			
Nefazodone (Serzone)	150 mg/d (divided)	300–500 mg/d (divided)	Inhibitor of CP450-3A4
Bupropion (Wellbutrin)	75 mg/d	75–300 mg/d	Inhibits CP450-2D6; high doses may cause seizures
Venlafaxine (Effexor)	25–37.5 mg/d (divided)	100–200 mg/d (divided)	Inhibits both reuptake of serotonin and norepinephrine; not well studied in elderly; requires blood pressure monitoring in elderly
Mirtazapine (Remeron)	7.5–15 mg/d	15–30 mg/d	Not well studied in the elderly; higher frequency of somnolence, dry mouth, and dizziness
Psychostimulants			Stimulants can be safe and well tolerated in medically compromised, frail elderly patients; the more important side effects include agitation, restlessness, confusion, increased paranoia, and cardiovascular stimulation (tachycardia, hypertension, arrhythmia, angina)
Methylphenidate (Ritalin)	5 mg/d	10–60 mg/d	
Dextroamphetamine (Dexedrine)	2.5 mg/d	5–30 mg/d	

ECG = electrocardiogram; TCAs = tricyclic antidepressants.

nausea, diarrhea, insomnia, headache, and agitation or restlessness (59). As stated above, SSRIs affect the CP450 enzyme system *in vitro*, so clinicians need to be aware of potential drug interactions. Therapeutic blood levels for SSRIs have not been established, and monitoring blood levels at this time is not recommended.

Getting well is not enough; it is *staying* well that counts. Data indicate that continuing antidepressant therapy with nortriptyline (a TCA) in combination with psychotherapy keeps geriatric depressed patients well, especially for patients between 60 and 69 years of age (75). Patients over 70 years of age have a more brittle course and more relapse risk within 1 year of successful recovery from an index depression episode (76). Testing the maintenance effectiveness of SSRIs has yet to occur for older adults. Controlled studies in middle-aged patients have provided support for the maintenance efficacy of paroxetine (75,76), citalopram (78), sertraline (79), and fluvoxamine (79). Despite the absence of controlled data from geriatric maintenance trials for SSRIs, the maintenance dose of SSRI is recommended to be the same as the acute therapy dose. Given the high rate of relapse reported in elderly patients with only one lifetime episode after discontinuing antidepressant medication, evidence also suggests that even these patients may be candidates for maintenance pharmacotherapy (80).

New Antidepressants Other Than Selective Serotonin-Reuptake Inhibitors
Antidepressants such as bupropion, venlafaxine, nefazodone, and mirtazapine have been less well studied in geriatric patients; therefore, recommendations about their clinical use are less firm. For a more detailed discussion of these drugs and their side effects, *see* Chapter 5.

Bupropion inhibits the reuptake of norepinephrine and dopamine and is a weak reuptake inhibitor of serotonin. Side effects of bupropion may cause restlessness, agitation, insomnia, anxiety, and akathisia. In younger patients, bupropion has caused seizures at high doses and therefore should be given in divided doses.

Venlafaxine inhibits the reuptake of both serotonin and norepinephrine. Data from the small subset receiving long-term treatment suggest that tolerability is equivalent to that in younger patients (81). Venlafaxine is a good option in elderly patients who fail to respond to other antidepressants but may cause hypertension at higher dose.

Nefazodone is a serotonin-reuptake inhibitor and potent antagonist of serotonin-2 (5-HT2) receptors. It has a suggested dosage range of between 300–500 mg/d and should be administered in divided doses.

Mirtazapine is a tetracyclic antidepressant and has presynaptic α-2-adrenergic antagonist effects that increase the release of norepinephrine and serotonin. It was somewhat less effective than TCAs in elderly depressed outpatients but was somewhat more effective than trazodone or placebo in another 6-week trial (82,83). In the latter study, mirtazapine was associated with a higher frequency of somnolence and dry mouth compared with placebo.

Treatment Resistance and Relapse

Despite advances in pharmacotherapy, longitudinal studies of late-life depression indicate a chronicity rate of 7% to 30%, which increases to 40% if partially remitted elderly depressed patients are included (84). Relapse rates in late-life depression range from 19% to 30% at 1 year (76,85,86) and come close to 50% at 2 years (87). For patients over 70 years of age, the relapse rate has been reported as being as high as 60% (76). Additionally, if a geriatric patient has a single relapse, he or she is significantly more likely to have multiple relapses. Risk factors for treatment resistance and relapse include history of frequent episodes, late onset of the illness, medical comorbidity, severity, and chronicity of the index depressive episode (84).

Treatment algorithms for treatment-resistant or relapse patients have not been well developed for geriatric patients (88). Treatment resistance or relapsing illness is a clear indication for referral to a psychiatrist with experience in treating geriatric patients. To help guide the medical decision making surrounding these difficult patients, the following sequence of questions are required:

1. **Is the patient's antidepressant dose adequate?** Concern over the side effects or tolerability of a particular antidepressant may lead to suboptimal dosing. For patients receiving nortriptyline or desipramine, blood levels should be obtained to see if the dosing scheme produces optimal levels. For patients receiving SSRIs, maximal titration doses should be given.

2. **Has the patient been on the medication long enough?** In geriatric patients, clinical response to antidepressant drug therapy depends not only on adequate dose and adequate blood levels but also on adequate length of treatment (59). A significant response often occurs later in elderly patients than in younger patients, often after 6 to 12 weeks of therapy.

3. **Are there compliance problems or difficulty maximizing the dose of the antidepressant because of side effects, medical comorbidity, or adverse drug interactions?**

4. **Should a new medication be tried?** Strategies such as switching medications within a single class or switching between classes of antidepressants should be considered, even though there are few published guidelines on how to do this for geriatric patients (especially the frail elderly) (88).

5. **Should augmentation strategies be tried?** Although the clinical evidence comes primarily from case reports or open-label trials, augmentation strategies (e.g., adding supplemental triiodothyronine or lithium, combining SSRIs and TCAs) can be tried in the elderly; however, results have been mixed (88). Psychostimulants such as methylphenidate or dextroamphetamine

have been shown to be effective in treating depressed frail elderly, either alone or in combination with other antidepressants (89,90). Monoamine oxidase inhibitors (MAOIs) such as phenelzine or parnate also have been shown to be helpful in treatment-resistant geriatric patients (91). However, MAOIs are associated with significant risks, including increased risk of orthostatic hypotension, hypertensive crises from dietary indiscretions, and potentially fatal drug interactions with SSRIs or meperidine.

6. **Should electroconvulsive therapy (ECT) be considered?**
ECT remains the most effective treatment for severe major depression in patients who have been treatment resistant or in those who have severe depressive symptoms (e.g., psychotic symptoms [delusions, hallucinations], severe psychomotor slowing, catatonic stupor, severe suicidality, refusal of oral intake). ECT should be considered for moderately or severely depressed patients who have been refractory to and/or intolerant of adequate trials of antidepressants. Geriatric patients with extensive periventricular white-matter disease (many of whom have been refractory to or intolerant of antidepressants) are also good candidates for ECT, with no evidence that ECT causes additional damage to brain structures (92,93).

ECT is effective, achieving acute remission rates for severely depressed geriatric patients of over 80% in recent studies (86). There is an increased risk of post-ECT confusion and memory impairment in the elderly, which can be reduced through unilateral, non–dominant-hemisphere, stimulus-titration methods (94,95). With appropriate precautions, ECT can be administered safely to patients with concurrent medical illnesses. Absolute contraindications for ECT in the elderly are few, the most notable being evidence of increased intracranial pressure. There is an increased risk of complications with recent myocardial infarction or severe hypertension. The most common post-ECT problems for patients over 85 years of age are delirium or confusion (32%), transient hypertension (67%), and reversible ectopy during treatment (18%) (96). Although controlled clinical trials have not been completed, maintenance ECT can be an effective strategy for preventing early relapse for geriatric patients who have been refractory to or intolerant of medication. Maintenance ECT is given generally as an outpatient procedure every month.

Choosing the Right Medication

Choosing the right medication for depressed geriatric patients requires an understanding of the "effectiveness" of antidepressants, i.e., efficacy plus performance under real-life circumstances (59). A major effectiveness consideration is compliance. Variables that impact compliance include such characteristics as a medication's tolerability, side-effect profile, drug-interaction potential, and cost. A medication's effectiveness also influences continuation and maintenance-treatment strategies, because compliance has a major role in treatment success.

Although TCAs and SSRIs have similar efficacy for elderly depressed outpatients, the SSRIs are likely to be somewhat more effective than TCAs because of their improved tolerability, which ensures adequate dosing, and their enhanced safety profile (97). This does not mean, however, that all depressed geriatric outpatients should be placed automatically on an SSRI. Physicians must match the choice of antidepressant to the symptoms of the patient's depression, medical comorbidity, compliance profile, and past treatment experience.

Role of Psychotherapy

Somatic therapies alone do not resolve many of the problems associated with late-life depression, including bereavement (*see* section on Recent Bereavement below), social isolation, physical disability, sensory impairments, dependency, loss of work or other meaningful activity, and unsatisfactory living arrangements. There is no basis for the belief that older patients are unlikely to accept or benefit from psychotherapy. Furthermore, some patients strongly prefer nonbiologic interventions, whereas others are not suitable candidates for somatic interventions because of side effects, concomitant illnesses, or other circumstances. Psychotherapy alone may be useful for outpatients with mild to moderate depression, and treatment studies have demonstrated that cognitive-behavioral therapy (CBT), brief psychodynamic therapy, and interpersonal therapy (IPT) work with elderly patients who have mild to moderate depression (98,99). Combined with pharmacotherapy, psychotherapy enhances medication compliance and reduces relapse rates in elderly depressed outpatients (75). Reminiscence therapy or psycho-educational interventions also help reduce depressive symptoms in elders with subclinical (or possibly dysthymic) forms of depression (98). Unfortunately, all of these studies used patient samples that lacked the medical, cultural, social, and/or clinical diversity typically seen in clinical practice and therefore may not be able to be generalized.

Depression in Special Geriatric Patient Populations

Patients with neurological disorders and those who have experienced recent bereavement are important subpopulations of geriatric patients who are vulnerable to depression. Detection of depression in geriatric neurological patients can be challenging because some neurological illnesses can cause somatic, motor, cognitive, and affective symptoms that may resemble depression symptoms (100). Bereavement, although considered a normal and expected reaction to the multiple losses experienced with age, is a significant risk factor for late-life depression.

Parkinson's Disease

Studies examining the prevalence of depression in Parkinson's disease vary considerably depending on the methodology used to ascertain each case. Most studies report the prevalence of major depression at rates between 35% and 50% (101,102). Longitudinal studies indicate that Parkinson's disease patients tend to segregate into either depressed or nondepressed groups, with little crossover (103). Mood disorders may precede motor symptoms in Parkinson's disease patients, and most reviews contend that depression is an expression of, not a psychological response to, the illness (104). However, some of the symptoms of Parkinson's disease (e.g., bradykinesia, flattened and restricted affect, bradyphrenia [slowed thinking], changes in the prosody of speech [the emotional coloring of speech]) may make an accurate detection of depression difficult.

Compared with patients who have major depression without Parkinson's disease, depressed Parkinson's disease patients tend to be less guilt-ridden or self-blaming, are more dysphoric, express higher levels of anxiety and suicidal ideation (although suicide attempts are less prevalent), and experience more cognitive deficits that correlate with the severity of the depression (101,104). The relationship between mood and motor abnormalities in Parkinson's disease patients is noteworthy. Patients with predominantly right-side symptoms have a higher prevalence of depression than patients with left-side symptoms (101). Greater bradykinesia, axial rigidity, and overall motor deterioration also have been associated with greater risk of depression (105). A relationship between the "on-off" phenomenon—the "on" phase being when patients have relatively good motor movement; the "off" phase being when they do not—and mood has been shown. Depressive symptoms are fewer during the "on" phase than during the "off" phase (101).

Depression treatment studies in Parkinson's disease patients, using a broad range of antidepressants, have shown medication response rates between 42% to 60% (101,104). Psychostimulants also have been used in Parkinson's disease patients to help relieve depression, but systematic trials are lacking. Extensive case report literature describing the efficacy of ECT in Parkinson's disease patients also exists. In general, ECT has been shown to improve both mood and motor symptoms, although improvement is short lived (101,104). ECT in Parkinson's disease is primarily indicated for those patients who are treatment refractory or intolerant of medication, especially those who are debilitated (106).

Stroke

Reviews of clinical studies suggests that between 20% and 50% of patients with cerebral vascular disease experience a depressive disorder (107,108). Recent epidemiologic studies, however, have failed to confirm the high incidence of post-stroke depression in community samples (109). In the original studies of stroke and depression, approximately 25% of post-stroke patients met criteria for major depression, whereas another 20% met criteria for minor depression (110). This high correlation between stroke and depression has been shown in both acute and chronic stroke patients and has been associated with increased mortality (111,112). The mechanisms behind post-stroke depression is not known but has been postulated to be secondary to the disruption of biogenic amine pathways from the brain stem into the frontal cortex (107).

The frequency of post-stoke depression cannot be explained as being due solely to an emotional reaction to disabling neurological sequelae, nor does the degree of disability predict which patients get depressed. However, neuroanatomical associations between stroke and depression have been found for the following (110,113):

1. Left anterior hemisphere stroke (in the region of the frontal dorsolateral cortex and head of the caudate nucleus)
2. Right parietal strokes
3. Significant subcortical atrophy and periventricular white-matter disease
4. Strong correlation between the severity of depression and the proximity of the stroke to the left frontal pole

Symptoms of post-stroke depression are similar to those found in older patients with major depression without stroke, except that post-stroke depression patients exhibit more psychomotor and cognitive slowing, more anxiety, and increased ideas of reference (the assumption by the patient that words or actions of others refer to himself or herself) (114,115). Patients with right hemispheric strokes may experience changes in the prosody of speech, making it difficult for them to express feelings of sadness or depression convincingly.

Treatment recommendations for post-stroke depressions are similar to treatment for other depressive disorders, although clinical trials are few. Nortriptyline has been found to be effective in post-stroke depression (116), but most experts recommend SSRIs as first-line medications because of their enhanced tolerability and safety profiles. Methylphenidate also has been found to be effective and exerted few side effects in depressed patients with depression following stroke (117). In patients who have failed, or who cannot tolerate antidepressant medications, ECT has been shown to be effective. ECT is not recommended for those patients who have suffered a recent hemorrhagic stroke or who demonstrate evidence for increased intracranial pressure.

Dementia

The relationship between late-life depression and dementia has been a major focus of clinical and epidemiologic research over the past two decades. The relationships are complicated and, for the purposes of this chapter, are organized as follows:

- Late-life depression as a risk factor for cognitive decline in the elderly
- Reversible cognitive impairment ("pseudodementia") in late-life depression
- Depression complicating dementia syndromes (both Alzheimer's disease and vascular dementia)

Depression as a Risk Factor for Cognitive Decline in the Elderly
Studies that have tried to establish a causal link between late-life depression and dementia have had discrepant results. A meta-analysis of case-control studies before 1990 suggested an elevated risk of developing Alzheimer's disease in individuals over 70 years of age if they had been treated for major depression at least 1 year before the dementia diagnosis (118). A recent community-based epidemiologic study from the United States supported the notion that depression presages future cognitive decline by finding a twofold risk of incident dementia in individuals with pre-existing depression (119). A second epidemiologic study, however, found that depressive symptoms predicted future cognitive losses in only those elderly with pre-existing moderate cognitive impairment and did not find an association between depressive symptoms and onset or rate of decline for cognitively intact elderly (120). Another study in France failed to find depression predictive of cognitive deterioration over a 3-year period (121). However, conclusions about the risk of developing dementia in depressed elderly from epidemiologic studies are problematic because they use only depression and cognitive screening instruments and fail to establish a clinical diagnosis (122).

The relationship between depression and the development of dementia is stronger in clinical studies in which clinical diagnoses have been determined. Elderly patients with "reversible dementia" may not achieve complete cognitive recovery after remission of depression (123). Between 11% and 23% of patients thought to have reversible dementia become irreversibly demented for each additional year of follow-up (124–128). Irreversible dementia begins to be diagnosed approximately 2 years after the initial recovery from depression (22). Conclusions from clinical studies must be tempered because of potential problems with selection and case-ascertainment biases. For example, more patients with cognitive impairment associated with depression may seek help because of the cognitive difficulties than patients who are depressed but not suffering from cognitive difficulties. The ongoing tension between epidemiologic and clinical studies over this issue will continue until more sensitive and specific measures can be developed common to both research activities (122).

Reversible Cognitive Impairment ("Pseudodementia") in Late-Life Depression

Reversible memory complaints characterize late-life depression. When severe, they have been described historically as "pseudodementia." More recently, this syndrome has been referred to as the "reversible dementia syndrome of depression" (22). Between 18% and 57% of depressed elderly patients present with memory complaints that improve after remission of the depression (129). As described in the previous section, however, many will go on to develop irreversible dementia syndromes. Elderly patients with depression and "reversible dementia" have a severe form of major depression that is characterized by motor retardation, hopelessness, helplessness, anxiety, and often delusions (130). The memory impairment is often accompanied by other cognitive deficits, including impairment of attention, free recall, motor speed, spontaneous elaboration of detail, word fluency, and syntactic complexity (23,129). A good bottom line for physicians to remember is never to hesitate to treat depression when it is accompanied by cognitive impairment. Patients and their families should be informed that successful treatment may improve cognition, but this should not be promised.

Depression Occurring with Dementia Syndromes (Alzheimer's Disease and Vascular Dementia)

Depression has long been recognized as a major comorbidity of dementia syndromes (131). Most studies report the prevalence of clinically significant depression in Alzheimer's disease between 17% and 29% (123). For vascular dementia, the prevalence rates are roughly similar (19% to 27%) (132). Dementia patients with depression may have a genetic vulnerability to depression (133).

Depressive symptoms in dementia patients often fluctuate and are difficult to identify in those patients with advanced dementia because of language impairments. Behavioral manifestations of depression (e.g., psychomotor slowing, emotional lability, crying spells, insomnia, anorexia, weight loss, apathy) can occur in dementia patients without depression (134). One study found that depressed Alzheimer's disease patients exhibited more self-pity, rejection sensitivity, anhedonia, and fewer neurovegetative signs than depressed older patients without dementia (135). Research-based depression rating scales for dementia patients have been developed to help discriminate between depressed and nondepressed dementia patients, but clinical applicability has not yet been established (136,137).

Dementia patients with co-existing depression can be treated effectively with antidepressants (138–140). Highly anticholinergic TCAs (e.g., amitriptyline, imipramine, doxepin) should be avoided because their anticholinergic side effects may impair cognition significantly (131).

In the final analysis, when it is unclear if a patient has dementia, depression, or both, it is often appropriate to treat him or her empirically with an antidepressant and then assess whether any improvement is achieved.

Recent Bereavement

Conjugal and other types of bereavement late in life are associated frequently with symptoms of major or minor depression. As many as 50% of recently bereaved older adults developed major depression within 1 year of the loss (141). Active intervention is recommended for individuals with prolonged grief or for those who show evidence of significant depressive symptomatology. Results of a recent controlled study support the effectiveness of combined pharmacotherapy and IPT for bereavement-related depression in the elderly (142). Given the fact that conjugal bereavement is a risk factor for suicide late in life, particularly for men, and given the greater safety of SSRIs in overdose, SSRIs are recommended as the first-line treatment for major and minor depression of bereavement (143). There is no evidence, however, that antidepressants are beneficial in normal grief, except when depression or pathological grief occurs.

Recommendations

Late-life depression should not be considered a natural part of the aging process. Clinically significant depression can be found in as many as 15% to 20% of community dwelling elderly, with higher rates found in primary care practices and institutional settings (12–15). Several features of late-life depression make accurate diagnosis a substantial clinical challenge. Brief depression-screening instruments are recommended for high-risk patients, such as patients with chronic medical illness, cognitive disturbances, or adverse life events.

An ideal treatment program integrates patient and family education, focused psychotherapy, and pharmacotherapy. Successful pharmacotherapy for depression in the elderly requires careful consideration of pharmacodynamic and pharmacokinetic actions of antidepressant medications. Because of these changes, lower doses of medication and more gradual titration schedules are required for elderly depressed patients. Clinicians should select TCAs that have minimal antihistaminic, anticholinergic, and α-adrenergic effects to minimize cognitive, cardiovascular, and autonomic side effects. The SSRIs have been shown to be effective in the elderly, and their side-effect profiles are generally milder than those of the older agents. The SSRIs affect the CP450 enzyme system, so clinicians need to be aware of potential drug interactions. Patients with treatment-resistant or recurrent late-life depression should be referred to a psychiatrist with experience in treating geriatric patients. Strategies for treatment-resistant or recurrent late-life depression have not been well studied. Recommendations are similar to those reported for younger adults and include optimizing medication dose, switching medication class, augmentation therapies, and ECT. Treatment for acute depressive episodes should last at least 6 to 8 months, and long-term maintenance treatment should be considered for individuals who have not experienced a full remission or who have relapsing illness.

Acknowledgments

This work was supported in part by the following grants: Dr. Reynolds—MH52247, MH37869, MH43832, MH00295, MH59318; Dr. Alexopoulos—MH49762, MH19132, MH51842, MH42819, MH59366; Dr. Katz—MH52129, MH19931, MH51247, MH538249, MH59380, SM52635.

Key Points

- Depression in late life is a serious illness that affects nearly five million of the 31 million U.S. citizens over 65 years of age; one million will suffer from major depression.

- Many elderly depressed patients will present initially to primary care practices.

- Failure to recognize late-life depression can lead to serious consequences, such as increased risk of suicide, worsening physical health and cognitive performance, poor compliance with medical treatment, increased health care use, and diminished quality of life.

- Detection of late-life depression can be improved if physicians systematically assess geriatric patients with depression-screening instruments, such as the Geriatric Depression Scale.

- Physicians also should have a high index of suspicion for depression in geriatric patients who have 1) memory complaints, 2) high use of medical care services (and who present with high levels of distress), 3) disability out of proportion to the severity of underlying diseases, 4) patterns of treatment noncompliance or refusal, and 5) hopelessness about the present and future.

- Antidepressant therapy is effective in a high proportion of depressed geriatric outpatients. Although TCAs and SSRIs have similar efficacy, SSRIs are recommended as first-line medications because of their side-effect profiles. Combining antidepressants and psychotherapy produces better outcomes as maintenance strategies than either modality alone.

- If geriatric patients do not experience a full remission or relapse, they should be maintained on medications indefinitely.

- For those patients who have serious depression, hospitalization and treatment with ECT may be required.

▒   ▒   ▒

REFERENCES

1. **National Institutes of Health.** *Diagnosis and Treatment of Depression in Late Life: Consensus Statement,* vol. 9, no. 6. Paper presented at National Institutes of Health Development Conference, November 4–6, 1991.

2. **Katz IR, Alexopoulos GS.** The diagnosis and treatment of late-life depression: consensus update conference. *Am J Geriatr Psychiatry.* 1996;4(Suppl 1):S1–2.

3. **Lebowitz BD.** Diagnosis and treatment of depression in late life: an overview of the NIH consensus statement. *Am J Geriatr Psychiatry.* 1996;4(Suppl 1):S3–6.

4. **Williams-Russo P.** Barriers to diagnosis and treatment of depression in primary care settings. *Am J Geriatr Psychiatry.* 1996;4(Suppl):S84–90.

5. **Koenig HG, Blazer D.** Minor depression in late life. *Am J Geriatr Psychiatry.* 1996;4(Suppl 1):S14–21.

6. **Broadhead EW, Blazer DG, George LK, et al.** Depression, disability days, and days lost from work in a prospective epidemiologic survey. *JAMA.* 1990;264:2524–8.

7. **Jaffee A, Froom J, Galambos N.** Minor depression and functional impairment. *Arch Fam Med.* 1994;3:1081–6.

8. **Unutzer J, Patrick DL, Simon G, et al.** Depressive symptoms and the cost of health services in HMO patients aged 65 years and older. *JAMA.* 1997;277:1618–23.

9. **U.S. Bureau of the Census.** *Current Population Reports, Special Studies P23–190, 65+ in the United States.* Washington, DC: U.S. Government Printing Office; 1996:3–13.

10. **Frasure-Smith N, Lesperance F, Talajic M.** Depression following myocardial infarction: impact on 6-month survival. *JAMA.* 1993;91:999–1005.

11. **Rovner BW, German PS, Brant LJ, et al.** Depression and mortality in nursing homes. *JAMA.* 1991;265:993–6.

12. **Blazer DG, Bachar JR, Manton KG.** The epidemiology of depression in an elderly community population. *Gerontologist.* 1987;27:281–7.

13. **Alexopoulos GS.** Geriatric depression in primary care. *Int J Geriatr Psychiatry.* 1996;11:397–400.

14. **Caine ED, Lyness JM, Conwell Y.** Diagnosis of late-life-depression: preliminary studies in primary care settings. *Am J Geriatr Psychiatry.* 1996;4(Suppl 1):S45–50.

15. **Parmelee PA, Katz IR, Lawton MP.** Depression among institutionalized aged: assessment and prevalence estimation. *J Gerontol.* 1989;44:M22-29.

16. **Katona C, Livingston G.** *Comorbid Depression in Older People.* London: Martin Dunitz Ltd; 1997:4.

17. **Koenig HG, Meador KG, Cohen HJ, et al.** Depression in elderly hospitalized patientrs with medical illness. *Arch Intern Med.* 1988;148:1929–36.

18. **Koenig HG, Meador KG, Shelp F, et al.** Major depressive disorder in hospitalized medically ill patients: an examination of young and elderly male veterans. *J Am Geriatr Soc.* 1991;39:881–890.

19. **Koenig HG, O'Connor CM, Guarisco SA, et al.** Depressive disorders in older medical inpatients on general medicine and cardiolgy services at a university teaching hospital. *Am J Geriatr Psychiatry.* 1993;1:197–210.

20. **Rabins PV.** Barriers to diagnosis and treatment of depression in elderly patients. *Am J Geriatr Psychiatry.* 1996;4(Suppl 1):S79–83.

21. **Reifler BV, Larson E, Hanley R.** Coexistence of cognitive impairment and depression in geriatric outpatients. *Am J Psychiatry.* 1982;139:623–6.

22. **Emery VO, Oxman TE.** Update on the dementia spectrum of depression. *Am J Psychiatry.* 1992;149:305–17.

23. **Gallo JJ, Rabins PV, Iliffe S.** The "Research Magnificent" in late life: psychiatric epidemiology and the primary care of older adults. *Int J Psychiatry Med.* 1997;27: 185–204.

24. **Wyshak G, Barksy A.** Satisfaction with and effectiveness of medical care in relation to anxiety and depression: patient and physician ratings compared. *Gen Hosp Psychiatry.* 1995;17:108–14.

25. **Yesavage JA, Brink TL, Rose TL, Adey M.** The geriatric rating scale: comparison with other self-report and psychiatric rating scales. In Crook T, Gerris S, Bartus R (eds). *Assessment in Geriatric Psychpharmacology.* New Canaan, CT: Mark Powley Associates; 1983:153–165.

26. **Radloff LS, Teri L.** Use of the Center for Epidemiologic Studies depression scale with older adults. *Clin Gerontol.* 1986;119–36.

27. **Lyness JM, Noel TK, Cox C, et al.** Screening for depression in elderly primary care patients: a comparison of the Center for Epidemiologic Studies depression scale and the geriatric depression scale. *Arch Intern Med.* 1997;157:449–54.

28. **Carpenter JS, Andrykowski MA, Wilson J, et al.** Psychometrics for two short forms of the Center for Epidemiologic Studies depression scale. *Issues Ment Health Nurs.* 1998;9:481–94.

29. **Burke WJ, Rangwani S, Roccaforte WH, et al.** The reliability and validity of the collateral source version of the geriatric depression rating scale administisterd by telephone. *Int J Geriatr Psychiatry.* 1997;12:288–94.

30. **Shah A, Herbert R, Lewis S, et al.** Screening for depression among acutely ill geriatric inpatients with a short geriatric depression scale. *Age Ageing.* 1997;26:217–21.

31. **Van Marwijk HW, Wallace P, de Bock GH, et al.** Evaluation of the feasibility, reliability, and diagnostic value of shortened versions of the geriatric depression scale. *Br J Gen Pract.* 1995;45:195–9.

32. **Stewart RB, Cooper JW.** Polypharmacy in the aged: practical solutions. *Drugs Aging.* 1994;4:449–61.

33. **Broderick E.** Prescribing patterns for nursing home residents in the US: the reality and the vision. *Drugs Aging.* 1997;11:255–60.

34. **Borson S, Doane K.** The impact of OBRA-87 on psychotropic drug prescribing in skilled nursing facilities. *Psychiatr Serv.* 1997;48:1289–96.

35. **Dubovsky SL.** Geriatric neuropsychophamacology. In Coffey CE, Cummings JL (eds). *Textbook of Geriatric Neuropsychiatry.* Washington, DC: American Psychiatric Press; 1994:596–631.

36. **Bergman U, Wilholm BE.** Patient medication on admission to a medical clinic. *Eur J Clin Pharmacol.* 1981;20:185–91.

37. **Salzman C.** Medication compliance in the elderly. *J Clin Psychiatry.* 1995;56 (Suppl 1):18–22.

38. **Richardson MA, Simons-Morton B, Annegers JF.** Effect of perceived barriers on compliance with antihypertensive medications. *Health Educ Q.* 1993;20: 489–503.

39. **Lamy PP, Salzman C, Nevis-Olesen J.** Drug prescribing patterns, risks, and compliance guidelines. In Salzman C (ed). *Clinical Geriatric Psychopharmacology.* New York: Williams & Wilkins; 1992:15–37.

40. **Young RC, Meyers BS.** Psychopharmacology. In Sadavoy J, Lazarus LW, Jarvik LF, Grossberg GT (eds). *Comprehensive Review of Geriatric Psychiatry,* 2nd ed. Washington DC: American Psychiatric Press; 1996:755–817.

41. **Richelson E.** Pharmacokinetic interactions of antidepressants. *J Clin Psychiatry.* 1998;59(Suppl 10):22–6.

42. **Nemeroff CB, Devane CL, Pollock BG.** Newer antidepressants and the cytochrome P450 system. *Am J Psychiatry.* 1996;153:311–20.

43. **Solai LK, Mulsant BH, Pollock BG, et al.** Effect of sertraline on plasma nortriptyline levels in depressed elderly. *J Clinical Psychiatry.* 1997;58:440–3.

44. **Alderman J, Preskorn SH, Greenblatt DJ, et al.** Desipramine pharmacokinetics when co-administered with paroxetine or sertraline in extensive metabolizers. *J Clin Psychopharmacol.* 1997;17:284–91.

45. **Veering BT, Burm AG, Souverijn JH et al.** The effect of age on serum concentration of albumin and alpha-1-acid glycoprotein. *Br J Clin Pharmacol.* 1990;29: 201–6.

46. **Woo J, Chan HS, Or KH, Arumanayagam M.** Effect of age and disease on two drug binding proteins: albumin and alpha-1-acid glycoprotein. *Clin Biochem.* 1994;27:289–92.

47. **Jackson PR, Tucker GT, Woods HF.** Altered plasma drug binding in cancer: role of alpha-1-acid glycoprotein and albumin. *Clin Pharmacol Ther.* 1982;32:295–302.

48. **Georgotas A, McCue RE, Hapworth W, et al.** Comparative efficacy and safety of MAOIs versus TCAs in treating depression in the elderly. *Biol Psychiatry.* 1986;21: 1155–66.

49. **Nelson JC, Jatlow P, Mazure C.** Desipramine plasma levels and response in elderly melancholic patients. *J Clin Psychopharmacol.* 1985;5:217–220.

50. **Flint A, Rifat S.** The effect of sequential antidepressant treatment on geriatric depression. *J Affect Disord.* 1996;36:95–105.

51. **Roose SP, Suthers KM.** Antidepressant response in late-life depression. *J Clin Psychiatry.* 1998;59(Suppl 10):4–8.

52. **Glassman AH, Rodriquez AI, Shapiro PA.** The use of antidepressant drugs in patients with heart disease. *J Clin Psychiatry.* 1998;59(Suppl 10):16–21.

53. **Roose SP, Laghrissi-Thode F, Kennedy JS, et al.** Comparison of paroxetine and nortriptyline in depressed patients with ischemic heart disease. *JAMA.* 1998;279: 287–291.

54. **Thapa PB, Gideon R, Cost TW, et al.** Antidepressants and the risk of falls among nursing home residents. *N Engl J Med.* 1998;339:872–5.

55. **Weiner DK, Hanlon JT, Studenski SA.** Effects of central nervous system polypharmacy on falls liability in community dwelling elderly. *Gerontology.* 1998; 44:217–22.

56. **Salzman C.** Pharmacological treatment of depression in the elderly. In Schneider LS Reynolds CF, Lebowitz BD, Friedhoff A (eds). *Diagnosis and Treatment of Depression in Late Life.* Washington, DC: American Psychiatric Press; 1994:181–244.

57. **NIH Consensus Development Panel on Depression in Late Life.** Diagnosis and treatment of depression in late life. *JAMA.* 1992;268:1018–24.

58. **Lebowitz BD, Pearson JL, Schneider LS, et al.** Diagnosis and treatment of depression in late life: consensus statement update. *JAMA.* 1997;278:1186–90.

59. **Schneider LS.** Pharmacologic considerations in the treatment of late-life depression. *Am J Geriatr Psychiatry.* 1996;4(Suppl 1):S51–65.

60. **Salzman C, Schneider L, Alexopoulos G.** Pharmacological treatment of depression in late life. In Bloom F, Kupfer D (ed). *Psychopharmacology: Fourth Generation of Progress.* New York: Raven Press; 1995:1471–7.

61. **Altamura AC, De Novellis F, Guercetti G, et al.** Fluoxetine compared with amitriptyline in elderly depression: a controlled clinical trial. *Int J Clin Pharmacol Res.* 1989;9:391–6.

62. **La Pia S, Giorgio D, Ciriello R, et al.** Evaluation of the efficacy, tolerability, and therapeutic profile of fluoxetine versus mianserin in the treatment of depressive disorders in the elderly. *Curr Ther Res.* 1992;52:847–58.

63. **Falk WE, Rosenbaum JF, Otto MW, et al.** Fluoxetine versus trazodone in depressed geriatric patients. *J Geriatr Psychiatry Neurol.* 1989;2:208–14.

64. **Fairweather DB, Kerr JS, Harrison DA, et al.** A double-blind comparison of the effects of fluoxetine and amitriptyline on cognitive function in elderly depressed patients. *Hum Psychopharmacol.* 1993;8:41–7.

65. **Feighner JP, Cohn JB.** Double-blind comparative trials of fluoxetine and doxepin in geriatric patients with major depressive disorder. *J Clin Psychiatry.* 1985;46:20–5.

66. **Schone W, Ludwig M.** A double-blind study of paroxetine compared with fluoxetine in geriatric patients with major depression. *J Clin Psychopharmacol.* 1993; 13(Suppl 2):S34-9.

67. **Geretsegger C, Bohmer F, Ludwig M.** Paroxetine in the elderly depressed patient: randomized comparison with fluoxetine of efficacy, cognitive and behavioral effects. *Int Clin Psychopharmacol.* 1994;9:25–9.

68. **Hutchinson DR, Tong S, Moon CAL, et al.** Paroxetine in the treatment of elderly depressed patients in general practice: a double-blind comparison with amitriptyline. *Int Clin Psychopharmacol.* 1992;6(Suppl 4):43–51.

69. **Geretsegger C, Stuppaeck CH, Mair M, et al.** Multicenter double-blind study of paroxetine and amitriptyline in elderly depressed inpatients. *Psychopharmacology.* 1995;119:277–81.

70. **Cohn CK, Shrivastava R, Mendels J, et al.** Double-blind, multicenter comparison of sertraline and amitriptyline in elderly depressed patients. *J Clin Psychiatry.* 1990;51(Suppl B):28–33.

71. **Finkel S, Richter EM, Clary CM.** Comparative efficacy and safety of sertraline versus nortriptyline in major depression in patients 70 and older. *Int Psychogeriatr.* 1999;11:85–99.

72. **Tollefson GD, Bosomworth JC, Heiligenstein JH, et al.** A double-blind, placebo-controlled clinical trial of fluoxetine in geriatric patients with major depression. *Int Psychogeriatr.* 1995;7:89–104.

73. **Kyle CJ, Petersen HE, Overo KF.** Comparison of the tolerability and efficacy of citalopram and amitriptyline in elderly depressed patients treated in general practice. *Depress Anxiety.* 1998;8:147–53.

74. **Gottfries CG, Pollock BG.** Citalopram: its use in elderly patients. *Ann Long Term Care.* 1999;7:181–9.

75. **Reynolds CF, Frank E, Perel JM, et al.** Outcomes of maintenance therapies for recurrent major depression in patients older than 59 years: randomized controlled trial of nortriptyline and interpersonal psychotherapy. *JAMA.* 1999;281:39–45.

76. **Reynolds CF, Frank E, Dew MA, et al.** The challenge of treatment with 70+ year olds with major depression: excellent short-term but brittle long-term response. *Am J Geriatr Psychiatry.* 1999;7:64–9.

77. **Montgomery SA, Dunbar G.** Paroxetine is better than placebo in relapse prevention and the prophylaxis of recurrent depression. *Int Clin Psychopharmacol.* 1993;8:189–95.

78. **Montgomery SA, Rasmussen JGC, Tanghoj P.** A 24-week study of 20-mg citalopram, 40-mg citalopram, and placebo in the prevention of relapse of major depression. *Int Clin Psychopharmacol.* 1993;8:181–8.

79. **Franchini L, Gasperini M, Perez J, et al.** A double-blind study of long-term treatment with sertraline or fluvoxamine for prevention of highly recurrent unipolar depression. *J Clin Psychiatry.* 1997;58:104–7.

80. **Flint A, Rifat S.** *Recurrence Following Discontinuation of Antidepressant Medication for First-Episode Geriatric Depression.* Paper presented at the American Association for Geriatric Psychiatry meeting, March 8, 1998, San Diego, CA.

81. **Schweizer E, Weise C, Clary C, et al.** Placebo-controlled trial of venlafaxine for the treatment of major depression. *J Clin Psychopharmacol.* 1991;11:233–6.

82. **Hoyberg OJ, Maragakis B, Mullin J, et al.** A double-blind multicentre comparison of mirtazapine and amitriptyline in elderly depressed patients. *Acta Psychiatr Scand.* 1996;93:184–90.

83. **Halikas JA.** Org 3770 (mirtazapine) versus trazodone: a placebo-controlled trial in depressed elderly patients. *Hum Psychopharmacol.* 1995;10:S125–33.

84. **Alexopoulos GS, Chester JG.** Outcomes of geriatric depression. *Clin Geriatr Med.* 1992;8:363–73.

85. **Burvill PN, Hall WD, Stampfer HG, et al.** The prognosis of depression in old age. *Br J Psychiatry.* 1991;158:64–71.

86. **Stoudemire A, Hill CD, Marquardt M, et al.** Recovery and relapse in geriatric depression after treatment with antidepressants and ECT in a medical-psychiatry population. *Gen Hosp Psychiatry.* 1998;20:170–4.

87. **Colenda CC, Trinkle D, Hamer RM, Jones S.** Hospital utilization and readmission rates for geriatric and young adult patients with major depression: results from a historical cohort study. *J Geriatr Psychiatry Neurol.* 1991;4:166–74.

88. **Bonner D, Howard R.** Treatment-resistant depression in the elderly. *Int Psychogeriatr.* 1995;7(Suppl):83–94.

89. **Kaplitz SE.** Withdrawn, apathetic geriatric patients responsive to methylphenidate. *J Am Geriatr Soc.* 1975;23:271–6.

90. **Satel SL, Nelson JC.** Stimulants in the treatment of depression: a critical overview. *J Clin Psychiatry.* 1989;50:241–9.

91. **Volz HP, Gleiter CH.** Monoamine oxidase inhibitors: a perspective on their use in the elderly. *Drugs Aging.* 1998;13:341–55.

92. **Coffey CE, Figiel GS, Djang WT, et al.** Leukoencephalopathy in elderly depressed patients referred for ECT. *Biol Psychiatry.* 1988;24:143–61.

93. **Coffey CE, Weiner RD, Djang WT, et al.** Brain anatomic effects of electroconvulsive therapy: a prospective magnetic resonance imaging study. *Arch Gen Psychiatry.* 1991;48:1013–21.

94. **McCall WV, Farah A, Reboussin D, Colenda CC.** Comparison of the efficacy of titrated and fixed-dose right-unilateral ECT in the elderly. *Am J Geriatr Psychiatry.* 1995;3:317–24.

95. **Colenda CC, McCall WV.** A statistical model predicting the seizure threshold for right unilateral electroconvulsive therapy in 106 patients. *Convuls Ther.* 1996;12:3–12.

96. **Tomac TA, Rummans TA, Pileggi TS, Li H.** Safety and efficacy of electroconvulsive therapy in patients over age 85. *Am J Geriatr Psychiatry.* 1998;5:126–30.

97. **Katona C, Judge R.** Antidepressants for elderly people: should selective serotonin reuptake inhibitors (SSRIs) be the first-line choice? *Prim Care Psychiatry,* 1996;2:123–30.

98. **Niederehe G.** Psychosocial treatments with depressed older adults: a research update. *Am J Geriatr Psychiatry.* 1996;4(Suppl 1):S66–78.

99. **Scogin F, McElreath L.** Efficacy of psychosocial treatments for geriatric depression: a quantitative review. *J Clin Consult Psychol.* 1994;62:69–74.

100. **Kahn DK.** Other dementias and mental disorders due to general medical conditions. In Sadavoy J, Lazarus LW, Jarvik LF, Grossberg GT (eds). *Comprehensive Review of Geriatric Psychiatry,* 2nd ed. Washington DC: American Psychiatric Press; 1996:497–528.

101. **Zesiewicz TA, Gold M, Chari G, Hauser RA.** Current issues in depression in Parkinson's disease. *Am J Geriatr Psychiatry.* 1999;7:110–8.

102. **Cummings JL.** Depression and Parkinson's disease: a review. *Am J Psychiatry.* 1992;149:443–54.

103. **Mayeux R, Stern Y, Sano M, et al.** The relationship of serotonin to depression in Parkinson's disease. *Mov Disord.* 1988;3:237–44.

104. **Koller WC, Megaffin BB.** Parkinson's disease and parkinsonism. In Coffey CE, Cummings JL (eds). *Textbook of Geriatric Neuropsychiatry.* Washington, DC: American Psychiatric Press; 1994:434–56.

105. **Huber SJ, Freidenberg DL, Paulson GW, et al.** The pattern of depressive symptoms with the progression of Parkinson's disease. *J Neurol Neurosurg Psychiatry.* 1990;53:275–8.

106. **Rasmussen K, Abrams R.** Treatment of Parkinson's disease with electroconvulsive therapy. *Psychiatr Clin North Am.* 1991;14:925–33.

107. **Robinson RG, Price TR.** Post-stroke depressive disorders: a follow up study of 103 outpatients. *Stroke.* 1982;13:635–41.

108. **Kramer SI, Reifler BV.** Depression, dementia, and reversible dementia. *Arch Geriatr Med.* 1992;8:289–97.

109. **House A, Dennis M, Warlow C, et al.** Mood disorders in the first year after stroke. *Br J Psychiatry.* 1991;158:83–92.

110. **Robinson RG, Starr LB, Kubos KL, et al.** A two-year longitudinal study of post-stroke mood disorders: findings during the initial evaluation. *Stroke.* 1983;14:736–44.

111. **Morris PLP, Robinson RG, Raphael B.** Prevalence and course of depressive disorders in hospitalized stroke patients. *Int J Psychiatry Med.* 1990;20:349–64.

112. **Morris PLP, Robinson RG, Andrezejewski P, et al.** Association of depression with 10-year post-stroke mortality. *Am J Psychiatry.* 1993;150:124–9.

113. **Morris PLP, Robinson RG, Ralphael B.** Lesion location and depression in hospitalized stroke patients: evidence supporting a specific relationship in the left hemisphere. *Neuropsychiatry Neuropsychol Behav Neurol.* 1992;3:75–82.

114. **Federoff JP, Starkstein SE, Parikh RM, et al.** Are depressive symptoms nonspecific in patients with acute stroke? *Am J Psychiatry.* 1991;148:1172–6.

115. **Lipsey JR, Spencer WC, Rabins PV, et al.** Phenonomenolgocial comparison of functional and post-stroke depression. *Am J Psychiatry.* 1986;143:527–9.

116. **Lipsey JR, Robinson RG, Pearlson GF, et al.** Nortriptyline treatment of post-stroke depression. *Lancet.* 1984;1:297–300.

117. **Lazarus LW, Winemiller DR, Lingam VR, et al.** Efficacy and side effects of methylphenidate for post-stroke depression. *J Clin Psychiatry.* 1992;53:447–9.

118. **Jorm AF, van Duijn CM, Chandra V, et al.** Psychiatric history and related exposures as risk factors for Alzheimer's disease: a collaborative re-analysis of case-control studies. *Int J Epidemiol.* 1991;20(Suppl):43–7.

119. **Devanand DP, Sano M, Tang MX, et al.** Depressed mood and the incidence of Alzheimer's disease in the elderly living in the community. *Arch Gen Psychiatry.* 1996;53:175–82.

120. **Bassuk SS, Berkman LF, Wypij D.** Depressive symptomatology and incident cognitive decline in an elderly community sample. *Arch Gen Psychiatry.* 1998;55:1073–81.

121. **Dufouil C, Fuhrer R, Dartigues JF, Alperovitch A.** Longitudinal analysis of the association between depressive symptomatology and cognitive deterioration. *Am J Epidemiol.* 1996;144:634–41.

122. **Meyers BS, Bruce ML.** The depression-dementia conundrum: integrating clinical and epidemiological perspectives. *Arch Gen Psychiatry.* 1998;1082–3.

123. **Reifler BV, Larson E, Teri L, Poulsen M.** Dementia of the Alzheimer's type and depression. *J Am Geriatr Soc.* 1986;34:855–9.

124. **Reding M, Haycox J, Blass J.** Depression in patients referred to a dementia clinic. *Arch Neurol.* 1985;42:894–6.

125. **Kral V, Emery O.** Long-term follow-up of depressive pseudodementia. *Can J Psychiatry.* 1989;34:445–7.

126. **Reynolds CF, Kupfer DJ, Hoch CC, et al.** Two-year follow-up of elderly patients with mixed depression and dementia: clinical and electroencephalographic sleep findings. *J Am Geriatr Soc.* 1986;34:793–9.

127. **Copeland JRM, Davidson IA, Dewey ME, et al.** Alzheimer's disease, other dementias, depression, and pseudodementia: prevalance, incidence, and three-year outcome in Liverpool. *Br J Psychiatry.* 1992;161:230–9.

128. **Alexopoulos GS, Meyers BS, Young RC, et al.** The course of geriatric depression with "reversible dementia": a controlled study. *Am J Psychiatry.* 1993;150:1693–9.

129. **Caine E.** Pseudodementia: current concepts and future directions. *Arch Gen Psychiatry.* 1981;38:1359–64.

130. **Reynolds CF III, Hoch CC, Kupfer DJ, et al.** Bedside differentiation of depressive pseudodementia from dementia. *Am J Psychiatry.* 1988;145:1099–103.

131. **Raskind M.** The clinical interface of depression and dementia. *J Clin Psychiatry.* 1998;59(Suppl 10):9–12.

132. **Fisher R, Simamyi M, Danielczyk W.** Depression indementia of the Alzheimer type and multi-infarct dementia. *Am J Psychiatry.* 1990;147:1484–7.

133. **Pearlson GD, Ross CA, Lohr WD, et al.** Association between family history of affective disorder and the depressive syndrome of Alzheimer's disease. *Am J Psychiatry.* 1990;147:452–6.

134. **McGuire MH, Rabins PV.** Mood disorders. In Coffey CE, Cummings JL (eds). *Textbook of Geriatric Neuropsychiatry.* Washington, DC: American Psychiatric Press; 1994:246–60.

135. **Greenwald BS, Kramer-Ginsberg E, Marin DB, et al.** Dementia with coexistent major depression. *Am J Psychiatry.* 1989;146:1472–8.

136. **Alexopoulos GS, Abrams RC, Young RC, et al.** Cornell scale for depression in dementia. *Biol Psychiatry.* 1988;23:271–84.

137. **Sunderland T, Alterman IS, Yount D, et al.** A new scale for the assessment of depressed mood in demented patients. *Am J Psychiatry.* 1988;145:955–9.

138. **Reifler BV, Teri L, Raskind MA, et al.** A double-blind trial of imipramine in Alzheimer's disease patients with and without depression. *Am J Psychiatry.* 1989;146:45–9.

139. **Nyth AL, Gottfries CG.** The clinical efficacy of citalopram in treatment of emotional disturbances in dementia disorders. *Br J Psychiatry.* 1990;157:894–901.

140. **Volicer L, Rheaume Y, Cyr D.** Treatment of depression in advanced Alzheimer's disease using sertraline. *J Geriatr Psychiatry Neurol.* 1994;7:227–9.

141. **Zisook S, Shuchter SR, Sledge PA, et al.** The spectrum of depressive phenomena after spousal bereavement. *J Clin Psychiatry.* 1994;55:29–36.

142. **Reynolds CF, Miller MD, Pasternak RE, et al.** Treatment of bereavement-related major depressive episodes in late life: a controlled study of acute and continuation treatment with nortriptyline and psychotherapy. *Am J Psychiatry.* 1999;156:202–8.

143. **Zygmont M, Prigerson HG, Houck PR, et al.** A post-hoc comparison of paroxetine and nortriptyline for symptoms of traumatic grief. *J Clin Psychiatry.* 1998;59:241–5.

KEY REFERENCES

Alexopoulos GS, Meyers BS, Young RC, et al. Vacular depression hypothesis. *Arch Gen Psychiatry.* 1997;54:915–22.

This paper reviews the evidence that cerebral vascular disease contributes significantly to some geriatric depressive syndromes. The "vascular depression hypothesis" is supported by comorbidity of depression, vascular disease, white-matter lesions in the brain, and distinctive behavioral syndromes associated with late-life depression. The authors point to disruption of prefrontal systems or their modulating pathways as directly contributing to patients' vulnerability to late-life depression. The authors present a rationale for using depression as an outcome measure in prevention studies for cerebral vascular disease. Additionally, the choice of antidepressants for vascular depression may be influenced by their effect on neurologic recovery from ischemic lesions.

Gallo JJ, Rabins PV, Iliffe S. The "Research Magnificent" in late life: psychiatric epidemiology and the primary care of older adults. *Int J Psychiatry Med.* 1997;27: 185–204.

This article highlights four themes crucial to understanding affective disorders in older adults: subsyndromal depression, co-existing depression and anxiety, comorbidity of depression and chronic medical conditions, and risk factors for cognitive impairment. The authors conclude that the primary care setting is an important venue for explaining mental health issues in aging and that the value of research in primary care settings has been undervalued in the past. The authors conclude that integration of mental health services into primary care can maximize the health and quality of life of older adults and their families.

Reynolds CF, Frank E, Perel JM, et al. Outcomes of maintenance therapies for recurrent major depression in patients older than 59 years: randomized controlled trial of nortriptyline and interpersonal psychotherapy. *JAMA.* 1999;281:39–45.

This article reports on one of the few studies examining the efficacy of maintenance strategies to prevent relapse in geriatric depression. Although the average age of the patient cohort was relatively young (67 years), the randomized control trial was designed to establish the efficacy of maintenance nortriptyline and interpersonal psychotherapy (IPT) in preventing recurrence of major depressive episodes in patients. The main outcome measure was recurrence of major depression. The results found that patients who have a combination of nortriptyline and IPT had a lower recurrence rate (20%) compared with nortriptyline alone (43%), IPT and placebo (64%), and placebo alone (90%). Additionally, patients over 70 years of age had a substantially higher and more rapid relapse rate than those between 60 and 69 years of age. This study was the first to demonstrate that combined therapy seems to be the optimal clinical strategy to prevent relapse among geriatric patients.

Schneider LS. Pharmacologic considerations in the treatment of late-life depression. *Am J Geriatr Psychiatry.* 1996;4(Suppl 1):S51–65.

This article summarizes the pharmacotherapy evidence supporting the efficacy of antidepressant medications in late-life depression. The article provides a comprehensive review of the available randomized control trial evidence supporting the efficacy of both tricyclic antidepressants and selective serotonin-reuptake inhibitors. The author also reviews the importance of understanding the difference between efficacy and effectiveness. Efficacy is the measure of the medication's action when given to a defined population, whereas effectiveness is efficacy plus performance under real-world circumstances.

9

■ ■ ■

Depression in Women

Susan G. Kornstein, MD
Barbara A. Wojcik, MD

With the increasing interest in women's health, there is a growing literature on gender differences in the prevalence, clinical presentation, and treatment response of various medical and psychiatric disorders. This chapter focuses on special considerations in the evaluation and management of depression in women. Following a general overview of epidemiology, symptoms, comorbidity, course, and treatment issues, we discuss various depressive syndromes that are unique to women (e.g., premenstrual dysphoric disorder, depression during pregnancy and the postpartum period, and depression around the time of menopause).

Epidemiology

Major depression is approximately twice as common in women as in men. In the National Comorbidity Survey—a large epidemiologic study in the United States—the lifetime prevalence of major depressive disorder was 21% in women compared with 13% in men (1). This gender difference in prevalence rates of depression has been found consistently across ethnic groups and in cross-national studies (2).

Sex differences in rates of depression vary across the life cycle. During childhood, boys and girls show similar rates of depression. According to National Comorbidity Survey data, the gender difference in rates of depression begins around 10 years of age and persists until mid-life, after which the rates are again similar in men and women (1). Thus, it is during the child-bearing years that women show the greatest risk for depression.

The sex difference in prevalence of depression may be caused by many factors, including biological, psychological, social, and environmental influences (3–5). Some have questioned whether diagnostic bias, the greater tendency for women to seek help, and the greater likelihood of women to report emotional distress could lead to artifactual differences in rates of depression. However, the consistency of findings across cultures—in community and clinical samples—argues against this artifact hypothesis (4). Biological differences that may differentially predispose women to depression include differences in brain structure and function, genetic transmission, and reproductive function (3). Estrogen and progesterone have been shown to influence serotonin, norepinephrine, and other neurotransmitters that seem to be involved in depression. Psychosocial factors (e.g., gender-specific socialization, role stress, victimization, an internalizing coping style, disadvantaged social status) also may contribute to women's increased vulnerability to depression (3).

Women seem to be more sensitive than are men to developing a depressive episode after a stressful life event (6). Seasonal changes may precipitate episodes of depression in women; nearly 80% of individuals with seasonal affective disorder are women (7). In addition, some women are prone to developing depression in relation to the reproductive cycle, such as premenstrually, during the postpartum period, and during the perimenopausal years (3). (These reproductive-related depressions are discussed in detail later in the chapter). Other reproductive experiences, including infertility, miscarriage or pregnancy loss, and various hormonal therapies (e.g., oral contraceptives, hormone replacement therapy [particularly, the progesterone component], hormones used in infertility treatment) also may be causes of depressive symptoms in women (3).

Assessment of Depression in Women

The diagnostic evaluation of depression in women requires some special considerations. First, there may be gender differences in symptom presentation. Although men typically exhibit classic neurovegetative features of depression (e.g., insomnia, weight loss), women are more likely to present with atypical or reverse neurovegetative features (e.g., increased appetite, weight gain) (8,9). In addition, depressed women tend to experience more anxiety and somatic symptoms (8,9) as well as a greater number of depressive symptoms compared with men (10) Women also are more likely to attempt suicide, although the rate of completed suicide is higher in men (11).

Second, depressed women often present with comorbid psychiatric or general medical conditions (3). The presence of such comorbid disorders may complicate both the diagnosis and treatment of depression and tends to be associated with a worse prognosis (12). Among psychiatric disorders, anxiety disorders are most frequently comorbid with depression in women (13). Other common comorbid psychiatric disorders in depressed women include eating disorders and borderline personality disorder. Although alcoholism is much more prevalent in men (in whom it usually precedes the onset of depression), women are more likely than men to develop alcoholism once they are depressed (14).

Comorbid general medical disorders common in depressed women include migraine headaches, thyroid disease, chronic fatigue syndrome, chronic pelvic pain, irritable bowel syndrome, and fibromyalgia (15). Women are nearly three times as likely as are men to experience depression and migraines together (16), and the lifetime incidence of major depression in fibromyalgia patients is reported to be as high as 50% (17). It is important to differentiate between a comorbid and a secondary depressive disorder. For example, thyroid disease may be either a cause of depression or a comorbid disorder. Thyroid screening generally is recommended for depressed women aged 45 years and over or for women with a personal or family history of thyroid disease (18).

It is important to consider the influence of the menstrual cycle when evaluating a female patient who presents with depression (3,19). Women should be asked where they are in their menstrual cycle at the time of assessment and at subsequent visits. If a patient's depression is occurring only during the premenstrual period and has a cyclical pattern, the diagnosis may be premenstrual dysphoric disorder rather than major depression. In addition, many women with an ongoing depressive disorder experience a worsening of symptoms during the premenstrual time (19,20). Knowing the patient's menstrual phase and symptom pattern throughout the cycle is important to assess accurately the severity of depression, suicide risk, and response to treatment. Similarly, it is important to consider a woman's menopausal status in evaluating her depression; for example, her symptoms of insomnia, depressed mood, and concentration difficulties may be due to perimenopausal changes rather than to depression.

Finally, it is important to assess carefully the psychosocial factors that may be contributing to either the onset or maintenance of depression in women (3). Although marriage is generally protective against depression, this is less true for women than for men; in unhappy marriages, women are much more likely than men to become depressed (21). A satisfying job outside the home may help to protect a woman from depression but only if she has chosen to work rather than being forced to do so by financial pressures. The presence of young children at home is also a risk factor for depression in women, especially if the woman works and has difficulty finding child care (22). A history of abuse or victimization is another important risk factor, for as many as 69% of abused women develop depression (23).

Treatment of Depression in Women

As for assessment, there are unique considerations for the treatment of depression in women. The array of treatment options includes pharmacotherapy, psychotherapy, and combination treatment. Selecting the appropriate treatment requires a careful assessment of the underlying causes, precipitating factors, and comorbid disorders as well as a consideration of the woman's reproductive stage of life (e.g., plans about pregnancy or breast-feeding). In addition, it is important to consider side-effect profiles; for example, many women will refuse to take an antidepressant that may cause weight gain or affect their sexual functioning.

Although most of psychotropic medications are prescribed to women, knowledge about how pharmacotherapy for depression in women differs from men is limited because of past exclusion of women from clinical trials. Sex differences in pharmacokinetics have been demonstrated, including differences in drug absorption, bioavailability, distribution, metabolism, and elimination (24). These differences may result in higher plasma levels and longer half-lives of drugs in women as well as in a greater sensitivity to side effects (24). Levels of antidepressant medications in women also may be affected by hormonal therapies, such as oral contraceptives (24). In addition, there is some evidence that drug levels may vary with the menstrual cycle (25) and during pregnancy (26).

There is a growing body of evidence suggesting that women may respond differently than do men to some antidepressants (3,27). For instance, several studies have shown that women respond less well to tricyclic antidepressants (TCAs) than do men (27,28) and may respond better to selective serotonin-reuptake inhibitors (SSRIs) (27). Differences in response in premenopausal versus postmenopausal women also have been suggested (27). Some researchers have noted that women may respond more slowly to pharmacotherapy and therefore may need a longer course of treatment (8) There also may be different considerations for augmentation strategies to enhance antidepressant response in women. For example, thyroid hormone augmentation has been shown to be more effective in women than in men (18), and some studies suggest that estrogen may be useful as an adjunct to antidepressant treatment in peri- and postmenopausal women (29). (*See* Chapter 7 for more information on augmentation strategies.)

Psychotherapy is an effective treatment for depression in women, both alone and in combination with pharmacotherapy. Individual therapies that have been proven to be helpful in women include cognitive-behavior therapy and interpersonal therapy (30). Group therapy and marital therapy are also important treatment options. Some researchers have emphasized that a combined treatment approach with medications and psychotherapy may be especially beneficial for depressed women (6).

Reproductive Mood Syndromes in Women

Various reproductive events (e.g., the premenstruum, pregnancy, the post-partum period, and the perimenopause period) may trigger the onset of depressive symptoms in some women (3). A history of one reproductive-related depression seems to be a risk factor for depression in association with other reproductive events (31). There may be a subgroup of women who are particularly vulnerable to the development of mood disturbances at times of hormonal fluctuation.

Premenstrual Dysphoric Disorder

Diagnosis
As many as 75% of women report some premenstrual symptoms (e.g., bloating, breast tenderness, mood swings) during their reproductive life-time (32,33). In 3% to 8% of menstruating women, the symptoms are se-vere enough to be diagnosed as premenstrual dysphoric disorder (PMDD) (32). PMDD has been classified as a psychiatric disorder, specifically as a mood disorder. It is classified in the *Diagnostic and Statistical Manual of Mental Disorders*, fourth edition (DSM-IV) as a depressive disorder not oth-erwise specified (34).

According to DSM-IV criteria, women with PMDD have symptoms showing a regular cyclical relationship to the luteal phase of the menstrual cycle (34). Symptoms typically begin 7 to 10 days before menses and remit within a few days after the onset of the follicular phase. PMDD differs from the broader category of premenstrual syndrome (PMS) in that it requires a mood disturbance (e.g., depressed mood, irritability, anxiety, mood labil-ity); in contrast, PMS may have either mood or physical symptoms or both. In addition to the specific symptom criteria, the diagnosis of PMDD re-quires that the symptoms must be severe enough to cause impairment in social or occupational functioning (34). Many women experience mildly unpleasant mood changes premenstrually, but they are not severe enough to interfere with their work, social activities, or relationships (33).

To meet criteria for PMDD, the symptoms must not represent merely an exacerbation of an underlying disorder (34). Premenstrual exacerbation of symptoms is seen commonly with many medical and psychiatric disorders, including asthma, seizures, migraines, and mood and anxiety disorders (20). Finally, DSM-IV requires that the diagnosis of PMDD must be con-firmed by at least two cycles of prospective daily ratings of mood changes (34). To qualify for the diagnosis, the charting must show severe symptoms during the late luteal phase of the cycle and few to no symptoms during the follicular phase (33). The Daily Record of Severity of Problems is one popular validated self-report instrument for prospective charting of symp-toms (35). Patients' retrospective reports of premenstrual symptomatology have been shown to be unreliable as a basis for diagnosis (36). Criteria for PMDD are summarized in Table 9.1.

Although numerous biological and psychosocial theories have been proposed, the pathogenesis of PMDD has not been explained definitively (33). The fall in estrogen and progesterone levels during the late luteal phase certainly may play a role in triggering symptoms in vulnerable women; however, recent attention has focused on a dysregulation of the serotonin system as a cause of PMDD (32). An association between PMDD and major depression has been described. In a study of women with PMDD, 78% were found to have a lifetime history of psychiatric disorder, with major depressive disorder being most common (37); moreover, a history of PMS has been shown to predict future major depressive episodes (38).

Treatment

Serotonergic antidepressants increasingly have been shown to be effective treatments for PMDD and depression (33). Fluoxetine, sertraline, paroxe-

---

Table 9.1   Criteria for Premenstrual Dysphoric Disorder

- Cyclic recurrence of symptoms during late luteal phase of menstrual cycle

- Few to no symptoms during follicular phase of menstrual cycle

- At least five of the following 11 symptoms are present, with at least one being a mood disturbance:

  Depressed mood

  Irritability

  Anxiety, tension

  Mood lability

  Decreased interest

  Concentration difficulties

  Fatigue

  Change in appetite or food cravings

  Changes in sleep

  Feeling out of control

  Physical symptoms (e.g., breast tenderness, bloating, headache)

- Symptoms cause functional impairment

- Not merely an exacerbation of another disorder

- Diagnosis confirmed by two cycles of prospective daily ratings

---

Adapted from American Psychiatric Association. *Diagnostic and Statistical Manual of Mental Disorders*, 4th ed. Washington, DC: American Psychiatric Press; 1994.

tine, and clomipramine all have demonstrated efficacy in placebo-controlled trials, using continuous dosing throughout the cycle (39–42). Other classes of antidepressants may not be equally effective; for example, bupropion (42a) and the noradrenergic compound maprotiline (42b) were less effective than SSRIs in placebo-controlled trials. Several preliminary studies suggest that SSRIs may be used only during the luteal phase with similar efficacy (39,43). A variable dosing strategy, with continuous treatment plus luteal-phase dose increases, may be useful in some cases. The SSRIs are currently the first-line treatment for PMDD.

Other treatments for PMDD include hormonal interventions, anxiolytics, and various other symptomatic treatments (33). Gonadotropin-releasing–hormone (GnRH) agonists, which essentially induce "medical menopause," have demonstrated effectiveness; however, their long-term use is limited by the resulting hypoestrogenism. Preliminary studies suggest that GnRH agonists combined with low-dose estrogen and progesterone "add-back" therapy may permit long-term use (44). Estradiol implants and transdermal patches and the synthetic androgen danazol also have been proven effective (33). Despite its popularity, progesterone has been shown to be ineffective in numerous placebo-controlled trials (45). For severe refractory cases, oophorectomy may be considered.

Alprazolam has been shown in several studies to improve premenstrual anxiety, tension, irritability, and insomnia when used during the late luteal phase (46); buspirone also has demonstrated efficacy in one trial (47). Diuretics and nonsteroidal anti-inflammatory agents may be helpful adjuncts for the relief of physical symptoms, such as fluid retention, cramps, and headaches (33,48). Bromocriptine may relieve premenstrual mastodynia (33). Lifestyle changes (e.g., dietary modifications, exercise, stress management) and nutritional supplements (e.g., vitamin B_6, calcium, magnesium), which have been used widely to treat mild premenstrual symptoms (despite lack of proven efficacy in many cases), have not been studied for PMDD (49).

Depression During Pregnancy

Contrary to popular belief, pregnancy is not protective against depression. The prevalence of depressive symptoms during pregnancy is approximately 25% to 35% (32), with approximately 10% of women meeting criteria for a major depressive disorder (rates are similar to nonpregnant women) (50). It is sometimes difficult to separate the neurovegetative signs and symptoms of depression (e.g., changes in sleep, changes in appetite, fatigue, decreased libido) from the normal experience of pregnancy (51). Symptoms that may be more specific to a depressive episode include lack of interest in the pregnancy, guilty rumination, and anhedonia (52). Depressive symptoms seem to be most likely to occur during the first or third trimester of pregnancy, although studies have shown conflicting results (53–55).

One of the major risk factors for depression during pregnancy is a previous history of depression. As many as 50% of women who discontinue an antidepressant before conception may experience a recurrence of the illness during the course of the pregnancy, requiring treatment (52). Other risk factors for depression during pregnancy include the following (51,56–58):

- Younger age
- Limited social support (especially from the father of the child)
- Living alone
- A greater number of children
- Marital conflict
- Ambivalence about the pregnancy
- Comorbid illness
- Closely spaced pregnancies
- Illness or death of a significant other
- Death of previous children
- Chronic stressors

In evaluating the risks versus benefits of treating depression during pregnancy, one must strongly consider the impact of untreated illness on the mother and fetus. Depression during pregnancy can lead to inadequate self-care, poor nutrition, smoking and substance abuse, failure to follow prenatal care guidelines, obstetric complications, increased risk of postpartum depression, and rarely suicide (51,52,59). As with depression at other times, mild to moderate symptoms may be addressed first with psychotherapy, such as cognitive or interpersonal therapy (30). However, in the case of moderate to severe depression, or when the illness poses a risk to mother or fetus, treatment with antidepressant medications should be considered (although the FDA has not approved any antidepressant medication for use during pregnancy) or even electroconvulsive therapy (ECT) in extreme or treatment-resistant depression (52).

Despite the lack of FDA approval, available data on the reproductive safety of antidepressant medications suggest relatively low teratogenic potential (52). It is important to educate the patient about known risks and benefits of treatment and to obtain informed consent, which should be documented carefully in progress notes. Because all psychotropic drugs cross the placenta to some degree via simple diffusion, it is preferable to wait until after the first trimester to institute therapy, if possible (32,60). Unfortunately, most women are not aware of their pregnancy for the first 6 weeks, which is also the period of greatest teratogenic risk (60). In addition to concerns about teratogenicity, other possible risks of prenatal exposure include direct toxicity to the fetus or neonate and long-term neurobehavioral sequelae (61).

The most extensive literature on reproductive safety exists for the TCAs and fluoxetine, which have shown no increased risk of teratogenicity after first-trimester exposure in both prospective and retrospective studies (52).

Desipramine and nortriptyline are preferred among the TCAs due to lower anticholinergic effects (60). A formal registry of 1900 cases exists for fluoxetine in pregnancy compared with only several hundred cases of TCA use in the literature (52). Safety data about the use of other SSRIs during pregnancy are insufficient; however, those with shorter half-lives may allow time for discontinuation after early documentation of pregnancy in women trying to conceive (52). The safety profiles for the monoamine oxidase inhibitors (MAOIs) bupropion, trazodone, venlafaxine, mirtazapine, and nefazodone are also unknown. In case reports, TCAs have been shown uncommonly to cause a neonatal withdrawal syndrome that consists of jitteriness, irritability, and seizures; functional bowel obstruction and urinary retention also have been described (61). With the exception of one case report of abruptio placentae, ECT is considered a safe and viable treatment option, especially for severe melancholic depression (Case 9.1) (62).

Patients taking antidepressant medications during pregnancy should be monitored closely for relapse, because antidepressant blood levels may decrease secondary to the physiologic changes of pregnancy (e.g., increased plasma volume, renal clearance, and liver enzyme activity); higher antidepressant doses may be required as the pregnancy progresses (26,63). Tapering the medication 1 to 2 weeks before delivery prevents potential maternal toxicity (due to restoration of physiologic function to pre-pregnancy levels) or withdrawal symptoms in the newborn (60). However, the increased risk of re-emergence of depression during the postpartum period also should be strongly considered, especially in women with previous postpartum depressive episodes.

CASE 9.1 *Major depression in pregnancy*

A woman 25 years of age who was 15-weeks' pregnant presented demanding an abortion for an unplanned pregnancy. The patient described a 6-month history of depressive symptoms, which had worsened over the 2 weeks before presentation. Symptoms included persistent low mood, tearfulness, decreased appetite with weight loss, poor sleep, social withdrawal, overwhelming anxiety, hopelessness, and worthlessness. The patient had been consistently noncompliant with recommendations for prenatal care. She was the primary caretaker of a 3-year-old son and reported feelings of inadequacy as a mother. Psychosocial stressors included marital conflict, financial difficulties, and recent loss of employment. Four months earlier, her primary care physician had prescribed bupropion, which was discontinued after evidence of the pregnancy.

At the time of presentation, the patient was started on fluoxetine but continued to worsen and required hospitalization due to cessation of oral intake. ECT was instituted, with subsequent dramatic improvement in both mood and neurovegetative symptoms.

On discharge from the hospital, the patient decided to continue her pregnancy and enrolled in prenatal care.

Postpartum Depressive Conditions

The postpartum period is an extremely vulnerable time for the onset of mood symptoms. Three primary conditions have been described: postpartum blues, postpartum depression, and postpartum psychosis (Table 9.2).

Postpartum Blues

The postpartum blues is a time-limited cluster of depressive symptoms occurring in new mothers during the first 2 weeks after delivery. The symptoms typically begin by the third postpartum day, with a peak in severity at days 4 or 5 and resolution by days 10 to 12 (64–66). Women usually complain of depressed mood, tearfulness, anxiety, irritability, emotional lability, sleep disturbance, and decreased appetite (67). Because approximately 50% to 80% of women will experience varying levels of the postpartum blues (66), this syndrome does not necessarily indicate psychopathology. However, up to 25% of those affected will experience persistence of symptoms and subsequent postpartum depression (65). Therefore, re-evaluation of the diagnosis is needed if the woman's distress persists beyond 2 weeks postpartum (64).

Although the pathophysiology of postpartum blues is unknown, several risk factors have been identified (66):

- Employment
- Interpersonal difficulties

Table 9.2   Characteristics of Postpartum Depressive Conditions

Postpartum Blues

- 50%–80% of new mothers
- Self-limited symptoms occurring during first 2 weeks postpartum
- Management is education and reassurance

Postpartum Depression

- 10%–15% of new mothers
- Past history of depression and depressive symptoms during pregnancy are major risk factors
- Symptoms and management similar to nonpostpartum major depressive episodes, except for considerations of breastfeeding

Postpartum Psychosis

- 0.1%–0.2% of new mothers
- Usually an affective disorder, with risk of suicide or infanticide
- Often requires psychiatric hospitalization

- Stressful life events (e.g., an infant with health problems)
- A personal or family history of depression
- A history of premenstrual depression
- Depressive symptoms during pregnancy
- Nighttime labor
- Sleep disruption late in pregnancy

Because most cases resolve spontaneously, management consists primarily of support, close monitoring, education, and reassurance as to the normality of the experience (66,67).

Postpartum Depression

The DSM-IV defines postpartum depression as a major depressive episode occurring within the first 4 weeks after childbirth (34); however, many researchers use 6 months or longer as the criterion for symptom onset. The symptoms experienced are those of major depression, often with prominent anxiety, ruminations and obsessions about the health of the infant, guilt, and agitation (66). Overall, suicidality is less common than with nonpostpartum depression (68). Symptoms often begin as early as the first week postpartum (66), with a peak in prevalence around the tenth week (67).

The incidence of postpartum depression in new mothers is 10% to 15% (64,66). Although a past history of major depression is associated with a 25% to 35% risk of postpartum depression, up to 50% of those affected are first-time sufferers (69). Once a woman has experienced postpartum depression, there is a 50% risk of subsequent puerperal episodes (57,64), and up to 40% will experience a nonpostpartum major depressive episode (67). Another strong predictor of postpartum depression is the presence of depressive symptoms during pregnancy, which is associated with a 35% risk (32,51). Additional risk factors for postpartum depression include family history of depression or postpartum depression, lack of social support (especially from the woman's spouse or partner), stressful life events in the year preceding delivery, and difficulties with the newborn (e.g., health problems, irritability) (51,70). It is interesting to note that age, multiparity, obstetrical complications, and breastfeeding do not increase a woman's risk of postpartum depression (71).

There are many proposed causes for postpartum depression, although none has been proven. A history of premenstrual syndrome may indicate a sensitivity to hormonal shifts, implicating the precipitous fall in estrogen postpartum (66). Hypothyroidism occurs in 10% of postpartum women, peaking at 4 to 5 months after delivery; decreased thyroid function has been found to correlate with decreased blood levels of serotonin (51,68). Investigation of other hormones, such as cortisol and prolactin, have found no consistent relationship with mood symptoms postpartum (66,68). Some researchers believe that hormonal changes contribute primarily to depression beginning in the early postpartum weeks, with psychosocial factors serving as the major precipitant for later-onset depression (66).

DIAGNOSIS AND TREATMENT

The importance of prompt diagnosis and treatment of postpartum depression deserves special emphasis. In addition to the impact of depression on the patient and family, untreated postpartum depression may have significant negative effects on infant development. Depressed mothers are often less responsive and affectionate toward their infants. Even after the mother's recovery, these children may show decreased developmental performance, less emotional responsiveness, behavioral problems, and cognitive deficits (66).

A general guideline is to treat depression that lasts for more than 2 weeks during the postpartum period. Education and support of both the patient and family are important aspects of treatment. Psychotherapy may be used either alone or in combination with medications and can address issues such as maternal guilt, poor self-esteem, and marital conflict (67). In addition to individual therapies, group, marital, or family therapy may be helpful (64,66).

For women who choose not to breastfeed, the pharmacologic approach to treatment of postpartum depression is similar to the treatment of nonpostpartum depressive episodes in terms of antidepressant choice, dosing, and duration of treatment (64,67). Preliminary studies suggest that antidepressants begun at the time of delivery may significantly protect against recurrence in women with a previous history of postpartum depression (72). A role for estrogen supplementation in both treatment and prophylaxis also has been suggested, but further study is needed (73,74). When discussing postpartum contraceptive options, patients should be counseled that oral contraceptives may exacerbate depressive symptoms (66).

The limited data available on the use of antidepressant medications during lactation confirm that they are excreted into breast milk; however, reports of adverse effects on nursing infants are few (60,61,75,76). Although the safety of the SSRIs has not been established clearly, most studies have found no adverse effects in mother or child (67,75). A recent study of sertraline reported infant blood levels below the level of detection (<1 ng/mL) in the majority of samples (76,77). There has been one case report of fluoxetine accumulating in the serum of an infant and causing symptoms of colic, gastrointestinal distress, irritability, and insomnia (78). Another case report described respiratory depression in an 8-week-old nursing infant that correlated temporally with an increase in the maternal dose of the tricyclic doxepin; the symptoms resolved within 24 hours of discontinuation of the medication (79).

As with the treatment of depression during pregnancy, the decision to use antidepressants in a woman who chooses to breastfeed should include evaluation of the risk-to-benefit ratio, especially the severity of the illness, the risk of harm to the mother and infant if no treatment is given, the mother's level of functional impairment, and the mother's preferences about treatment. Because no single antidepressant seems to be safer than the others, the clinician is advised to choose a medication based on previous treatment response and side effects experienced by the mother (64,76). Among the TCAs, the secondary amines (e.g., desipramine, nortriptyline) are preferred (60). Medications with a short half-life and few active metabolites are recommended; medication doses should be kept as low as possible and feeding and dosage schedules adjusted to minimize infant exposure (66,69). Close communication with the involved pediatrician is advised (76).

PREVENTION AND SCREENING

Attention to both prevention and screening for postpartum depression is important. Psychoeducational groups during the pregnancy and postpartum periods have been shown to decrease the incidence of postpartum depression (64). Women who take 3 to 6 months of maternity leave have been found to experience fewer depressive symptoms than those who must return to work sooner (58). All women should be monitored carefully and screened for depression during the postpartum period; routine follow-up visits with the obstetrician or pediatrician may provide this opportunity (64). The Edinburgh Postnatal Depression Scale has been validated for use as a screening instrument during this time (80); the Beck Depression Inventory also is used frequently (64).

Postpartum Psychosis

Postpartum psychosis is believed to be a variant of bipolar disorder, with prominent cognitive impairment and bizarre behavior (67). Symptoms include severe dysphoria or elated mood, mood lability, disorganized behavior, delusions, hallucinations, feelings of depersonalization, confusion, disorientation, and agitation. Women with postpartum psychosis may pose a threat to themselves and their infant and almost always require hospitalization and aggressive treatment. The onset of symptoms is usually within 2 weeks and often as early as 2 to 3 days after delivery (64,66).

The incidence of postpartum psychosis is 0.1% to 0.2% of new mothers, with 78% of cases occurring after a woman's first delivery (66). Approximately 50% of those affected will experience a recurrence with subsequent deliveries (52); the relapse rate for those who deliver again within 24 months of the index episode is as high as 70% (64). Other major risk factors for postpartum psychosis are a personal or family history of psychosis or major affective disorder, especially bipolar disorder (66). Although the great majority of episodes of postpartum psychosis are severe mood disorders, the clinician must rule out organic causes, including postpartum thyroiditis, Sheehan's syndrome, or intracranial mass (66).

The standard for pharmacologic treatment of postpartum psychosis is mood stabilizers (lithium, valproic acid, or carbamazepine), with benzodiazepines as needed for agitation and neuroleptics for psychotic symptoms. Care should be taken to minimize the dose and duration of neuroleptic use, because young women with mood disorders are at increased risk of developing tardive dyskinesia (67). Antidepressants should be avoided if possible, because they may induce rapid cycling. In severe cases (e.g., when suicide or infanticide is a concern), ECT may be the treatment of choice (67). If the patient has no previous psychiatric history, mood stabilizers and antipsychotics may be tapered safely and discontinued after a 9- to 12-month symptom-free period (66).

The severity of this disorder makes prevention a key concern. All women with a past history of bipolar disorder should have a prepartum evaluation. Prophylaxis with a mood stabilizer within 24 hours of delivery should be strongly considered (66). Otherwise, symptoms should be monitored closely and therapy instituted immediately with the occurrence of even mild symptoms (66,67).

The American Academy of Pediatrics considers both valproic acid and carbamazepine to be compatible with breastfeeding (66). Valproic acid accumulates less in breast milk than carbamazepine, with infant serum levels at 1.5% to 6.0% of maternal levels compared with 15.0% for carbamazepine (81). There have been reports of transient hepatotoxicity in neonates with carbamazepine, consisting of cholestasis and elevated levels of gamma-glutamyl transferase (75). The current recommendation when using either anticonvulsant is to monitor the infant's liver function tests, bilirubin, and white blood cell count (66,76).

Lithium, on the other hand, is not recommended for use during lactation (76). Its levels in breast milk closely approach maternal serum levels, with subsequent infant serum levels ranging from 18% to 65% of maternal levels (66). This concern is further complicated by significantly decreased renal clearance in infants under 5 months of age (66). If lithium must be used, the mother should not breastfeed. If she is nonadherent to this recommendation, the infant should be monitored closely for hypotonia, lethargy, cyanosis, and hydration status, because dehydration can increase the concentration of lithium in the blood and increase the risk of toxicity (76).

Menopause and Depression

Causes and Diagnosis

Occurring at a mean age of 51 years among U.S. women, natural menopause is defined as the cessation of menses for 1 year, with a follicle-stimulating–hormone (FSH) level consistently greater than 40 IU/L and an estradiol level less than 25 pg/mL (82). Menopause also may be induced surgically in younger women through oophorectomy.

Although menopause was once thought to cause a specific depressive disorder, which was termed "involutional melancholia," current research indicates that the onset of menopause is not associated with an increased risk of depression (83). However, minor mood symptoms that do not meet criteria for major depression are seen commonly during the perimenopause period—the 5 to 7 years preceding menopause (82). Women who experience a protracted perimenopause or have a surgically induced menopause seem to be at higher risk for depressive symptoms (32,83). In addition to these minor symptoms, women with a history of major depressive disorder show an increased risk of recurrence during the perimenopausal years (1). Women who experience depression during this time are likely to have had a past history of reproductive-related depression, such as PMDD or postpartum depression (31).

At times, the psychological symptoms of perimenopause (e.g., dysphoria, impaired concentration, irritability, emotional lability, anxiety, insomnia, decreased libido) may be difficult to distinguish from the manifestations of a depressive disorder. Women who seek help from a menopause clinic are likely to be those who suffer from psychological symptoms; at least 65% of patients who seek treatment for menopausal symptoms have symptoms of a major or minor depression (84–86).

There are three main theories about the possible cause of depressive symptoms during the perimenopause. First, the symptoms may result from changes in reproductive hormone production (82,86,87). Estradiol, a product of the ovary, is the primary premenopausal estrogen. Postmenopausally, the primary circulating hormone is estrone, a weaker estrogen that results from peripheral conversion. This shift may alter possible antidepressant effects of estrogen on neurotransmitters (e.g., norepinephrine, serotonin, acetylcholine). In addition, postmenopausal testosterone production is one third the premenopausal level (87). A second theory is that depressive symptoms may be caused or exacerbated by the primary somatic symptoms of menopause (82,87). For example, hot flushes, which occur primarily at night, may disturb sleep and consequently affect mood.

A psychosocial explanation for the depressive symptoms during the perimenopausal period is that the symptoms result from the stress of role changes that women experience during mid-life, such as taking care of elderly parents, children leaving home, and increased personal health problems (82). In addition, a woman's expectations of menopause may profoundly affect her experience and adjustment. For example, women who expect disturbing hot flushes have been found to have higher levels of depressive symptoms postmenopausally. In contrast, women who expect benefit from menopause, or who feel that education and a positive outlook will result in a positive experience, seem to have higher levels of support and fewer symptoms (85).

Treatment

Hormone replacement therapy, which can effect dramatic improvements in the somatic symptoms of menopause, has been shown to improve both quality and length of life (85,87). In addition, it has been shown to have positive mood effects in women with or without mild depressive symptoms (87–89). For women who have not undergone a hysterectomy, estrogen replacement therapy must be balanced with progesterone, which has been known to cause dysphoria (86,87). There is some evidence that androgens may be useful both for mood symptoms and for postmenopausal sexual dysfunction, especially decreased libido (86,89).

All middle-aged women who meet criteria for a major depressive episode should be treated with antidepressants, psychotherapy, or both (Case 9.2) (82). Replacement doses of estrogen are ineffective as monotherapy for major depression (32,82,87). However, recent studies do suggest a possible role for estrogen as an augmentation strategy in peri- and postmenopausal women with refractory depression (28,90,91).

For a middle-aged woman who presents with mild depressive symptoms, FSH and estradiol levels should be checked to determine menopausal status. If the woman is premenopausal, she should be referred for psychotherapy, antidepressant treatment, or both. If she is perimenopausal or menopausal, a trial of hormonal therapy is warranted, especially if somatic and vasomotor symptoms are prominent. If this approach is not effective, it is reasonable to add antidepressant therapy and psychotherapy.

CASE 9.2 *Depression in menopause*

A woman 50 years of age presented with menstrual cycle changes, hot flushes, insomnia, and low mood. Further history revealed a postpartum major depressive episode after the birth of her first child and a recent diagnosis of degenerative joint disease. The patient also noted that she recently had become the primary caretaker for her mother, who had suffered a cerebrovascular accident 4 months earlier. A detailed interview with the patient revealed a major depressive episode with crying spells, decreased appetite, guilty rumination about her mother, feelings of hopelessness, and suicidal ideation.

FSH and estradiol levels were drawn, which indicated early menopausal status. The patient was started on hormone replacement therapy and an SSRI and was referred for individual psychotherapy. Vasomotor symptoms, depressed mood, and insomnia resolved after 6 weeks.

■ ■ ■

Recommendations

- The diagnosis and treatment of women with depression should include consideration of gender differences in symptomatology, comorbid disorders, hormonal factors, and differences in pharmacokinetics and treatment response.
- Mild premenstrual mood symptoms should be managed with lifestyle changes and a symptom-oriented approach. For moderate to severe symptoms that meet criteria for premenstrual dysphoric disorder, a trial of an SSRI should be instituted as a first-line agent, using month-long or possibly luteal-phase dosing.
- Although minor self-limited depressive symptoms are common during the immediate weeks postpartum, depressive symptoms that persist for more than 2 weeks constitute a major depressive episode and should be treated as such.
- Hormonal therapy effectively relieves minor depressive symptoms associated with the perimenopause; however, symptoms that satisfy criteria for a major depressive episode require antidepressant treatment, psychotherapy, or both.

■ ■ ■

Key Points

- Women show a greater prevalence rate of depression than do men, especially during the child-bearing years; in addition, gender differences have been demonstrated in both presentation and treatment response.
- Depressive symptoms in women commonly occur in association with reproductive events, such as premenstrually, during pregnancy and the postpartum period, and during the perimenopausal years.
- Although the exact cause of premenstrual dysphoric disorder remains elusive, effective treatments are available, including antidepressant medications and hormonal therapies.
- Available data suggest that many antidepressants may be used with minimal risk in pregnant or breast-feeding mothers. The risks of untreated illness or relapse should be strongly considered in the decision about whether to treat in such cases.

• Although the onset of menopause is not associated with an increased risk of major depression, hormonal fluctuations and changing life roles may contribute to minor depressive symptoms during the perimenopausal period as well as to an increased likelihood of recurrence among women with previous depressive episodes.

▦   ▦   ▦

REFERENCES

1. **Kessler RC, McGonagle KA, Swartz M, et al.** Sex and depression in the National Comorbidity Survey. Part I: Lifetime prevalence, chronicity, and recurrence. *J Affect Disord.* 1993;29:85–96.

2. **Weissman MM, Bland R, Joyce PR, et al.** Sex differences in rates of depression: cross-national perspectives. *J Affect Disord.* 1993;29:77–84.

3. **Kornstein SG.** Gender differences in depression: implications for treatment. *J Clin Psychiatry.* 1997;58(Suppl 15):12–8.

4. **Wolk SI, Weissman MM.** Women and depression. In *Annual Review of Psychiatry*, vol. 14. Washington, DC: American Psychiatric Association Press; 1995:59–95.

5. **Blehar MC, Oren DA.** Women's vulnerability to mood disorders: integrating psychobiology and epidemiology. *Depression.* 1995;3:3–12.

6. **Karp JF, Frank E.** Combination therapy and the depressed women. *Depression.* 1995;3:91–8.

7. **Leibenluft E, Hardin TA, Rosenthal NE.** Gender differences in seasonal affective disorder. *Depression.* 1995;3:13–9.

8. **Frank E, Carpenter LL, Kupfer DJ.** Sex differences in recurrent depression: Are there any that are significant? *Am J Psychiatry.* 1988;145:41–5.

9. **Kornstein SG, Schatzberg AF, Yonkers KA, et al.** Gender differences in presentation of chronic major depression. *Psychopharmacol Bull.* 1996;31:711–8.

10. **Angst J, Dobler-Mikola A.** Do the diagnostic criteria determine the sex ratio in depression? *J Affect Disord.* 1984;7:189–198.

11. **Isometsa ET, Henriksson MM, Aro HM, et al.** Suicide in major depression. *Am J Psychiatry.* 1994;151:530–6.

12. **Keitner GI, Ryan CE, Miller IW, et al.** Twelve-month outcome of patients with major depression and comorbid psychiatric or medical illness (compound depression). *Am J Psychiatry.* 1991;148:345–50.

13. **Regier DA, Burke JD, Burke KC.** Comorbidity of affective and anxiety disorders in the NIMH Epidemiologic Catchment Area Program. In Maser JD, Cloninger CR (eds). *Comorbidity of Mood and Anxiety Disorders.* Washington, DC: American Psychiatric Press; 1990:113–22.

14. **Hanna EZ, Grant BF.** Gender differences in DSM-IV alcohol use disorders and major depression as distributed in the general population: clinical implications. *Compr Psychiatry.* 1997;38:202–12.

15. **Moldin SO, Scheftner WA, Rice JP, et al.** Association between major depressive disorder and physical illness. *Psychol Med.* 1993;23:755–61.
16. **Breslau N, Merikangas K, Bowden C.** Comorbidity of migraine and major affective disorders. *Neurology.* 1994;44(Suppl 7):17–22.
17. **Clauw DJ.** Fibromyalgia: more than just a musculoskeletal disease. *Am Fam Phys.* 1995;52:843–51.
18. **Whybrow PC.** Sex differences in thyroid axis dysfunction: relevance to affective disorder and its treatment. *Depression* 1995;3:33–42.
19. **Endicott J.** The menstrual cycle and mood disorders. *J Affect Disord.* 1993;29: 193–200.
20. **Kornstein SG, Yonkers KA, Schatzberg AF, et al.** *Premenstrual Exacerbation of Depression.* Paper presented at the American Psychiatric Association 149th Annual Meeting, 1996.
21. **Wu X, DeMaris A.** Gender and marital status differences in depression: the effects of chronic strains. *Sex Roles.* 1996;34:299–319.
22. **Ross CE, Mirowsky J.** Child care and emotional adjustment to wives' employment. *J Health Soc Behav.* 1988;29:127–38.
23. **Carmen E, Rieker PP, Mills T.** Victims of violence and psychiatric illness. *Am J Psychiatry.* 1984;141:378–83.
24. **Jensvold MJ, Halbreich U, Hamilton JA, eds.** *Psychophamacology of Women: Sex, Gender, and Hormonal Considerations.* Washington, DC: American Psychiatric Association Press; 1996.
25. **Kimmel S, Gonsalves L, Youngs D, et al.** Fluctuating levels of antidepressants. *J Psychosom Obstet Gynecol.* 1992;13:277–80.
26. **Wisner KL, Perel JM, Wheeler SB.** Tricyclic dose requirements across pregnancy. *Am J Psychiatry.* 1993;150:1541–2.
27. **Kornstein SG, Schatzberg AF, Thase ME, et al.** Gender differences in treatment response to sertraline and imipramine in chronic depression. *Am J Psychiatry.* In press.
28. **Hamilton JA, Grant M, Jensvold MF.** Sex and treatment of depressions: When does it matter? In Jensvold MJ, Halbreich U, Hamilton JA (eds). *Psychophamacology of Women: Sex, Gender, and Hormonal Considerations.* Washington, DC: American Psychiatric Association Press; 1996:241–57.
29. **Schneider LS, Small GW, Hamilton SH, et al.** Estrogen replacement and response to fluoxetine in a multicenter geriatric depression trial. *Am J Geriatr Psychiatry.* 1997;5:97–106.
30. **Seligman ME.** The effectiveness of psychotherapy. *Am Psychol.* 1995;50:965–74.
31. **Stewart DE, Boydell KM.** Psychological distress during menopause: associations across the reproductive cycle. *Int J Psychiatry Med.* 1993;23:157–162.
32. **Steiner M, Yonkers K.** *Depression in Women.* London: Martin Dunitz; 1998.
33. **Kornstein SG.** Premenstrual syndrome: an overview. *Primary Psychiatry.* 4:56–60, 1997.
34. **American Psychiatric Association.** *Diagnostic and Statistical Manual of Mental Disorders,* 4th ed. Washington, DC: American Psychiatric Press; 1994.
35. **Endicott J, Harrison W.** *The Daily Record of Severity of Problems.* Available by writing to Dr. Endicott, New State Psychiatric Institute, Biometrics Unit, 722 West 168th Street, New York, NY 10032.

36. **Rubinow DR, Roy-Byrne P.** Premenstrual syndromes: overview from a methodological perspective. *Am J Psychiatry.* 1984;141:163–72.

37. **Pearlstein TB, Frank E, Rivera-Tovar A, et al.** Prevalence of axis I and axis II disorders in women with late luteal phase dysphoric disorder. *J Affect Disord.* 1990;20:129–134.

38. **Graze KK, Nee J, Endicott J.** Premenstrual depression predicts future major depressive disorder. *Acta Psychiatr Scand.* 1990;81:201–6.

39. **Yonkers KA.** Antidepressants in the treatment of premenstrual dysphoric disorder. *J Clin Psychitry.* 1997;58(Suppl 14):4–10.

40. **Freeman EW.** Premenstrual syndrome: current perspectives on treatment and etiology. *Curr Opin Obstet Gynecol.* 1997;9:147–53.

41. **Steiner M, Steinberg S, Stweart D, et al.** Fluoxetine in the treatment of premenstrual dysphoria. *N Engl J Med* 1995;332:1529–34.

42. **Yonkers KA, Halbreich U, Freeman E, et al.** Symptomatic improvement of premenstrual dysphoric disorder with sertraline treatment: a randomized controlled trial. *JAMA.* 1997;278:983–8.

43. **Steiner M, Korzekwa M, Lamont J, Wilkins A.** Intermittent fluoxetine dosing in the treatment of women with premenstrual dysphoria. *Psychopharm Bull.* 1997;33: 771–4.

44. **Mezrow G, Shoupe D, Spicer, D, et al.** Depot leuprolide acetate with estrogen and progestin add-back for long-term treatment of premenstrual syndrome. *Fertil Steril.* 1993;62:932–7.

45. **Freeman E, Rickels K, Sondheimer S, et al.** Ineffectiveness of progesterone suppository treatment for premenstrual syndrome. *JAMA.* 1990;264:349–53.

46. **Harrison WM, Endicott J, Nee J.** Treatment of premenstrual dysphoria with alprazolam: a controlled study. *Arch Gen Psychiatry.* 1990;47:270–5.

47. **Rickels K, Freemen E, Sondheimer S.** Buspirone in the treatment of premenstrual syndrome. *Lancet.* 1989;1:777.

48. **Kornstein SG, Parker AJ.** Menstrual migraines: pathophysiology, treatment, and relationship to premenstrual syndrome. *Curr Concepts Obstet Gynecol.* 9:154–158, 1997.

49. **Pearlstein T.** Nonpharmacologic treatment of premenstrual syndrome. *Psychiatr Ann.* 1996;590–4.

50. **O'Hara MW, Schlechte JA, Lewis DA, Varner MW.** Controlled prospective study of postpartum mood disorders: psychological, environmental, and hormonal factors. *J Abnorm Psychol.* 1991;100:63–73.

51. **Altshuler LL, Hendrick V, Cohen LS.** Course of mood and anxiety disorders during pregnancy and postpartum period. *J Clin Psychiatr.* 1998;59(Suppl 2):29–33.

52. **Cohen LS, Rosenbaum JF.** Psychotropic drug use during pregnancy: weighing the risks. *J Clin Psych.* 1998;59(Suppl 2):18–28.

53. **Kumar R, Robson KM.** A prospective study of emotional disorders in childbearing women. *Br J Psychiatry.* 1984;144:35–47.

54. **O'Hara MW, Zekoski EM, Phillips LH, et al.** Controlled prospective study of postartum mood disorders: comparison of childbearing and nonchildbearing women. *J Abnorm Psychol.* 1990;1:3–15.

55. **Kitamura T, Shima S, Sugawara M, Toda MA.** Psychological and social correlates of the onset of affective disorders among women. *Psychol Med.* 1993;23:967–75.

56. **Miller IJ.** Psychiatric disorders during pregnancy. In Stewart DE, Stotland NL (eds.). *Psychological Aspects of Women's Healthcare: The Interface Between Psychiatry and Obstetrics and Gynecology.* Washington, DC: American Psychiatric Press; 1993:55–70.

57. **O'Hara MW.** *Postpartum Depression: Causes and Consequences.* New York: Springer-Verlag 1995.

58. **Szewczyk M, Chennault SA.** Women's health: depression and related disorders. *Primary Care.* 1997;21:83–101.

59. **Steer RA, Scholl TO, Hediger ML, et al.** Self-reported depression and negative pregnancy outcomes. *J Clin Epidemiol.* 1992;45:1093–9.

60. **Stowe ZN, Nemeroff CB.** Psychopharmacology during pregnancy and lactation. In Schatzberg AF, Nemeroff CB (eds). *The American Psychiatric Press Textbook of Psychopharmacology.* Washington, DC: American Psychiatric Press; 1995:823–37.

61. **Cohen LS, Altshuler LL.** Pharmacologic management of psychiatric illness during pregnancy and the postpartum period. *Psych Clin North Am.* 1997;4:21–60.

62. **Miller IJ.** Use of electroconvulsive therapy during pregnancy. *Hosp Community Psychiatry.* 1994;45:444–50.

63. **Altshuler LL, Hendrick V.** Pregnancy and psychotropic medication: changes in blood levels. *J Clin Psychopharmacol.* 1996;16:78–80.

64. **Nonacs R, Cohen LS.** Postpartum mood disorders: diagnosis and treatment guidelines. *J Clin Psych.* 1998;59(Suppl 2):34–40.

65. **O'Hara MW, Schlechte JA, Lewis DA, Wright EJ.** Prospective study of postpartum blues: biological and psychosocial factors. *Arch Gen Psychiatr.* 1991;48:801–6.

66. **Suri R, Burt VK.** The assessment and treatment of postpartum psychiatric disorders. *J Practical Psychiatr Behav Health.* 1997;3:67–77.

67. **Pariser SF, Nasrallah HA, Gardner DK.** Postpartum mood disorders: clinical perspectives. *J Womens Health.* 1997;6:421–34.

68. **Hendrick V, Altshuler LL, Suri R.** Hormonal changes in the postpartum period and implications for postpartum depression. *Psychosomatics.* 1998;39:93–101.

69. **Stowe ZN, Nemeroff CB.** Women at risk for postpartum-onset major depression. *Am J Obstet Gynecol.* 1995;173:639.

70. **O'Hara MW, Swain AM.** Rates and risk of postpartum depression: a meta-analysis. *Int Rev Psychiatry.* 1996;8:37–54.

71. **Righetti-Veltema M, Conne-Perreard E, Bousquet A, Manzano J.** Risk factors and predictive signs of postpartum depression. *J Affect Disord.* 1998;49:167–180.

72. **Wisner KL, Wheeler SB.** Prevention of recurrent postpartum major depression. *Hosp Community Psychiatry.* 1994;45:1191–6.

73. **Sichel DA, Cohen LS, Robertson LM, et al.** Prophylactic estrogen in recurrent postpartum affective disorder. *Biol Psychiatry.* 1995;38:814–8.

74. **Gregoire AJP, Kuman R, Everitt B, et al.** Transdermal oestrogen for treatment of severe postnatal depression. *Lancet.* 1996;347:930–3.

75. **Wisner KL, Perel JM.** Psychopharmacological treatment during pregnancy and lactation. In Jensvold MF, Halbreich U, Hamilton JA (eds). *Psychopharmacology and Women: Sex, Gender, and Hormones.* Washington, DC: American Psychiatric Press; 1996:191–224.

76. **Llewellyn A, Stowe ZN.** Psychotropic medications in lactation. *J Clin Psychiatry.* 1998;59:41–52.

77. **Stowe ZN, Owens MJ, Landry JC, et al.** Sertraline and desmethylsertraline in human breast milk and nursing infants. *Am J Psychiatry.* 1997;154:1255–60.

78. **Lester BM, Cucca J, Andreozzi L, et al.** Possible association between fluoxetine hydrochloride and colic in an infant. *J Am Acad Child Adolesc Psychiatry.* 1993;32: 1253–5.

79. **Matheson I, Pande H, Alertsen AR.** Respiratory depression caused by *N*-desmethyldoxepin in breast milk (Letter). *Lancet.* 1985;2:1124.

80. **Murray L, Carothers A.** The validation of the Edinburgh Postnatal Depression Scale on a community sample. *Br J Psychiatry.* 1990;157:288–90.

81. **Wisner KL, Perel JM.** Serum levels of valproate and carbamazepine in breastfeeding mother-infant pairs. *J Clin Psychopharmacol.* 1998;18:167–9.

82. **Burt VK, Altshuler LL, Rasgon N.** Depressive symptoms in the perimenopause: prevalence, assessment, and guidelines for treatment. *Harvard Rev Psychiatry.* 1998;6:121–32.

83. **Avis NE, Brambilla D, MsKinlay SM, Vass K.** A longitudinal analysis of the association between menopause and depression: results from the Massachusetts Women's Health Study. *Ann Epidemiol.* 1994;4:214–20.

84. **Sherwin BB.** Menopause: myths and realities. In Stewart DE, Stotland NL (eds.). *Psychological Aspects of Women's Health Care: The Interface Between Psychiatry and Obstetrics and Gynecology.* Washington, DC: American Psychiatric Press; 1993: 227–48.

85. **Matthews KA.** Myths and realities of menopause. *Psychosomatic Med.* 1992;54: 1–9.

86. **Pearlstein T, Rosen K, Stone AB.** Mood disorders and menopause. *Endocrinol Metab Clin North Am.* 1998:26:279–94.

87. **Sherwin BB.** Menopause, early aging, and elderly women. In Jensvold MF, Halbreich U, Hamilton JA (eds). *Psychopharmacology and Women: Sex, Gender, and Hormones.* Washington, DC; American Psychiatric Press; 1996:225–37.

88. **Ditkoff EC, Clary WG, Cristo M, et al.** Estrogen improves psychological function in asymptomatic postmenopausal women. *Obstet Gynecol.* 1991;78:991–5.

89. **Zweifel JE, O'Brien WH.** A meta-analysis of the effect of hormone replacement therapy upon depressed mood. *Psychoneuroendocrinology.* 1997;22:189–212.

90. **Halbreich U, Rojansky N, Palter S, et al.** Estrogen augments serotonergic activity in postmenopausal women. *Biol Psychiatry.* 1995;27:434–41.

91. **Stahl SM.** Basic psychopharmacology of antidepressants. Part 2: Estrogen as an adjunct to antidepressant treatment. *J Clin Psychiatry.* 1998;58(Suppl 4):15–24.

KEY REFERENCES

Burt VK, Altshuler LL, Rasgon N. Depressive symptoms in the perimenopause: prevalence, assessment, and guidelines for treatment. *Harvard Rev Psychiatry.* 1998;6:121–32.

Comprehensive review of both cross-sectional and longitudinal studies of depressive symptoms during the perimenopause and of the effectiveness of ERT in treating mood symptoms.

Cohen LS, Rosenbaum JF. Psychotropic drug use during pregnancy: weighing the risks. *J Clin Psychiatry.* 1998;59(Suppl 2):18–28.

Provides summary of safety studies of antidepressants, antipsychotics, mood stabilizers, anxiolytics, and electroconvulsive therapy. Reviews risks and benefits of treatment and provides clear guidelines for treatment of mood, anxiety, and psychotic disorders during pregnancy.

Kornstein SG. Gender differences in depression: implications for treatment. *J Clin Psychiatry.* 1997;58(Suppl 15):12–8.

Comprehensive review of literature on gender differences in depression, including differences in symptoms, comorbidity, course, and treatment response. Provides gender-specific guidelines for assessment and treatment of depression.

Kornstein SG. Premenstrual syndrome: an overview. *Primary Psychiatry.* 1997;4: 56–60.

Detailed review of current literature on PMS and PMDD, including symptoms, etiology, assessment, and comprehensive discussion of management options.

Llewellyn A, Stowe ZN. Psychotropic medications in lactation. *J Clin Psychiatry.* 1998;59:41–52.

Detailed review of lactation studies using various psychotropics, including antidepressants, anxiolytics, antipsychotics, sedative-hypnotics, and mood stabilizers.

10

Depression in
Children and Adolescents

Aradhana A. Sood, MD
Rakesh K. Sood, MD

n contrast to depressive disorders in adults, depression in children and
adolescents is a relatively new concept. Over the past 25 years, childhood depression has been recognized as a distinct entity, one that is
characterized by a specific symptom complex and that follows a defined
clinical course with a predictable response to treatment. Before this period,
some clinicians argued that children lacked the capability of experiencing
depression because of cognitive and psychological immaturity. Others con-
ceived depression so broadly that it encompassed symptoms as diverse as
enuresis, hyperactivity, and separation anxiety. In its revised versions of the
early 1980s, the *Diagnostic and Statistical Manual of Mental Disorders*
(DSM) (1) began to acknowledge that children can experience depression.
Over the past decade, it has become evident that children and adolescents
with depression have some distinct differences in their clinical presentation
compared with adults. This chapter highlights some of these differences.

Currently, the DSM's fourth edition (DSM-IV) states that children can be
diagnosed with depression using the same criteria used for diagnosing depression in adults. However, a developmental framework is necessary
when assessing children. For example, children rarely have the cognitive
sophistication to identify irritable mood as "depression," but they may be
able to acknowledge feeling "down in the dumps."

Epidemiology

The prevalence and incidence of depression varies with the methodology and the populations sampled. In children and adolescents in the community, the prevalence of major depressive disorder (MDD) varies between 1% and 2%, with some symptoms of depression endorsed by up to 17% (2). In older adolescents, the point prevalence rates are similar to the adult rates of 2% to 5% (3). In hospitalized pediatric populations, approximately 7% meet criteria for major depression (4). In psychiatric outpatient settings, the figure rises to 20%; in inpatient settings, 23% to 59% of psychiatrically ill children show depressive symptoms. Boys seem to be overrepresented in the prepubertal age group with major depression, but by late adolescence girls approach the adult pattern of women outnumbering men (5,6). Separation anxiety symptoms have a strong correlation with depressive symptoms (7). In view of its high prevalence, the diagnosis of childhood MDD should be explored actively in primary care and general pediatric practices in which children are most commonly assessed and treated.

Phenomenology

The general consensus in the mental health field is that the diagnostic criteria for major depression in adults (DSM-IV) are applicable to children and adolescents. Clinicians have long been aware that children and adolescents may not exhibit the full-blown constellation of major depression according to the adult criteria, but they seem depressed, exhibit signs and symptoms not typical of adult-onset depression, and are impaired significantly in their functioning. Furthermore, there are higher rates of depression in relatives of depressed child probands. A recent cluster analysis of depressive symptoms in an inpatient population could separate a group of depressed adolescents from a nondepressed psychiatrically ill group (8). The depressed adolescents could be divided further into clusters similar to the pattern seen in adults. Follow-up studies of children with depressive disorders indicate that as adults they are at higher risk for subsequent depression than are nondepressed controls and that this increased risk at follow-up is specific for depression and no other psychiatric disorder (9). These factors underscore the idea that childhood-onset and adulthood depression are a continuum of the same disorder across the lifespan. However, the application of adult criteria for major depression to children has been challenged by researchers who have attempted to refine our understanding of the developmental psychopathology of childhood depression (10). Unfortunately, stringent research into the phenomenology of childhood depression has yielded results that allow us to make only general statements about the differences between childhood and adult depression (11).

Chapter 3 discusses the diagnostic criteria for MDD in adults in detail. We highlight the differences between MDD in adults and childhood depression based on 1) clinical observations and case vignettes, and 2) current research. Although the current classification does not make any distinctions between adult, childhood, and adolescent depression, the DSM-IV does acknowledge some age-specific associated features that differ across these age ranges (Table 10.1). Irritable mood is the predominant presentation in both children and adolescents. In younger children, irritability, agitation coupled with somatic complaints—headaches, stomach aches, and hallucinations depressive in theme—are common. The hallucinations may be amorphous, half-formed, or clear. They may consist of voices telling the child that they are ugly and fat and that they should die. School performance gradually declines, so much so that an honor roll student may struggle to make passing grades. Social isolation and low self-esteem develop. Some older children are able to recognize the depression as sadness, hopelessness, and helplessness and may use these terms to describe themselves. Suicidal ideation is relatively rare in children but, if expressed, must be considered seriously. Suicidal children, in contrast with adolescents may lack the cognitive capabilities to devise successful suicide attempts. Case 10.1 illustrates the symptoms of MDD in a child.

CASE 10.1 *Child with symptoms of major depressive disorder*

FD is a boy 8 years of age brought in by his mother and his mother's boyfriend (who is also the child's biological father) after two school suspensions for insubordination to the principal and for pulling a girl's hair. He is described as a wonderful child one day and an angry boy who will fight other kids at the slightest provocation the next day. FD has been having considerable difficulty with behavior at home and in church, with defiance and kicking, hitting, biting, and scratching others. The school has been concerned because he has begun to talk about death. On one occasion, FD asked a teacher to bring a gun to school and kill him. On another, he ignored the teacher completely and refused to do class work. FD states that he hates school and would rather be dead than be there. His grades have dipped from the honor roll down to C's and D's. Social withdrawal has been noted. There is no change in his appetite. The only way he will go to sleep is with his sister, but he wakes up at 4 AM. His mother notes that he complains of his leg hurting all the time. She notes an exacerbation of the leg pain when he is particularly stressed (e.g., when parental discord erupts over child-care arrangements). He is tiny for his age and has a deadpan expression that shifts to sadness when he is unaware that he is being observed.

Table 10.1   DSM-IV Criteria for Major Depressive Disorder

	In Adults	*In Children*	*In Adolescents*
1	Depressed mood for at least 2 weeks Irritable mood for at least 2 weeks	Usual presentation	Usual presentation
2	Weight or appetite loss Weight or appetite gain	Loss of appetite rare in younger children	Weight gain more common in both children and adolescents
3	Insomnia Hypersomnia		Hypersomnia more common in adolescents
4	Decreased interest or pleasure in activities	Withdrawal from friends	Lack of interest in socializing, sports
5	Decreased or lack of energy	Similar to adults	Similar to adults
6	Psychomotor retardation or agitation	Hyperactivity in classroom	Decreased activity
7	Inability to think or concentrate	Declining academic performance	Declining academic performance
8	Feelings of worthlessness, guilt	Somatic symptoms (e.g., headaches, stomach aches) common Delusions rare but hallucinations common in younger children (12)	Delusions more common than hallucinations
9	Suicidal thoughts	Suicidal thoughts, plans, and gestures relatively rare	Common in adolescents

In adolescents, the depression may be difficult to distinguish from normal developmental struggles. Symptoms may include threats to run away, aggression, grouchiness, restlessness, and a refusal to take part in family activities. When these behavioral problems are accompanied by neurovegetative symptoms such as appetite and sleep disturbance, a MDD should be considered. In comparison with childhood, suicidal thoughts and gestures rise dramatically in adolescence. Adolescents often are able to identify their irritability as stemming from sadness and hopelessness about the future (Case 10.2). Guilt feelings are common. Remorse after an episode of out-of-control behavior may signal a mood disorder rather than a conduct disorder.

CASE 10.2 *Adolescent with symptoms of major depressive disorder*

Becky is a high school freshman 14 years of age who is rude and argumentative with family members and teachers. She had been diagnosed previously with ADHD and has been prescribed methylphenidate. She told her father that he was horrible and that she hated him. She feels her sister attacks her verbally; in retaliation, she dipped her sister's favorite blouse in paint and hid it. She also has become more isolated and angry. She has visualized her own death, seeing images of her own body lying on the floor. On a rating scale for depression, she endorsed items such as "she was so sad and unhappy she could not stand it, she felt the future was hopeless, she saw herself as a failure, does not get satisfaction from anything, feels she is unworthy, feels she is better off dead." She has lost interest in her friends, and they shun her because she is always "so tense."

Causes

As in adults, the cause of childhood depression is best understood as being multifactorial, stemming from such factors as genetic vulnerability and other biological aspects, temperament, adverse life events, and chronic stress. A combination of predisposing and precipitating factors in a vulnerable individual can initiate psychological and biological phenomena that then culminate in depression.

Predisposing Factors

Biological Factors
Genetic vulnerability is supported by the often familial pattern of childhood depression. Affective disorders occur at a higher frequency in the first-degree relatives of children with MDD. Children of parents with affective disorders are at a much higher risk for depression. The risk of developing an affective disorder before the age of 18 years doubles if one parent suffers from major depression and quadruples if both parents suffer from major depression. However, familial transmission may occur through environmental, not just genetic mechanisms. Genetic risk does not guarantee phenotypic expression; some children have unknown resilience factors that protect them from the illness (12).

Studies of neurotransmitter systems in children have been performed infrequently and are complicated by the ongoing maturation of the nervous system. There is some evidence that cortisol secretion rhythm may be abnormal in children and adolescents, as it may be in adults. The literature indicates that the increase in gonadotropins in puberty cannot account for the increase in depressive symptoms in adolescents (compared with children); however, the rise in gonadotropins in combination with adverse life events may precipitate depression (13). Unlike in adults, studies have not been able to demonstrate sleep architecture abnormalities in children or adolescents.

Other predisposing influences include several interrelated factors such as child and maternal temperament, parenting style, and environmental stressors.

Temperament

Children with "difficult" or "slow-to-warm-up" temperaments seem to be at higher risk for developing psychiatric disorders, including depression (14). Parents may react to a difficult child in a critical and punitive manner, producing feelings of worthlessness and hopelessness. Temperamental difficulties may mediate an effect by 1) eliciting negative and critical reactions from others (e.g., caregivers), and 2) impeding the ability of the child to adapt to normal stressors as well as traumatic events. From a biological standpoint, differences in temperament may reflect differences in neuroendocrine systems implicated in depression. Case 10.3 illustrates temperament problems in a child in whom depression should be suspected.

CASE 10.3 *Child with temperamental difficulties*

JK is a boy 7 years of age in the first grade who is fidgety and disruptive in his classroom. Recently, he has become sassy to his teachers and has temper tantrums at home—a direct contrast to his usually quiet but sad demeanor. His teacher left on maternity leave 2 weeks ago, and he hates his substitute teacher. He was retained in kindergarten because of "social immaturity." If previously made plans are canceled unavoidably, he regresses to screaming, sobbing, and flailing around on the floor. Mother walks on "eggshells" around him. As an infant, he was colicky and had his nights and days mixed. In preschool, he had few friends and was not invited to any neighborhood birthday parties because of his bossiness. His mother feels exhausted and admits to spanking him when she gets frustrated. Both mother and JK end up feeling unhappy after these episodes.

The pervasiveness of dysfunction at this stage points to the development of depression. An unusual degree of hypersensitivity to environmental changes in the past has given way to constant behavioral problems without any external provocation. Recent stressors and negative feedback from caregivers may have precipitated this episode. Children who have only temperamental difficulties and intermittent periods of normal functioning may not suffer from depression and usually regress when faced with transitions. In this case, further enquiry should be directed toward eliciting neurovegetative symptoms of depression.

Social Bonding and Cognitive Styles

Social relationships of children with depression have been shown to be impaired across several domains (15). Although relationships are often impaired in children with any psychiatric illness, there are certain deficits that are specific to depressed children (e.g., lack of warmth, poor communication), and they may not improve fully when the depressive episode subsides. The social behavior of depressed children seems to lack the qualities that allow for lasting friendships. There is poor understanding of whether the lack of social competence leads to a lack of friends and thereby produces depression or whether depression produces a sense of poor self-esteem and deepening isolation. It is clear from clinical experience that depressed children have a difficult time both making and retaining friends. As with adults, having a close relationship with parents or peers (in which the sharing of emotions can occur freely) has a protective effect against the development of depression.

Depressed youngsters tend to have negative appraisals of themselves, often attributing negative events to internal, uncontrollable causes, which engenders a sense of hopelessness and powerlessness. For example, a depressed teenager may interpret a date being postponed because of an illness in the girlfriend's family as a rejection (i.e., "Why would anyone want to go out with a loser like me?"). This negative world view or cognitive style can be a stable personality trait (leading to depression), can result from chronic depression itself, and/or can arise from negative interactions with peers or family.

Precipitating Events

Usually, acute life stresses (e.g., parental divorce) in children occur against the backdrop of chronic stresses such as marital discord. These events carry with them other adversities with which the child is faced (e.g., lack of emotional availability of parents, change in lifestyle, economic hardship, parental distress) (Case 10.4). Stressors such as the birth of a sibling, death of a parent, parental psychopathology, and chronic abuse and neglect may precipitate the development of depression in a vulnerable child. Hence, it becomes difficult to tease out the impact of these events on the child's psychopathologic development. Although, depressive symptoms such as sad mood or sleep disturbance may be frequent, the development of a full depressive syndrome (constellation of symptoms meeting DSM-IV criteria) is rare in the majority of children faced with adversity. Some children seem to have competencies that allow them to withstand stresses. Those parents who develop psychiatric symptoms in the aftermath of an adverse event (e.g., a divorce) may be emotionally unavailable to their children and may indirectly precipitate impairment or distress in a vulnerable child. There does seem to be a nonspecific link between depression and the various trauma to which a child may be exposed. Stressful events such as bereavement, divorce, and sexual and physical abuse may produce varied psychiatric syndromes, including posttraumatic stress disorder, anxiety, or depression. However, many depressed children do experience traumatic effects of adverse life events, either preceding their illness or during it.

CASE 10.4 *Adolescent with acute life stresses*

JG is a high school junior 16 years of age with chronic depression. He is currently in a school for the gifted and is struggling with a 2.8 average GPA, which is not consistent with his tested IQ of 130. He has no learning disabilities. His symptoms started 4 years ago and include moderate weight gain, irritability, initial insomnia, poor concentration, and lack of interest in any activity except video games, which keep him house-bound. He has been treated with methylphenidate for a diagnosis of ADHD for the past 5 years because of disruptiveness at school; improvement has been modest with persistent irritability. His parents divorced 3 years ago after the family relocated. Before the move, the parents fought openly with each other. At the same time, JG's older brother (now age 24) was kicked out of the home because of active alcoholism. JG claims that he hates his new home and that, because he is overweight, he has no friends. He gets testy with his mother during the interview.

ADHD is one of the most frequent diagnoses given to children with disruptive disorders, usually after brief evaluations that may be inaccurate. As a differential diagnosis, depression is often missed. Subsequent treatment with stimulant medications may postpone detection of depression. However, nonresponsiveness to treatment or side effects of increasing irritability should be evaluation thoroughly for accuracy of diagnosis compared with mere side effects of the psychotropic agent. Onset of mood symptoms after initiation of medications point to iatrogenic mood disorder (i.e., side effects from stimulants). Presence of neurovegetative symptoms and onset of irritability and mood symptoms before treatment of ADHD point to a mood disorder.

Assessment

A good clinical interview remains the cornerstone for diagnosing depression in children. How does one obtain useful and clinically meaningful information from children about abstract issues such as psychiatric symptoms? Are children capable of giving accurate information about how they are feeling, or should one rely on parents and teachers only? Twenty years of research supports the acceptance of children as accurate reporters of their feelings. Parents are better at describing overt behaviors, such as hyperactivity, oppositionality, distractibility, declining school performance and changes in appetite. Children are more accurate at reporting their internal or feeling states, such as anger, fear, sadness, and hopelessness. Interviewing techniques of both children and adolescents have shifted from the observational, play therapy model to a more direct interview model in which the child is asked specific questions pertaining to mood and other associated features of depression. Adequately assessing children for depression requires a developmental approach. Kovacs (16) describes the following three developmental dimensions when assessing children:

1. **Knowledge of emotions and mood:** By approximately 5 years of age, children begin to recognize the connection between situations and feelings in themselves and begin to have a vocabulary for basic emotions in others. By approximately 10 years of age, they develop an understanding that facial expressions may not be congruent with internally felt emotions. Younger children tend to link feelings to emotionally laden situations and should be asked questions temporally connected with specific events. They cannot name internal feelings such as sadness or anxiety, expressing these feelings instead as somatic complaints such as stomach aches. Furthermore, children with depression and other psychiatric illnesses seem to have a poorer understanding of psychological issues than their non-ill counterparts, tend to be more concrete, and cannot identify emotions accurately. Therefore, corroborative information or double-checking answers is recommended.

2. **Understanding of self:** Up to 7 or 8 years of age children understand themselves in terms of concrete attributes such as color of skin, hair, name, friends, or the activities in which they are involved. After this age, children begin to describe the "self" in more psychological terms and compare their own competencies to other children. Statements such as "I am no good at baseball; I suck" or "No one likes me because I am fat" are heard from children after the age of seven. Hence, with the capacity for self reflection comes the vulnerability to experience depressive feelings.

3. **Time concepts and memory:** Children younger than 8 years of age have difficulty with calendar time and the temporal sequencing of events; only after 12 years of age can they describe the duration of an event with any accuracy. Questions about time have to be tailored to the child's developmental stage; hence, for children, questions such as "Did this happen around Christmas?" are better than "Did this happen six months ago?"

Clinical Interview

Children do not respond well to the abstract language that most adults are comfortable using. With appropriate language, style, and rapport, the process of obtaining a history and eliciting symptoms to generate a diagnosis is generally easy. An informal, conversational, age-appropriate style of interviewing helps build rapport.

Mood Questions

Avoid jargon and abstractions. Instead of asking "Are you depressed?", it is better to ask "Are you sad, empty, down in the dumps, or blah?" Children (especially when depressed) may have a difficult time responding to open-ended questions such as "How do you feel?" It is preferable to provide them with a framework such as "If I had something like this happen to me [i.e., a mother who is gravely ill], I'd be sad. How are you feeling?" It may be useful to provide them with a Likert-style scale to rank their mood. Adolescents and children over 8 years of age have no difficulty understanding the question "On a scale from one to ten, with ten being that you have no problems at all and you feel good, and one being that you feel life is awful and you feel like crying all the time, how would you rate yourself since you went back to school this week?" This helps determine the severity of the mood disturbance and also provides a measure of response to treatment. With children under 8 years of age, using photographs or sketches of varied facial expressions, such as happy, sad, angry, or worried (visual analogue), and having them choose the one that matches their own mood state will produce an accurate response. Changes in mood states throughout a single day should be elicited by anchoring time to a regular event in the schedule, such as "from the time when you wake up to when you come back home from school." In adolescents, one must differentiate normal mood lability from depression. The nondepressed adolescent will not have a pervasive mood disturbance, crying spells, or lack of energy to socialize with peers. They also do not exhibit neurovegetative symptoms of depression, such as sleep or appetite disturbance.

Guilt Feelings

The paraphrasing of questions elicits meaningful responses from children. For example, asking a child "How do feel after you have done something wrong?" is better than asking "Do you feel guilty?", which may be more appropriate for adolescents. Other variations may include asking "Are there many times when you feel that another person did something wrong but you ended up feeling it was your fault?" Provide the child with hypothetical examples liberally.

Suicidal Ideations

Physicians and parents are reluctant to broach the issue of suicide with children. There is no evidence to support the fear that asking about suicidal ideations puts children (or adults) more at risk. Depressed children and adolescents, like adults, are relieved that someone is concerned and understands how badly they are feeling. Physicians should develop a standard way of inquiring about suicidality. A useful framework is to ask about suicidal thoughts (e.g., "Have things ever been so bad for you that you have thought life was not worth living?") or suicide attempts (e.g., "Have you ever tried to do anything to hurt yourself? What have you tried? What were you thinking would happen? Did you think you were going to die or did you feel that this was a good way to let other people know how bad you were feeling?"). Prepubertal children may not have an accurate understanding of the lethal consequences of an attempt (Case 10.5). Children under 6 years of age view death as being reversible. By 8 years of age, they begin to understand that death is irreversible. Between 10 and 12 years of age, the cognitive understanding of death is accurate but has not achieved the abstract thinking typical of adolescents who pose philosophical questions about death or engage in risky behaviors to test their own invulnerability. A combination of strong suicidal intent and accurate cognitive understanding of the lethal consequences of various methods (e.g., the adolescent who had access to a *Physicians' Desk Reference* and took enough acetaminophen to destroy his liver) poses the greatest risk for young people and must be explored actively.

CASE 10.5 *Child in whom suicidal ideation is suspected*

KJ is a boy 7 years of age who was admitted to an inpatient psychiatric unit after an escalation of acting-out behavior (e.g., playing with knives, poking holes in clothes, hitting other kids) and poor sleep with nightmares of his mother being abused. He had watched his mother's now ex-boyfriend abusing her repeatedly for 4 years. The admission was precipitated by the child's attempt to use his mother's umbrella as a parachute to "fly" out of a second-story window. However, on interview it became clear that, although profoundly depressed, this child had thought that nothing harmful would happen to him if he had jumped from the window with the umbrella and that he would be a "hero."

HALLUCINATIONS AND DELUSIONAL THINKING

Hallucinations are more common in prepubertal depressed children than in adolescents who may present with delusional thinking. These perceptual and thought distortions are usually "mood congruent," i.e., typically involve morbid, sad themes that go along with their depressed mood (e.g., "I heard my grandmother's voice tell me that I must kill myself"). Limited hallucinatory experiences, such as hearing one's name being called or hearing noises in an empty house, are normal developmental phenomena, not pathologic.

NEUROVEGETATIVE SYMPTOMS

Because depression is an episodic illness, appetite or sleep disturbances resulting from depression should be established as a change from baseline. They must be distinguished from normal habit patterns, such as always being a late sleeper or a finicky eater.

SOCIAL WITHDRAWAL AND SOMATIC SYMPTOMS

Social withdrawal and somatic symptoms, such as headaches and stomach aches, are strong markers for depression in children. Somatic complaints usually are connected temporally to stressful events and social withdrawal.

Parent Interview

Parent and other adult informants are of great importance in assessing the depressed child. As stated earlier, parents are accurate reporters of observable behaviors such as loss of appetite, school attendance, irritability, and loss of friendships. They are much more accurate with time concepts and cross-situational variations in their child (e.g., at school, with friends, at home) and can clarify stressors or other life events for the family. Often, it is not depression but rather ancillary symptoms such as fatigue or stomach aches that bring the family in to seek help. Parents may be vaguely aware that their child "is not the same" but may not recognize depression. In some situations, the parents may be depressed themselves as a cause and effect of the child's behavior and mood and may need assessment and treatment themselves. Depressed parents seem to be more sensitive to depression in their child.

The sequencing of who to interview first depends on the age of the patient. For the initial few minutes, it is appropriate to have the parent and child in the room to explain how the interview will proceed and to get the parent's view of the problem. Adolescents to whom privacy, independence, and respect are critical should be interviewed alone unless they opt to have the parent in the room. With younger children, the initial questions should be addressed to the child; however, if the child cannot or will not respond, their parents should then be interviewed. After obtaining information from the adolescent or child, the parent, and the teacher, the clinician needs to sort through any discrepancies in the information and come up with the best estimate of positive symptoms present.

Self-Report or Other Structured Rating Scales

Supplementing the clinical interview with self-report or other structured rating scales is a technique used in all psychiatric research and in many clinical psychiatric settings. Their usefulness in a primary care clinical setting, is determined in large part by what additional information they will provide that will be clinically useful. The other issues are the availability of personnel to administer them and the willingness of the family to participate in a process that is time consuming.

As stated earlier, a categorical diagnosis of depression is generated by the clinical interview only. In a busy primary care office, the purpose of including structured interviews is to screen for depression and to obtain a

Table 10.2   Rating Scales for Childhood Depression

	Rating Scale	Informant	Items	Comments
1	Children's Depression Inventory (CDI + CDI-P) (17)	Child self-report Parent report	27 items	Takes 10–20 minutes; is the most widely used scale; can identify children who are distressed
2	Beck's Depression Inventory (BDI) (18)	Adolescent	21 items	Can identify adolescents with depression
3	Mood and Feelings Questionnaire (MFQ) (20)	Parent report of 8–18-year-olds	2 forms (32 & 11 items)	Has good discriminating power; has been used in primary care settings; uses a DSM-III-R item format
4	Reynolds Adolescent Depression Scale (RADS) (19)	Adolescent	30 items	Uses DSM-III format; has good psychometric properties
5	Child Behavior Checklist (CBCL) (21)	Parent and child versions	100 items	Is not specific for depression; computer version is available; breaks symptoms down to "internalizing" and "externalizing"; depression scale has good psychometric properties

severity measure for the depression if necessary. Table 10.2 briefly summarizes select rating scales that could be adapted for use in a primary care setting. This list is by no means exhaustive and does not include the structured rating scales that are more appropriate for psychiatric settings.

These types of rating scales do not require extensive preparation or training time because they are self-report measures. Accompanying manuals have scoring instructions that are relatively simple. They use cut-off scores to identify clinically depressed individuals, and the numerical score also provides a measure of severity.

Comorbidity and Differential Diagnosis

Most children who have MDD meet criteria for one or more nondepressive diagnoses as well (8). The depression is usually missed because the symptoms of the comorbid diagnosis overlap with symptoms seen in depression. This could be seen as true comorbidity or could be accounted for by conceptualizing psychiatric symptoms as part of a continuum of disorders rather than as categorical diagnoses. Just as fever and arthralgia can be a part of rheumatic fever, they also can be prodromal of systemic lupus erythematosus. Similarly, individuals with eating disorders present with weight loss and may have significant dysphoria; however, the primary clinical focus remains the eating disorder.

Anxiety Disorders

Anxiety disorders are the most common comorbid disorders associated with MDD in children. Separation anxiety disorder co-occurs in approximately 58% of prepubertal depressed children, decreasing to 37% by adolescence; phobias occur in 45% of prepubertal depressed children, decreasing to 27% by adolescence (22). On the other hand, 30% of children with anxiety disorders exhibit depressive symptoms. Anxiety coupled with depression usually is associated with more dysfunction than pure depression.

Conduct Disorder

Conduct problems often may be the manifestation of depression in a child. A depressed child can lie, steal, or be aggressive as a result of the pervasive sense of hopelessness he or she may feel. These behaviors are followed frequently by guilt and withdrawal, unlike in the conduct disordered child who has no remorse or concern about violating other people's rights. Conduct disorder may be comorbid with depression, which puts the young person at a higher risk for substance abuse and risk-taking behavior than the child with pure depression.

Substance Abuse

Nearly half the children with severe depression are substance abusers (23). Depression is strongly associated with substance dependency. Frequently, the substance abuse is an attempt to self-medicate the depression. The sequence of appearance of depression compared with the substance abuse determines whether the disorders are comorbid or causative.

Attention-Deficit–Hyperactivity Disorder

Although attention-deficit–hyperactivity disorder (ADHD) frequently is confused with depression, it can co-occur with MDD. The symptoms of ADHD (e.g., distractibility, problems with concentration and the resulting academic difficulties, disruptive behavior) overlap with the symptoms of a depressive syndrome. Furthermore, attention difficulties and hyperactivity often precede the onset of depression.

The 16-year-old high school junior discussed in Case 10.4 is an example of a missed diagnosis of depression because of overt irritability and inattention.

Notably, the diagnosis of ADHD is the second most common diagnosis (after depression) in the children of depressed mothers (24).

Academic or Learning Disabilities

In broad terms, a discrepancy of two standard deviations between the child's innate potential as measured by the Intelligence Quotient (IQ) and Achievement tests signifies learning disabilities (LD). A child with LD, who has not been identified correctly can struggle in the classroom, get bored, disrupt the class, and also become reactively depressed because of a repeated lack of success. The presence of neurovegetative symptoms along with academic difficulties should lead to active consideration of the diagnosis of depression.

Bipolar Mood Disorder

There is good evidence to contradict previously held beliefs that children and adolescents cannot suffer from bipolar disorder. However, children younger than 8 years of age exhibit bipolar disorder primarily as irritability, aggression, and mood lability. This frequently is confused with conduct disorder and ADHD. By adolescence, the symptomatology may resemble more classic adult mania. However, adolescents with bipolar disorder may start using illicit substances to medicate their disorder, creating the classic conduct-disordered teenager. Children and adolescents with a family history of affective disorder who present in their first episode of depression with an abrupt onset, psychomotor retardation, mood congruent delusions or hallucinations, and antidepressant-induced hypomania are at high risk for the eventual development of a bipolar disorder (25). Such individuals may need to be on mood stabilizers.

Clinical Course

Young people with MDD are at high risk for developing subsequent episodes of depression. In contrast to adjustment disorder, children with dysthymic disorder (chronic depression) and MDD are at much higher risk for MDD as adults (26). Risk factors for recurrent MDD are shown in Table 10.3.

Follow-up studies of children with depressive disorders indicate that as adults they are at higher risk for subsequent depression than nondepressed

---

Table 10.3   Risk Factors for Major Depressive Disorder in Children

Severe index episode

Dysthymia (chronic depression)

Older age

Family history of depression, especially maternal

Chronic adverse family environment

Table 10.4   Risk Factors for Suicide in Children and Adolescents

Aggression

Substance abuse; propensity to engage in risky behavior

Hopelessness

Severe depression

Previous attempt and severity

Presence of precipitant to which child is historically sensitive

Comorbidity

Easy access to means, especially firearms

---

controls and that this increased risk at follow-up is specific for depression and no other psychiatric disorder (27).

Suicide is the third most common cause of death in people aged 15 to 24 years (28). Although suicide is rare in younger children, children as young as 7 years of age have committed suicide successfully. Sixty percent of children and adolescents with MDD have suicidal ideation, and 40% actually make an attempt. Suicide attempts in young people usually occur after a disciplinary event or relationship breakup but are symptomatic of deeper problems. As stated earlier, a strong suicidal intent coupled with an accurate understanding of the lethal consequences of the method poses the greatest risk. Risk factors for suicide attempts in children and adolescents are shown in Table 10.4.

Management

It is important to establish that the child or adolescent is in no danger at the time of assessment. If there are any concerns about suicidal behaviors that put the child at risk, then the physician should refer the patient to a child psychiatrist who can further assess whether the child needs to be in a safe setting (e.g., a hospital) or whether stabilization can be achieved by outpatient therapy and medication management. Factors that could be assessed in a primary care setting are the following

1. Will the child be safe at home?
2. Is the adolescent or child agreeing not to harm self?
3. Is there an appropriate degree of supervision on returning home?
4. Is the family supportive?
5. Have there been any previous suicide attempts? If so, how did the child and family deal with the incident? How quickly can arrangements be made for therapy or professional support ?
6. Is the child honest or is he guarded, hostile, and responding compliantly to questions just to get the interviewer "off his back"?

Some initial clinical pitfalls include 1) conceptualizing the depressive symptoms as a "normal" reaction to phase-of-life problems in adolescents, 2) not talking to the child individually, and 3) conducting a superficial evaluation that misses comorbid diagnoses and underlying dynamics, leading to premature closure and simplistic interventions. The notion that "all adolescents get depressed" lulls parents and clinicians alike into a false sense of ease while the child may be contemplating suicide.

As in adults, depression in children is a heterogenous disorder, and the treatment is therefore multimodal. The following section highlights the focal points in managing childhood depression.

Somatic Treatments

Tricyclic Antidepressants

Although tricyclic antidepressants (TCAs) have had proven efficacy in adult depression, 11 controlled trials in children and adolescents show no statistical difference between placebo and active drug (29). This could be an artifact of small samples, problems with diagnostic validity, inadequate dosing, or a pharmacodynamic difference between children and adults. Children and adolescents seem to have a much higher placebo response than do adults (70% vs. 30%) (30). Despite the paucity of supporting data, clinical experience suggests that TCAs do have a place in selected children and adolescents with the following characteristics:

- Comorbidity with ADHD, enuresis, separation anxiety disorder
- Failure on a selective serotonin-reuptake inhibitor (SSRI)
- Behavioral disinhibition or hypomania on SSRI
- Excessive aggression at baseline

Of major concern is the potential TCA cardiotoxicity (e.g., exacerbation of cardiac conduction defects as well as their lethal consequences in an

Table 10.5   Tricyclic Antidepressants

Generic	Brand	Dose	Comments
Nortriptyline	Pamelor	3–5 mg/kg body weight or 25–200 mg	Initial: gradual increase of doses; less sedating and anticholinergic; available in liquid preparation; most reliable blood levels
Imipramine	Tofranil	25–200 mg	Strongly anticholinergic, sedating; may be useful when insomnia is a major problem
Desipramine	Norpramin	25–200 mg	Metabolite of imipramine; case reports of sudden death, but no causal link established
Amitriptyline	Elavil	25–200 mg	Strongly sedating and anticholinergic

overdose). Standard work-up before and during the use of TCAs in children includes the following:

- Obtain an electrocardiogram (ECG)
- Rule out history of sudden cardiac death in family and, if positive, choose another agent
- Repeat ECG after TCA dosage of more than 100 mg/d
- Administered TCAs within a dosage range of 3–5 mg/kg body weight

Characteristics of TCAs are shown in Table 10.5.

Selective Serotonin-Reuptake Inhibitors
Open studies of the use of fluoxetine have been promising with up to 70% to 90% response rates in adolescents (31,32). However, only one double-blind placebo-controlled study (33) showed a significant improvement on active drug (56%) compared with placebo (33%) in depressed adolescents. Many patients showed partial response to fluoxetine. Clearly, more controlled studies in children and adolescents are needed before conclusive statements can be made about efficacy.

Starting and maximum dosages of SSRIs are shown in Table 10.6. These drugs are widely used in adolescents and to a lesser extent in children. Insomnia and weight gain or loss are common side effects. An underrecognized side effect of SSRIs in children is the behavioral disinhibition syndrome, which is characterized by a worsening of behavior with hyperactivity, irritability, and insomnia in an individual who had responded initially to the medication (Case 10.6). Clinicians frequently mistake this for recrudescence of the depressive syndrome and increase the SSRI dose. Accurate recognition and reduction of the dose leads to improvement of be-havior. However, the dose decrease may cause resurgence of depressive symptoms, and another antidepressant (e.g., a TCA or bupropion) may be a better choice. When symptoms of irritability, hyperactivity, and insomnia do not remit with reduction of the SSRI dose, a switch to hypomania should be suspected. Antidepressants should be discontinued, and, if symptoms of hypomania persist, a mood stabilizer such as valproate or car-bamazepine should be considered.

CASE 10.6 *Behavioral disinhibition syndrome in a child on a SSRI regimen*

DW is girl 11 years of age who has been depressed for 6 months and now has command auditory hallucinations that tell her to jump out of a window. She has no other psychotic symptoms. She describes feeling "yucky and sad." Her ap-petite is poor, and she has initial and middle insomnia. Fluoxetine 10 mg in the morning was prescribed. After a month, her grandmother stated that DW was like her old self again. As episodic dysphoria continued, the fluoxetine was in-creased to 20 mg. After 2 weeks, her grandmother became frantic because the school was threatening to suspend DW because she was becoming unmanage-able: incessant talking, hyperactivity, and irritability. The fluoxetine was decreased to 10 mg/d. The adverse effects resolved, but depressive symptoms recurred, so fluoxetine was replaced with nortriptyline.

Electroconvulsive Therapy

In children and adolescents, anecdotal reports indicate that electroconvul-sive therapy (ECT) may be helpful in refractory depression (34). ECT is usually considered for adolescents when the depression is chronic and nonresponsive to antidepressants and psychosocial interventions and when there is grave concern about chronic suicidality. (*See* Chapter 4 for a more detailed discussion of ECT.)

Psychosocial Interventions

Psychosocial interventions are strongly indicated when there are identifi-able environmental stressors and long-standing deficits in functioning.

Individual Therapy

A large controlled study of depressed adolescents comparing cognitive-be-havioral therapy (CBT), nondirective supportive therapy, and systemic fam-ily therapy showed that, although the subjects responded to all the

Table 10.6   Selective Serotonin and Other Reuptake Inhibitors

Generic Name	Brand Name	Dosage*	Comments
Fluoxetine	Prozac	5–20 mg/d in children 10–60 mg/d in adolescents (once-daily dose)	Good anti-anxiety properties; one trial (33) showed drug to be better than placebo in adolescent depression; long half-life; watch for drug interactions
Sertraline	Zoloft	25–100 mg/d in children 50–200 mg/d in adolescents (divided doses)	Less activating; shorter half-life than fluoxetine
Paroxetine	Paxil	10–20 mg/d in children 10–40 mg/d in adolescents	Similar profile as fluoxetine but shorter half-life
Fluvoxamine	Luvox	50–100 mg/d in children 50–200 mg/d in adolescents (divided doses)	Useful in depression with comorbid obsessive-compulsive symptoms; no pediatric research data
Citalopram	Celexa	10–20 mg/d in children 10–40 mg/d in adolescents (once-daily dose)	Anti-anxiety component; new; little clinical pediatric data; less effect on P450 enzyme systems; fewer drug interactions claimed
Venlafaxine	Effexor	18.75–75.0 mg/d in children 37.5–150.0 mg/d in adolescents (divided or once-daily dose)	Both noradrenergic and serotonergic effects; well tolerated; no pediatric data
Nefazadone	Serzone	100–300 mg/d in children 200–600 mg/d in adolescents (divided doses)	5HT-2–receptor and serotonin-reuptake block; no pediatric data
Bupropion	Wellbutrin	75–250 mg/d in children 75–400 mg/d in adolescents (divided doses)	Useful in comorbid attention-deficit–hyperactivity disorder

therapies at a 70% rate, the CBT group showed the quickest response (35). CBT is useful with adolescents and children who are 10 years of age or older because it requires verbal skills and a capacity for abstract thinking. The focus of treatment is to modify the child's or adolescent's negative view of self, others, and the future and to decrease errors in logic that maintain depression. The interaction between the therapist and the child is usually active and didactic, with an emphasis on a "Socratic" dialogue during which the therapist asks questions about assumptions (both false and depressogenic), thereby forcing the child to acknowledge the fallacies in his or her perceptions and interpretations of the world. As these assumptions disappear, the child becomes more optimistic and less helpless and hopeless.

Preschool children respond well to play therapy. Play materials are used to elicit the underlying feelings of conflict. As the child, under the supervision of the therapist, repeatedly re-enacts the memories of traumatic events in his play, depressive or acting-out behavior decreases. Children and adolescents should be referred for psychotherapy when there are:

- Identifiable stresses in the environment to which the child is reacting (e.g., divorce, death, peer-related problems).

- Long-standing problems that are interfering with functioning (e.g., difficulty with anger management, aggression towards peers or siblings, isolation because of poor social skills).

In practice, psychotherapy may be more effective in conjunction with medication because, as the depression lifts, the individual has more energy to work on psychological issues. An important focus of treatment should be the recognition of precipitating factors and the learning of compensatory strategies to ward off depressive feelings when faced with varied stressors. For example, teaching time-management skills to the disorganized child or conflict-resolution skills to the irritable child decreases the impact of external triggers for depression.

Family Interventions

Family therapy is based on the assumption that childhood depression occurs in the context of parent-child problems. The family is considered a homeostatic system, and the child who is identified as the patient is merely a symptom bearer of the distress within the family. In practical terms, the therapist faces the task of identifying occult family conflicts, advising and counseling the family members about depression, and convincing the family to become actively involved as a treatment agent.

In addition, because depression clusters in families, other affected individuals—siblings or parents—can be identified. Their diagnosis and treatment may enhance family functioning significantly. If there is strong genetic loading for depression, this knowledge can be used 1) to intervene proactively in unaffected individuals who are beginning to show depressive symptoms, and 2) to pre-empt any recrudescence of symptoms in affected individuals by seeking treatment before full-blown depression occurs.

School-Based Interventions

Depressed children are often quiet and go unnoticed by teachers; if irritable, they are labeled "troublemakers." Such mislabeled or "missed" children continue to function poorly, leading to complications such as educational skill deficits, low self-esteem, substance abuse, and suicidal tendencies. Identification of such children can occur only if clinicians make an effort to educate school personnel about depression. Raising awareness by seminars on childhood depression and making available screening questionnaires for use in suspected cases can lead to appropriate intervention and decreased morbidity for a treatable disorder.

Conclusions

Childhood depression is a poorly recognized disorder. It is frequently missed, because children suffering from depression often present with irritability, somatic complaints, and failing grades. Psychosocial stressors, genetic vulnerability, and underlying temperament all may contribute to the onset of depression. Depression is often comorbid with other psychiatric disorders such as anxiety and conduct disorders and, if untreated, can lead to academic failure, skill loss, substance abuse, and suicide. Childhood depression responds to antidepressant medications and psychotherapy. Appropriate education and skill development to manage depressive triggers improve the prognosis for children with depression.

Recommendations

- *Acute Care*
  Protection of child
  Symptomatic relief of depression with medications
  Assess need for other treatments
- *Continued Care*
  Maintain remission
  Improve and maintain functioning in school, home, and social settings
  Liaison with the school

Key Points

- Childhood depression is a poorly recognized disorder because children and adolescents with depression often present with irritability, somatic complaints, behavioral disturbance, and failing grades rather than with sadness.
- Psychosocial stresses may precipitate depression in genetically and temperamentally vulnerable children and adolescents.
- Childhood depression is a treatable disorder that is responsive to psychotherapy and medications.
- If untreated, childhood depression can lead to academic failure, suicide, or substance abuse.

■   ■   ■

REFERENCES

1. **American Psychiatric Association.** *Diagnostic and Statistical Manual of Mental Disorders*, 3rd ed. Washington, DC: American Psychiatric Press; 1980.
2. **Kashani JH, Beck NC, Hoeper EW, et al.** Psychiatric disorders in a community sample of adolescents. *Am J Psychiatry.* 1987;144,584–9.
3. **Verhulst FC.** Childhood depression: problems of definition. *Israel J Psychiatry Related Sci.* 1989;26:3–11.
4. **Kashani JH, Guiliano B, Bolender F.** Depression in hospitalized pediatric patients. *J Am Acad Child Adolesc Psychiatry.* 1981;20:123–34.
5. **Rutter M.** The developmental psychopathology of depression: issues and perspectives. In Rutter M, Izard CE, Read PB (eds). *Depression in Young People: Developmental And Clinical Perspectives.* New York: Guildford; 1986:3–30.
6. **Fleming JE, Offord DR, Boyle MH.** Prevalence of childhood and adolescent depression in the community: Ontario Child Health Study. *Br J Psychiatry.* 1989;155: 647–54.
7. **Puig-Antich J, Gittleman R.** Depression in childhood and adolescence. In ES Paykel (ed). *Handbook of Affective Disorders.* Edinburgh: Churchill Livingston; 1982:379–92.
8. **Carmanico SJ, Erickson MT, Singh NN, et al.** Diagnostic subgroups of depression in adolescents with emotional and behavioral disorders. *J Emotional Behav Disord.* 1988;6:222–32.
9. **Harrington RD, Fudge H, Rutter M, et al.** Adult outcomes of childhood and adolescent depression. Part I: Psychiatric status. *Arch Gen Psych.* 1990;47:465–73.
10. **Angold A.** Childhood and adolescent depression. Part II: Research in clinical populations. *Br J Psychiatry.* 1988;153:476–92.
11. **Chambers WJ, Puig-Antich J, Tabrizi MA, Davies M.** Psychotic symptoms in prepubertal major depressive disorder. *Arch Gen Psychiatry.* 1982;39:921–7.

12. **Hammen C.** *Depression Runs in Families: The Social Context of Risk and Resilience in Children of Depressed Mothers.* New York: Springer-Verlag; 1991.

13. **Brooks-Gunn J, Warren MP.** Biological and social contributions to negative affect in young adolescent girls. *Child Dev.* 1989; 60:40–55.

14. **Chess S, Thomas A, Hassibi M.** Depression in childhood and adolescence: prospective study of six cases. *J Nerv Ment Dis.* 1983;171:411–20.

15. **Puig-Antich J, Lukens E, Davies M, et al.** Psychosocial functioning in prepubertal major depressive disorders. Part II: Interpersonal relationships after sustained recovery from affective episode. *Arch Gen Psychiatry.* 1985;42:511–7.

16. **Kovacs M.** A developmental perspective on methods and measures in the assessment of depressive disorders: the clinical interview. In Rutter M, Izard CE, Read RB (eds). *Depression in Young People: Developmental and Clinical Perspectives.* New York: Guildford; 1986:435–65.

17. **Kovacs M.** *The Children's Depression Inventory.* Unpublished manuscript. Pittsburgh, PA: University of Pittsburgh; 1982.

18. **Beck AT, Ward CH, Mendelsohn M, et al.** An inventory for measuring depression. *Arch Gen Psychiatry.* 1961;4:53–63.

19. **Reynolds WM.** *Reynolds Adolesc Depression Scale.* Odessa, FL: Psychological Assessment Resources; 1987.

20. **Angold A, Costello EJ, Pickles A, Winder F.** *The Development of a Questionnaire for Use in Epidemiological Studies of Depression in Children and Adolescents.* Unpublished manuscript. London: London University; 1987.

21. **Achenbach TM, Edelbrook CS.** *Manual for the Child Behavior Checklist and the Revised Child Behavior Profile.* Burlington, VT: University Associates in Psychiatry; 1983.

22. **Ryan ND, Puig-Antich J, Ambrosisni P, et al.** The clinical picture of major depression in children and adolescents. *Arch Gen Psychiatry.* 1987;44:854–61.

23. **Greenbaum PE, Prange ME, Friedman RM, Silver SE.** Substance abuse prevalence and comorbidity with other psychiatric disorders among adolescents with severe emotional disturbances. *J Am Acad Child Psychiatry.* 1991;30:575–83.

24. **Weissman MM, Gammon D, John K, et al.** Children of depressed parents: increased psychopathology and early onset of major depression. *Arch Gen Psychiatry.* 1987;44: 847–53.

25. **Strober M, Lampert C, Schmidt S, Morrell W.** The course of major depressive disorder in adolescents. Part 1: Recovery and risk of manic switching in a follow-up of psychotic and nonpsychotic subtypes. *J Am Acad Child Adolesc Psychiatry.* 1993;32:34–42.

26. **Kovacs M, Feinberg TL, Craus-Novak M, et al.** Depressive disorders in childhood. Part II: A longitudinal study of the risk for subsequent major depression. *Arch Gen Psychiatry.* 1984;41:643–9.

27. **Weissman MM, Wolk S, Goldstein RB, et al.** Depressed adolescents grown up. *J Am Med Assoc.* 1999;281:1707–13.

28. **Holinger PC, Offer D, Barter JT, Bell CC.** *Suicide and Homicide Among Adolescents.* New York: Guildford; 1999.

29. **Birmaher B, Ryan ND, Williamson DE, et al.** Childhood and adolescent depression: a review of the past 10 years. Part II. *J Am Acad Child Adolesc Psychiatry.* 1996;35:1575–83.

30. **Burke MJ, Preskorn SH.** Short-term treatment of mood disorders with standard antidepressants. In Bloom FE, Kupfer DJ (eds). *Psychopharmacology: The Fourth Generation of Progress.* New York: Raven Press; 1995:1053–65.

31. **Boulos C, Kutcher S, Gardner D, Young E.** An open naturalistic trial of fluoxetine in adolescents and young adults with treatment resistant major depression. *J Child Adolesc Psychopharmacol.* 1992;2:103–11.

32. **Colle LM, Belair JF, DiFeo M, et al.** Extended open-label fluoxetine treatment of adolescents with major depression. *J Child Adolesc Psychopharmacol.* 1994;4: 225–32.

33. **Emslie G.** A double-blind, randomized, placebo-controlled trial of fluoxetine in children and adolescents with depression. *Arch Gen Psychiatry.* 1997;54:1031–7.

34. **Ghaziuddin N, Kine C, Naylor M, et al.** *Electroconvulsive Therapy in Refractory Adolescent Depression.* Paper presented at the 42nd Annual Meeting of the Academy of Child and Adolescent Psychiatry, New Orleans, 1995.

35. **Brent DA, Birmaher B, Holder D, et al.** *A Clinical Psychotherapy Trial for Adolescent Major Depression.* Paper presented at the 42nd Annual Meeting of the Academy of Child and Adolescent Psychiatry, New Orleans, 1995.

KEY REFERENCES

Birmaher B, Ryan ND, Williamson DE, et al. Childhood and adolescent depression: a review of the past 10 years. Part I. *J Am Acad Child Adolesc Psychiatry.* 1996;35: 1427–39.

A review summarizing the literature on the prevalence and symptomatology of major depression in children and adolescents.

Kovacs M. Presentation and course of major depressive disorder during childhood and later years of the lifespan. *J Am Acad Child Adolesc Psychiatry.* 1996;35:705–15.

A review and critical analysis of data-based findings on the presentation of major depressive symptoms and the clinical course of the illness from ages 6 to 80 years.

11

■ ■ ■

Depression in the Terminally Ill

Thomas S. Zaubler, MD, MPH

A lthough most patients who are critically ill do not suffer from depression, they are at significantly increased risk for developing a clinical depression compared with patients who have less severe medical illnesses. The importance of diagnosing depression in this population is underscored by the effectiveness of various pharmacologic and therapeutic interventions. If left untreated, depression may impair a patient's competence to make treatment decisions, which often are of a life-and-death nature in the critically ill. Depression and feelings of hopelessness in patients with terminal illness also may lead to an increased risk of suicide and requests for assistance in suicide.

Prevalence

Depression is a common problem in patients who are terminally ill. Between 13% and 26% of terminally ill patients have been found to have major depression (1). Prevalence rates of depression may vary depending on the stringency of the criteria used to diagnose depression, the type and severity of illness a patient may have, hospitalization status, and time since diagnosis of a patient's medical illness (2). The frequency of depression increases with the severity of terminal illness symptoms experienced by pa-

251

tients. In one study, more than 40% of patients with advanced cancer were found to have a major depression (3). Given such exceedingly high rates of depression, it is essential that clinicians thoroughly evaluate all patients with terminal illness for depression.

It is also important that clinicians neither expect all patients with terminal illness to be depressed nor assume that all depression in the terminally ill is "normal." Most studies have shown that fewer than one third of these patients suffer from clinical depression. Those caring for the critically ill may tend to assume incorrectly that anyone with a severe, life-threatening illness must be depressed and therefore should be treated for depression. Alternatively, clinicians may dismiss depressive symptomatology as sadness or demoralization perceived as a natural consequence of severe illness that does not merit treatment. Clinicians should avoid these perspectives. Although depression may be a consequence of severe or terminal illness, it is neither an inevitability nor a transient emotional state considered to be a "normal" response to difficult circumstances.

Diagnosis

Patients with terminal illness have feelings of sadness and despondency, often in the absence of a clinical depression, as they grieve the loss of their health, autonomy, life, friends, and family (4). Some individuals may be very forthcoming and demonstrative with these feelings. Conversations with them may reflect a tendency toward introspection and communication of emotions. Others may be much more reserved about discussing their thoughts and feelings. They may focus on how those around them are coming to terms with their demise. Stoic extroversion may characterize the coping mechanism of such individuals.

It is best to be respectful of different personality styles and to avoid imposing a single or rigid prescription for how one should come to terms with dying. Feelings of sadness, despondency, and demoralization should be respected and validated. One challenge for clinicians who care for the terminally ill is to avoid conflating healthy and appropriate responses to a tragic circumstance with a clinical depression. For example, because patients with a terminal illness often benefit from reassurance and support, an inappropriate diagnosis of depression in a patient in whom a healthy expression of sadness is pathologized may erode the supportive relationship between patient and health care providers. Receiving such a diagnosis is likely to increase their feelings of being out of control, not only of their bodies but also of their minds. Conversely, failing to diagnose clinical depression leads to unnecessary suffering, may cause increased morbidity and premature mortality, and may deprive an individual of a dignified death.

Distinguishing Clinical Depression from Subclinical Depressive Symptoms

One of the greatest challenges in diagnosing depression in the terminally ill is distinguishing clinical depression from normal reactive symptoms, such as feelings of demoralization or sadness (5). There are quantitative and qualitative distinctions that may help. Quantitatively, the severity with which patients experience feelings of dysphoria (e.g., sadness, irritability) may help to distinguish a treatable clinical depression from emotional responses that are within a normal range. The number of depressive symptoms distinguishes major from minor depressions (see Chapter 3). Qualitatively, it is important to pay close attention to the consistency and intensity of a patient's affect. Patients with clinical depression are likely to have a consistently constricted, irritable, and/or sad affect. They are less likely to be able to engage in conversation and express feelings of hope, interest, or future plans than those who may be discouraged but not clinically depressed. The patient with clinical depression typically expresses feelings of hopelessness, helplessness, and worthlessness that can be severe and unremitting. Although many patients with a terminal illness lose hope of a cure, they do not lose hope of the possibility of amelioration of pain and suffering before their death. A pervasive sense of hopelessness accompanied by feelings of despair indicates a depressive disorder (6). Clinical depression may lead to maladaptive coping with the illness, such as noncompliance with palliative treatment or severing contact with friends and family.

Bereavement Versus Depression

Although bereavement typically refers to a grieving process experienced in response to the death of others, dying patients may experience bereavement as they grieve the losses they experience as a result of their illness. These may include the loss of self; relationships with friends, family, and loved ones; bodily function; independence and autonomy; professional identity; financial stability; and self-esteem. Distinguishing between clinical depression and a grief reaction to critical illness is often difficult; in fact, both may occur simultaneously.

The patient who grieves for the losses associated with dying may experience psychological symptoms such as intermittent feelings of helplessness, hopelessness, worthlessness, and anger. Somatic symptoms of depression (e.g., changes in sleep pattern, appetite, concentration, memory, and energy level) are also fairly common (7). It is common for dying patients to experience these symptoms up until the time of their death.

A "normal" grief response to a terminal illness may be distinguished by the intensity and persistence of various psychological and somatic symptoms. Patients with depression may have persistent guilty ruminations about not being sufficiently available to help provide for family and friends over the course of their lifetime. Patients experiencing a grief reaction, on the other hand, may have feelings of guilt that are more circumscribed and focused on how they will not be available to others after they have died. Although grief may be associated with fleeting suicidal thoughts, pervasive thoughts of killing one's self are associated more typically with major depression. Patients with a grief reaction have been found to have occasional limited hallucinations, such as hearing the voice or seeing an image of a deceased friend or relative; however, more extensive hallucinations or delusions are psychopathologic.

Overlapping Symptoms of Medical Illness and Depression

Many symptoms of depression, somatic symptoms in particular, also are associated with medical illness, and it may be exceedingly difficult to determine their cause (8,9). For example, symptoms such as fatigue, poor sleep, anorexia, or psychomotor retardation—all of which are associated with depression—may be the direct result of a medical illness. Among patients with terminal illness, it is more likely than not that they will experience one or several of these symptoms as a direct effect of the illness itself. The diagnosis of depression in patients with critical illness is, therefore, confounded by this effect.

Given the difficulty of discerning whether symptoms are due to depression or medical illness, several approaches have been proposed to diagnose depression in the medically ill. The *inclusive approach* entails counting all symptoms toward a diagnosis of depression, whether or not they may be due primarily to a medical problem. Another approach, the *etiologic approach*, attempts to determine the etiology of symptoms and counts symptoms toward a diagnosis of depression only if they clearly are not due to a physical illness (10). A third approach, known as the *substitutive approach*, suggests that when a determination cannot be made about whether symptoms are due to depression or a physical illness, they should be substituted with ones that can be attributed more clearly to depression. For example, Endicott (11) suggests that symptoms such as brooding, pessimism, social withdrawal, decreased talkativeness, seeming depressed, and an unreactive mood (i.e., inability to be cheered up) should be used as substitutes for the somatic symptoms of depression to facilitate the accuracy and validity of the diagnosis of depression in the medically ill. A fourth diagnostic approach simply entails the exclusion of depressive symptoms that may be attributed to physical illness. This *exclusive approach* clearly maximizes the specificity of the diagnosis of depression but may decrease the sensitivity, resulting in possible false-negative diagnoses of depression (3).

Several studies have explored systematically the effect of each of these diagnostic approaches on prevalence rates of depression in the medically ill. There is a reduction of approximately 1.5% to 8.0% in the prevalence of major depression among medically ill patients when comparing the inclusive approach with the exclusive approach (12,13). When stringent criteria are used to diagnose major depression in patients who are critically ill, there is a negligible difference in the prevalence rates of depression when comparing an inclusive approach with a substitutive approach (1,5). There is little information about the effect of the etiologic approach on prevalence rates of major depression among the medically ill; however, a problem with this approach is the difficulty inherent in being able to infer whether or not a somatic symptom is due to depression or physical illness. For example, it simply may be impossible to know whether fatigue is due to an underlying malignancy or whether it is a symptom of depression. Ultimately, this determination may be contingent on whether or not the fatigue responds to antidepressant treatment.

An Inclusive Approach to Diagnosis

Clinicians must decide which approach they will use when diagnosing depression in the medically ill. Whichever approach is used, it is important to bear in mind that, although major depression tends to be underdiagnosed in the medical setting (14), some authors have suggested that studies exploring rates of major depression in the medically ill may overestimate the prevalence of depression given the methodologic problems of diagnosing depression in this setting (1,5). In order for a diagnosis of depression to be made, the *Diagnostic and Statistical Manual of Mental Disorders*, fourth edition (DSM-IV) states that "depressive symptoms must not be due to a general medical condition" (15). This is largely consistent with an etiologic approach; however, given the lack of validity and reliability inherent in the etiologic and substitutive approaches, I do not recommend them. The exclusive approach may be particularly useful for research purposes in which it is important to maximize diagnostic specificity rather than sensitivity. In the clinical setting, however, it is critical to diagnose and treat major depression. The inclusive approach clearly maximizes the chance that depression will be diagnosed by counting all somatic symptoms toward a diagnosis of major depression. I, therefore, recommend using an inclusive diagnostic approach and disregarding the DSM-IV requirement that clinicians infer whether symptoms are due directly to depression or a medical illness.

Psychological Symptoms

When diagnosing depression in the critically ill, clinicians must pay close attention to the psychological symptoms of depression. Feelings of hopelessness, helplessness, worthlessness; loss of self-esteem; persistent dysphoria; and suicidal ideation are often telltale diagnostic symptoms of depression. Given the limitations of using somatic symptoms when diagnosing depression in the medically ill, many recommend for diagnostic purposes that more weight be given to the psychological symptoms of depression because they may reflect the presence of a clinical depression in the critically ill more accurately (Case 11.1) (6,8,9,11,12,16,17).

CASE 11.1 *Assessment of psychological symptoms in a terminally ill patient with depression*

A man 53 years of age with metastatic lung cancer complains of fatigue, poor appetite, decreased concentration, and insomnia. These symptoms initially are attributed to the lung cancer; however, his family comments that his symptoms are persistent even after receiving successful palliative chemotherapy to relieve tumor burden. Although the patient has not discussed being depressed with either his family or his physicians, when he is questioned specifically about his mood, he describes feelings of emptiness, helplessness, hopelessness, and worthlessness that have persisted for over 3 months.
He is diagnosed with major depression.

Screening

To facilitate the detection of depression in the terminally ill, clinicians should screen all terminally ill patients for clinical depression. This may be accomplished simply by asking patients if they are depressed. A study that specifically examined various screening measures for depression in the terminally ill found that asking a patient "Are you depressed?" had the highest correlation with a full depression inventory (18). This simple query may be the most efficient and effective screen for depression in the terminally ill. If a patient responds affirmatively, the clinician should perform a full diagnostic interview using the inclusive approach to determine if a patient meets the full criteria for clinical depression. (For a more detailed discussion of screening instruments, *see* Chapter 3.)

Treatment of Depression in the Critically Ill

The treatment of depression in patients with terminal illness is similar to the treatment of depression in the medical setting in general. There are various modalities of treatment, including individual and group psychotherapy and antidepressant medications, all of which are known to be helpful and effective. (*See* also Chapters 5 and 6.)

Pharmacologic Management

The efficacy of antidepressant medication in the treatment of depression in the critically ill is well established (6,19,20). Among the antidepressants, the selective serotonin-reuptake inhibitors (SSRIs) venlafaxine, trazadone, nefazadone, and bupropion are often the best tolerated in terms of side effects. This is particularly important because patients with critical illness may be especially sensitive to the side effects from the older tricyclic antidepressants or monoamine oxidase inhibitors. The anticholinergic side effects of these older medications may lead to a worsening of cognitive function and delirium. Their antihistaminic properties may lead to excessive sedation, and their alpha-adrenergic–blocking properties can cause orthostatic hypotension. Because patients who are terminally ill are likely to be on many other medications, it is important to minimize the possibility of drug interactions. Some antidepressants are less likely to cause drug interactions mediated by the hepatic cytochrome P450 system than others. For example, citalopram, venlafaxine, mirtazapine, and bupropion are not known to have any significant effects on the cytochrome P450 isoenzymes and may be especially safe to use in patients who are on multiple medications that are metabolized by this cytochrome system. (For more information on drug interactions, *see* Chapter 13.)

Psychostimulants

The psychostimulants (dextroamphetamine and methylphenidate) are an extremely useful and effective alternative to other antidepressants for the treatment of depression in the critically ill. Because the onset of action of most antidepressants is generally between 2 to 4 weeks (sometimes longer), it may take an unacceptably long period of time before depression is treated in an individual who has only days or weeks to live. The psychostimulants, however, have a nearly immediate onset of action. Patients typically respond with significantly improved mood and energy level within 1 or 2 days after psychostimulant treatment is initiated (21). Psychostimulants have been shown to improve attention, concentration, and overall neuropsychological function (22). At a low dose, they also may stimulate appetite and ameliorate feelings of fatigue and lethargy that can be particularly problematic in depressed patients who are terminally ill (Case 11.2). Because of their activating properties, the psychostimulants are particularly useful in depressed patients who are anergic, unmotivated, and anhedonic, but they may aggravate insomnia or anxiety.

It also has been shown that the psychostimulants can potentiate the analgesic properties of narcotic medications while counteracting unwanted sedation (23). Patients with depression who are being treated concurrently for pain with narcotics such as methadone or morphine may derive an additional benefit of enhanced analgesia with the psychostimulants.

CASE 11.2 *Benefit of a psychostimulant in a terminally ill woman with depression*

A woman 41 years of age with melanoma that has metastasized to her bones and mediastinum describes feeling very depressed and hopeless. She says that she has not been able to get pleasure out of anything for several weeks and spends almost all her time lying in bed watching television. She describes having very little energy and poor concentration. Her appetite is markedly diminished, and she has lost almost 20 lb in the past 3 weeks.

She is diagnosed with major depression and is treated with Ritalin titrated to a dosage of 10 mg twice daily. Within days, her mood improves. She seems visibly brighter and more energetic and spontaneous. Her appetite also improves, and she gains 10 lb over the next 3 weeks.

Although they generally are not associated with adverse effects, psychostimulants may cause reversible dose-related central nervous system, cardiovascular, and gastrointestinal side effects. Psychostimulants should be used with caution in patients with uncontrolled cardiac arrhythmias, severe hypertension, and delirium because these conditions can be exacerbated. Although psychostimulants (primarily at higher doses) can lead to craving and compulsive use, the abuse potential in the medical setting is extremely low and is far outweighed by the potential benefits for patients with depression and terminal illness (24). Addiction to stimulants (like opiates) is an irrelevant concern in the terminally ill.

Dosing

The dosing of the psychostimulants is fairly straightforward (Table 11.1). Methylphenidate is generally begun at a dose of 5 mg at 8 AM. Pulse and blood pressure should be checked approximately 1 hour after the dose to see if there are significant elevations. If not, the dose can be titrated up as needed. Typically, the dose is increased by 5 mg every 2 to 3 days. Patients generally do not require a dosage that exceeds 30 mg/d (divided into AM and Noon-time doses). Dextroamphetamine is typically started at 2.5 mg at 8 AM and increased by 2.5 to 5.0 mg every 2 days. Patients generally do not require a dosage of greater than 30 mg/d. Some patients may benefit from an additional dose of dextroamphetamine in the afternoon; however, because of its longer half-life this is often unnecessary. Doses after 4 PM should be avoided in the administration of either of these medications because insomnia can occur.

Psychostimulants also may be given adjunctively with other antidepressants in the early phases of treatment. When this is done, the psychostimulant helps to treat the acute phase of depression, whereas the other antidepressant may take several weeks to become effective. Eventually, the psychostimulant may be tapered and discontinued, and the additional antidepressant will continue to treat the depression and prevent a recurrence of depressive symptoms.

Table 11.1   Psychostimulants and the Treatment of Depression

Drug	Dosage	Peak Plasma Level (hours)	Half-Life (hours)
Methylphenidate (Ritalin)	5–30 mg/d divided in twice-daily doses at 8 AM and Noon	0.3–4.0	1.0–7.0
Dextroamphetamine (Dexedrine)	2.5–30 mg/d in once-daily dose at 8 AM; sometimes patients benefit from an additional afternoon dose	1.0–4.0	11.5

In some cases, patients may experience only a partial response to an antidepressant and may require ongoing augmentation with a psychostimulant.

Psychotherapy

The importance of providing dying patients an opportunity to discuss their thoughts and feelings about death and dying cannot be underestimated. Too often, patients with a terminal illness are not questioned sufficiently about their views of the dying process. Health care providers, family, and friends frequently are uncomfortable talking about death, perhaps because of fears of their own mortality (25). The dying patient is likely to feel even more isolated as the subject of their death is conspicuously avoided in conversation. Health care providers may tend to distract themselves unwittingly from anxieties about death and dying by focusing on a patient's acute medical problems and by providing treatment and symptomatic relief (26). When there are multiple physicians from different disciplines consulting on a patient's care, it is not uncommon for that care to become fragmented, with the emphasis on treating organ systems, not on the patient as a unique individual facing the prospect of an imminent demise.

One obstacle to discussing death and dying with a terminally ill patient is the concern that the health care provider will not know what to say. Furthermore, the fear of not knowing how to respond to a patient may be compounded by feelings that the health care provider has given insufficient or inadequate care that was not able to treat the patient's underlying medical illness effectively. It is critical for health care providers who treat terminally ill patients to be aware of the feelings of inadequacy engendered by medical treatment failures and to avoid emotionally distancing themselves from their dying patients. Moreover, what is most important in discussions with the dying patient is not providing advice or profound insight into the dying process but simply listening to what the patient has to say (27). Listening to a patient talk about death can provide support, empathy, and compassion, which can be enormously therapeutic.

Supportive Psychotherapy

Supportive psychotherapy plays an important role in the care of the terminally ill patient with depression. Depression among the terminally ill may lead to increased social withdrawal and poor communication with family, friends, and health care providers. The isolation often associated with the dying process is magnified by depression, which has a profound effect on quality of life and may deprive an individual of a graceful, dignified death. Supportive psychotherapy attempts 1) to bolster the patient's coping styles and defenses; 2) provides him or her with an opportunity to ventilate feelings of rage, anger, guilt, and humiliation; and 3) helps him or her come to terms with the process of dying (28). Usually, the most effective treatment for depression in the terminally ill is a combination of medication and psychotherapy.

There is considerable evidence supporting the effectiveness of psychotherapy for depression in the terminally ill (29). Studies have shown that individual psychotherapy in patients with a critical illness can help treat depression, decrease psychological distress, and improve the patient's quality of life and ability to cope with medical problems (30–32). Supportive group psychotherapy for patients with critical illness also has been shown to be effective in treating depression, improving coping skills and pain control, and decreasing social isolation; it may even improve survival rates (29,33–36). One study of patients with metastatic breast cancer showed that survival for patients in the support group was a mean of 36.3 months compared with 18.9 months in the control group (35).

Depression and Competence

Inevitably, terminally ill patients are faced with critical decisions about their medical care on a continuum of treatment options from aggressive interventions to comfort care. Patients must decide whether invasive or aversive treatments (e.g., chemotherapy, dialysis, ventilator) are desired, including resuscitation or intubation in the event of cardiac or respiratory arrest. Clinicians face particularly challenging ethical and clinical problems when a terminally ill patient who has depression is faced with critical treatment decisions. The clinician should attempt to establish whether a patient's treatment preferences are characteristic of values and beliefs held before the onset of the depression or a distorted product of the depression itself.

How Depression May Impair Competence

Depression may lead to an impairment of competence that should be neither assumed nor overlooked in patients with critical medical illnesses. The depressed patient may be able to understand the facts of his or her treatment, including the risks and benefits of treatment, but often has difficulty appreciating how treatment may be helpful (37). The translation of an abstract, factual understanding of information to an appreciation of how this information applies to one's life may be very difficult for the patient with depression.

In particular, it may be helpful to focus on the psychological symptoms of depression rather than somatic symptoms when evaluating competence (38,39). Feelings of hopelessness may lead patients to underestimate the benefits and overestimate the risks of treatment. Hopelessness may make it impossible for patients to imagine an improved quality of life and a reasonable balance of benefits and burdens associated with treatment. Worthlessness and guilt may lead to a perception that suffering and even death are deserved and should not be prevented (Case 11.3). Guilty feelings of being a burden on others may result in patients refusing treatment. Anhedonia may make it impossible for patients to imagine ever again experiencing pleasure, thereby leading to a sense that medical treatment and its indignities are not worth pursuing. Apathy may lead to a perception that any painful or labor-intensive treatment intervention is intolerable. Conversely, apathy also may result in patients passively acquiescing to their physician's treatment plans, which may be overly aggressive. All of these symptoms may make it very difficult for patients to develop a trusting rapport with their health care providers. Finally, suicidal thoughts may lead patients to refuse prematurely any life-saving or -sustaining treatment.

CASE 11.3 *Effect of depression on the competence of a terminally ill patient*

A man 38 years of age with AIDS is refusing to take medications (e.g., protease inhibitors) that will likely help prolong his life. He describes feeling overwhelmed by his medical problems and that he has nothing to which to look forward in the future. He comments that he may deserve his illness because of things he has done in the past, which he is too embarrassed to discuss. On further examination, the patient is diagnosed with a major depression.

After receiving treatment with antidepressant medication, his mood brightens, he is hopeful about the future, stops dwelling on misdeeds in the past, and agrees to take his medications.

Effect of Depression on Preferences for Life-Sustaining Treatment

Surveys of treatment preferences of older patients have found no consistent association between the severity of depressive symptoms and preferences for life-sustaining treatment (40,41). One study in elderly patients showed that severe depression was associated with a desire for *more* treatment in hypothetical treatment scenarios (42). However, another study found that elderly patients with mild to moderate depression were more likely to choose *less* aggressive treatment in hypothetical treatment scenarios than elderly subjects who were not depressed (43). The effect of depression, however, was limited to scenarios in which the prognosis was good and depression accounted for only 5% of the variance in subjects' treatment preferences. Patients' assessments of quality of life were far more likely than depression to predict desire for life-sustaining treatment. A follow-up study showed that treatment of mild to moderately severe major depression did not affect treatment preferences about life-sustaining treatment (43). Treatment of patients with severe depression has resulted in an increased desire for life-sustaining treatment; once their depression resolved, some patients who refused lifesaving treatment while severely depressed wound up grateful that their treatment preferences were overridden (44,45).

Although it is hard to draw definitive conclusions from these studies collectively, it does seem that severe depression and the hopelessness often associated with it may lead patients to refuse or have a decreased desire for life-sustaining treatment. One possible explanation for this is that patients with severe depression may be pessimistically inclined to overestimate the risks of treatment and underestimate the benefits. Mild to moderate depression does not seem to have a significant effect on desire for life-sustaining treatment.

Determining Whether Depression Affects Patient Competence

Although there may be a differential effect of depression on treatment preferences depending on depression severity, it may be very difficult for clinicians to determine which requests for do-not-resuscitate orders or refusal of life-sustaining treatment should be honored and which should not in patients with depression. In contrast to schizophrenia, mania, dementia, and delirium, depression (without psychotic features) is unlikely to affect a patient's ability to offer "rational" explanations for treatment preferences (46). Physicians also may be inclined to perceive depression and the attendant feelings of hopelessness or helplessness as appropriate responses to severe medical illness. This "pseudo-empathy" leads to a disregard for distortions of judgment and decision making that may be associated with depression (39). Another factor that also undermines the appropriate detection of judgment and decision-making problems due to depression in the terminally ill is that physicians are likely to underestimate quality of life and desire for life-sustaining treatment in their patients with severe medical illness (41).

The determination of when depression is adversely affecting a patient's ability to make decisions about treatment is best determined by a thorough and systematic assessment of competence (39). Competence refers to a patient's ability to make an informed, rational choice about treatment. The doctrine of informed consent mandates that we must respect patients' competent decisions about their treatment, even when these may include refusal of life-saving treatment. Depression may lead to impairment of competence; however, depressed patients are often capable of making competent decisions. Depression, even when severe and accompanied by suicidal ideation, does not automatically preclude some capacity for decision making.

When evaluating competence, clinicians must assess the patient's thought process that leads to a particular decision about treatment. The decision itself should not form the basis for establishing whether or not a patient has made a competent choice (although some choices naturally raise more concerns than others). Patients certainly have a right to make treatment decisions that conflict with their physicians' recommendations. The assessment of competence focuses on one particular decision a patient must make about treatment. A patient, for example, may be deemed competent to make some decisions about treatment, whereas other decisions may be judged as too complex for him or her. Technically, competence refers to a legal determination of a patient's decision-making process and must be adjudicated in a court of law. In the clinical setting, physicians are actually assessing patients' decision-making capacity. The distinction between capacity and competence is largely procedural, and in this chapter both are used interchangeably.

Standards Used To Evaluate Competence

In general, four standards are used to evaluate competence (47) (Table 11.2). The least rigorous standard entails ascertaining whether a patient has *expressed a clear and consistent choice* about his or her treatment. Patients who are severely aphasic or so ambivalent that they constantly change their mind fail to meet this standard. A second standard involves determining whether a patient understands the nature of his or her medical condition, the treatment that is being recommended (and its risk and benefits), and alternative treatment options. Evaluation of patient *understanding* of these issues, of course, presupposes that there has been sufficient disclosure of information about their medical condition and treatment options from their physicians. A third standard focuses on patient *appreciation* of their medical illness and treatment needs. Appreciation involves the capacity to apply facts about medical illness or treatment options to one's own life and circumstances. Patients may be able to elaborate on their understanding about their medical condition but fail to appreciate the personal significance and impact of this information on their lives. It is as though they were talking about a third person or hypothetical scenario. The fourth standard entails an assessment of patient *rationality*—whether a patient is

Table 11.2   Standards Used To Assess Competence To Make Treatment Decisions

Standard	Definition	Level of Stringency
Expressing a choice	The ability to express a clear, unambiguous, and consistent choice about treatment	Easiest of the standards to meet
Understanding	The ability to understand the nature and purpose of the treatment being recommended, its risks and benefits, and any alternatives	More difficult to meet than "expressing a choice" but less difficult than "appreciation" or "rationality"
Appreciation	The ability to apply the facts about medical illness or treatment to one's own life	Along with "rationality," this is more difficult to meet; patients also may be able to understand information about their treatment but fail to appreciate its significance on a personal level
Rationality	The ability to reason clearly and logically about medical illness and the risks and benefits of treatment	Along with "appreciation," this is more difficult to meet

able to provide a clear, logical reasoning process that supports their decisions about treatment. These last two standards—appreciation and rationality—generally are considered to be more rigorous than an understanding of or an ability to express a choice about treatment.

The application of these standards of competence involves an assessment of the risk-to-benefit ratio of the treatment decision a patient has made (48). A patient who is refusing a life-sustaining treatment probably should meet all four standards of competence before accepting the refusal as competent. On the other hand, a patient refusing a treatment that has many risks associated with it and may be of questionable benefit may need to meet only one or two of the less rigorous competence standards, such as "expressing a choice" or "understanding," before a refusal can be accepted. Hence, assessments of competence depend the unique circumstances that a patient faces about a particular treatment decision. The stringency of the threshold used to determine whether a patient should be deemed competent or incompetent is set in part by the rigor of the competence standard used and by a determination to use one, all, or a combination of the competence standards. From a legal perspective, there may be case law or statutory definitions of competence that specify the application of these standards, which may vary among different jurisdictions.

When To Evaluate Competence

When assessing competence, the burden of proof is on the clinician, not the patient. All patients, depressed or not, should be treated with the presumption that they are capable of making competent decisions about treatment. If the psychological symptoms of depression seem to affect a patient's judgment in such a way that he or she is making treatment decisions that seem out of character, odd, or unreasonable, then a competency evaluation should be set in motion. The clinician must demonstrate clearly which standards of competence the patient fails to meet and make an ultimate determination about competence based on the patient's decision-making process rather than the decision's outcome. The doctrine of informed consent clearly provides patients with the right to make treatment decisions that may seem inappropriate or unreasonable to their health care providers so long as the decision-making process reflects the reasoning of a competent individual.

Advance Directives for Patients with Impaired Competence

If a patient is found to be incompetent due to depression, it is extremely helpful if an advance directive expresses the patient's preferences about treatment and choice of a surrogate decision maker. If an advance directive is not available, decisions about treatment should be deferred to family and friends. Steps also should be taken to restore the patient's competence by treating depression. Competence is not a static determination. It may change with a patient's mental status and course of depression.

The Challenge of Evaluating Competence in the Terminally Ill

It may be especially difficult to determine whether depression is sufficiently impairing competence to justify overriding a patient's treatment preferences. If, for example, a patient refuses life-sustaining treatment, determining whether depression is affecting his or her decision-making ability may be extremely difficult. For a patient who is not critically ill, a typically viable option (e.g., to postpone the decision, treat the depression, and reassess competence at a later time) will not be possible for a patient who is terminally ill because he or she may die before an antidepressant takes effect. Moreover, sometimes depression in the terminally ill may be treatment resistant. Clinicians must be cognizant of the unique circumstances in evaluating competency in patients with terminal illness; they must be open to the possibility that there are times when it is better to respect rather than to override a patient's decision, even if it means the patient might die prematurely (i.e., days, weeks, or months before death is ultimately inevitable) (39).

Suicide and Terminal Illness

The risk of suicide is much higher among patients with terminal illness than in the general population. In patients with cancer, the relative risk of suicide is twice that of the general population. Among patients with AIDS, the rate of suicide may be 66 times as high as in the general population (49). Although depression is a risk factor for both attempted and completed suicides, little is known about the association between suicide and depression in the terminally ill.

Most of the literature on depression and suicidality is based on psychological postmortem reviews of individuals who have completed suicide but were not critically ill at the time of their deaths. These "psychological autopsies" reveal that, in more than 90% of all suicides, individuals were suffering from a psychiatric disorder such as depression at the time of the suicide (50–52). Given the unique circumstances surrounding terminal illness, it is problematic to extrapolate from the association between depression and suicidality in the medically well and postulate a similar association in the terminally ill (53). Only two studies have examined explicitly this association in the terminally ill. One study found that 10 of 44 patients with terminal illness were suicidal or desired an early death, and all 10 were suffering from clinical depression (54). Another study found that 17 out of 199 (8.5%) terminally ill patients had a "serious and pervasive desire" for death (55). Of these 17 patients, 10 (58%) had a clinical depression. These results suggest that, although depression may be a risk factor for suicide among the terminally ill, it is certainly not always associated with suicidal ideation in this population. Moreover, studies have shown that feelings of hopelessness and assessments of poor quality of life may play a far more important role than depression in mediating suicidal feelings among the terminally ill (38,56).

Physician-Assisted Suicide

Given the increased risk of suicide among terminally ill patients, their physicians are likely to encounter requests by patients for assistance in suicide. Although patients may be capable of attempting suicide on their own without any assistance, they may approach their physicians to ensure that their suicides will be effective in a quick and comfortable manner. It is critical that health care providers be familiar with some of the legal, ethical, and clinical issues pertaining to the physician-assisted suicide debate before responding reflexively to patient requests for assistance in suicide.

From a legal perspective, Oregon is the only state that has legalized physician-assisted suicide. Physicians who assist in their patients' suicides elsewhere are risking the possibility of a criminal conviction and jail sentence. Ethically, there is much debate about the appropriateness of physician-assisted suicide. Some argue that out of respect for patient autonomy, patients should be permitted the opportunity to commit suicide and seek their physician's assistance if so desired. From this point of view, for a physician to refuse such a request is tantamount to abandoning a suffering patient when they are at their greatest need of help (57). Others argue that it is never ethically acceptable for a physician to participate in an activity that directly and intentionally leads to the ending of a human life. To do so not only may violate the sanctity of life but also the integrity of the medical profession. Some also have postulated a slippery slope, i.e., a scenario in which the actions or policies that legitimate or legalize physician-assisted suicide lead to abuses wherein vulnerable patients are pressured, coerced, or even forced to die (58).

Responding to Requests for Physician-Assisted Suicide

From a clinical perspective, it is critical that health care providers explore the possibility that requests for assisted suicide are mediated by treatable clinical conditions such as depression. It is certainly possible that, after receiving appropriate treatment for depression, patients may change their minds about ending their lives prematurely. Some argue that physicians should come to an agreement with patients who request assistance in suicide to have this decision postponed for a period of time that would allow for the depression treatment to take effect; however, this may not always be feasible in terminally ill patients who face an imminent natural death (59). Furthermore, it is critical that clinicians assess a patient's competence to make a decision about assisted suicide given the distinct possibility that there may be clinical factors such as depression that are impairing competency.

When responding to requests for assistance in suicide among the terminally ill, physicians should look for other underlying, potentially remediable problems in addition to depression (60). Changes in a patient's social support system and relationships with friends, family, and health care providers may play a role in the development of suicidal thoughts. Poor control of pain or other symptoms (e.g., nausea, delirium) may lead to a desire for death. An individual's perspectives on the dignity versus the sanctity of life and the meaning of suffering may be important determinants in the development of suicidal ideation. Studies have shown that the most common reasons why patients request or receive assistance in suicide pertain to concerns about "physical disintegration, dependence, being a burden, extreme fatigue, and lack of meaning" (61). Therefore, in responding to requests for assisted suicide, it is critical that health care providers involve family and friends whenever possible, ensure that pain and other symptoms are well treated, and contact the patient's spiritual or religious advisors when appropriate.

Exploring the underlying motivations and personal meaning of patient requests for assistance in suicide is a critical role for health care providers who care for terminally ill patients. Although the expression of suicidal ideation among the terminally ill may reflect a rational decision to avoid the ravages of a progressive illness and to die a dignified death, it also may convey unarticulated psychological conflicts and needs to health care providers (62). Suicide may reflect a desire by patients to wrest some control over their destiny and their deteriorating physical health away from the irrevocable course of their terminal illness. A skillful clinician may help to redirect a desire for an early death by attempting to restore a sense of control over the symptoms associated with the illness and over treatment choices patients can make. Sometimes when patients are given the option of suicide, they lose interest in committing suicide and achieve a renewed sense of mastery over their circumstances. However, too-rapid agreement by the physician may dangerously demoralize patients who were hoping to be reassured and talked out of their pessimism by their doctor. Suicidality may represent an expression of rage that patients are experiencing over their prognosis, failed treatment, or disappointing relationships. It also may signify the guilt that patients are experiencing about 1) the previous behavior that caused or contributed to their illness, and/or 2) their inability to continue to be available for family or friends. Furthermore, patients may consciously believe that suicide is a way of coping with the difficult circumstances of dying (e.g., physical deterioration, pain, loss of dignity). However, patients actually may be displacing fears of death unconsciously onto these circumstances (63). Therefore, it is important to ask patients about their fears of death and to facilitate discussion about this.

In responding to requests for assisted suicide, physicians must avoid reflexive responses that cut off further discussion. Physicians should listen sympathetically and provide patients with an opportunity to discuss suicidal thoughts openly and freely. There is no reason to believe that inquiring about suicidal thoughts will somehow put the idea of suicide in the patient's head. It is critical to explore the *meaning* of the requests for assistance in suicide, rather than to take them literally, and to examine the role that untreated depression may play. With appropriate intervention, suicidality usually will wane and patients will be able to live out their final days with dignity. It is often helpful to seek psychiatric consultation when patients express suicidal ideation, but this consultation should not supplant ongoing discussion between patients and their primary physicians. Actions to take and issues to consider and discuss with the patient are summarized in Table 11.3.

Table 11.3   Responding to Requests for Physician-Assisted Suicide

- Supportive and compassionate response—avoid reflexive, overly judgmental responses

- Discuss suicidal thoughts with the patient

- Explore alternatives to suicide

- Evaluate for clinical depression

- Evaluate for uncontrolled physical symptoms

- Address with the patient any problems in relationships with family, friends, and/or significant others

- Explore underlying motivations and personal meaning of requests for assisted suicide

- Explore fears about death and the dying process

- Consider a referral to a mental health professional

- Evaluate competence if concerns are raised about the patient's decision-making capacity

---

■   ■   ■

Recommendations

- To maximize the chance of diagnosing depression in the terminally ill, clinicians should focus on the psychological symptoms of depression (e.g., feelings of hopelessness, helplessness, worthlessness) and should count all physical symptoms (e.g., problems with sleep, appetite, energy) toward the diagnosis, whether or not they may be attributable to the underlying medical illness.

- There is a risk of over- and under-diagnosing and -treating depression in the critically ill. Most patients with critical illness are not depressed, but depression is not a normal and inevitable consequence.

- Although antidepressants are a safe and effective treatment for depression in critical illness, they may take too long to work in patients who may have only days or weeks to live. Psychostimulants are equally safe and effective treatments for depression in this setting, and their onset of action may occur within hours after treatment has been initiated. Psychotherapy also may be very helpful for critically ill patients with depression.

- Depression may compromise a patient's decision-making ability and may lead the patient to refuse life-saving or -sustaining treatments. A patient with depression who must make critical treatment decisions should be evaluated to determine whether he or she is competent. Competence evaluations entail the assessment of the patient's ability to make a choice about treatment and to understand, appreciate, and reason rationally about the purpose, risks, and benefits of and alternatives to the recommended treatment.

- Clinicians should respond to requests for assisted suicide in critically ill patients in a supportive, compassionate manner that provides patients with the opportunity to discuss thoughts and feelings about death and dying. It is important to explore the underlying meaning of these requests as well as the roles that depression, pain, other distressing symptoms, and relationships play in the development of suicidal thoughts.

Key Points

- 13% to 26% of terminally ill patients suffer from major depression.
- The diagnosis of major depression in the terminally ill may be difficult to determine because of the overlapping symptoms in psychiatric and medical illness.
- Effective treatments for depression in the terminally ill include antidepressant and psychostimulant medication and psychotherapy.
- Depression may impair a patient's competence to make treatment decisions.
- Terminally ill patients are at relatively high risk for suicide and may request assistance from their physicians to commit suicide. Depression is often, but not always, a key factor underlying such requests.

1. **Chochinoc HM, Wilson KG, Enns M, et al.** Prevalence of depression in the terminally ill: effects of diagnostic criteria and symptom threshold judgments. *Am J Psychiatry*. 1994;151:537–40.

2. **McDaniel JS, Musselman DL, Porter MR, et al.** Depression in patients with cancer. *Arch Gen Psychiatry.* 1995;52:89–99.

3. **Bukberg J, Penman D, Holland J.** Depression in hospitalized cancer patients. *Psychosom Med.* 1984;43:199–212.

4. **Schwab JJ, Bialow MR, Clemmons RS, et al.** The affective symptomatology of depression in medical patients. *Psychosomatics.* 1996;7:214–7.

5. **Kathol RG, Musselman DL, Porter MR, et al.** Diagnosing depression in patients with medical illness. *Psychosomatics.* 1990;31:434–40.

6. **Massie MJ, Holland JC.** Depression and the cancer patient. *J Clin Psychiatry.* 1990; 51:12–7.

7. **Clayton PJ, Darvish HS.** Course of depressive symptoms following the course of bereavement. In Barrett JE, Rose RM, Klerman GL (eds). *Stress and Mental Disorder.* New York: Raven Press; 1979:121–39.

8. **Cavanaugh S, Clark DC, Gibbons RD.** Diagnosing depression in the hospitalized medically ill. *Psychosomatics.* 1983;24:809–15.

9. **Schwab JJ, Clemmons RS, Bialow M, et al.** A study of the somatic symptomatology of depression in medical inpatients. *Psychosomatics.* 1965;6:273–7.

10. **Spitzer RL, Endicott J, Robbins E.** Research diagnostic criteria. *Arch Gen Psychiatry.* 1978;35:773–82.

11. **Endicott J.** Measurement of depression in patients with cancer. *Cancer.* 1983;53: 2243–8.

12. **Kathol RG, Mutgi A, Williams J, et al.** Major depression diagnosed by DSM-III, DSM-III-R, RDC, and Endicott criteria in patients with cancer. *Am J Psychiatry.* 1990;147:1021–4.

13. **Federoff JP, Starkstein SE, Parikh RM, et al.** Are depressive symptoms non-specific in patients with acute stroke? *Am J Psychiatry.* 1991;148:1172–6.

14. **Koenig HG, Meador KG, Cohen HS.** Detection and treatment of depression in older medically ill hospitalized patients. *Int J Psychiatry Med.* 1988;18:17–31.

15. **American Psychiatric Association.** *Diagnostic and Statistical Manual of Mental Disorders,* 4th ed. Washington, DC: American Psychiatric Association; 1994:327.

16. **Mermelstein HT, Lesko L.** Depression in patients with cancer. *Psychooncol.* 1992; 1:199–215.

17. **Plumb MM, Holland JC.** Comparative studies of psychological function in patients with advanced cancer. *Psychosom Med.* 1977;39:264–76.

18. **Chochinov HM, Wilson KG, Enns M, Lander S.** "Are you depressed?": screening for depression in the terminally ill. *Am J Psychiatry.* 1997;154:674–6.

19. **Popkin MK, Callies AL, Mackenzie TB.** Outcome of antidepressant use in the medically ill. *Arch Gen Psychiatry.* 1985;42:1160–3.

20. **Rifkin A, Reardon G, Siris S.** Trimipramine in physical illness with depression. *J Clin Psychiatry.* 1985;46:4–8.

21. **Wallace AE, Kofoed LL, West AN.** Double-blind, placebo-controlled trial of methylphenidate in older, depressed, medically ill patients. *Am J Psychiatry.* 1995; 152:929–31.

22. **Fernandez F, et al.** Cognitive impairment due to AIDS related complex and its response to psychostimulants. *Psychosomatics.* 1988;29:38–46.

23. **Masand PS, Tesar GE.** Use of stimulants in the medically ill. *Psychiatr Clin North Am.* 1996;19:515–47.

24. **Angrist B, D'Hollosy M, Sanfilipo M, et al.** Central nervous stimulants as symptomatic treatments for AIDS-related neuropsychiatric impairment. *J Clin Psychopharmacol.* 1992;12:268–72.

25. **Gerber I.** Medical care of the dying patient: physicians' attitudes and behavior. In Klagsburn SC, Goldberg IK, Rawnsely MM, et al. (eds). *Psychiatric Aspects of Terminal Illness.* Philadelphia: The Charles Press; 1988:13–24.

26. **McCue JD.** The naturalness of dying. *JAMA.* 1995;273:1039–43.

27. **Cassem NH.** The dying patient. In Cassem NH, Stern TA, Rosenbaum JF, Jellinek MS (eds). *Massachusetts General Hospital Handbook of General Hospital Psychiatry.* St. Louis: Mosby; 1997:605–36.

28. **Muslim HL.** Psychiatric assessment and management of the dying patient. In Klagsburn SC, Goldberg IK, Rawnsely MM, et al. (eds). *Psychiatric Aspects of Terminal Illness.* Philadelphia: The Charles Press; 1988:101–8.

29. **Fawzy FI, Fawzy NW, Arndt LA, Pasnau RO.** Critical review of psychosocial interventions in cancer care. *Arch Gen Psychiatry.* 1995;52:100–13.

30. **Greer S, Moorey S, Baruch JDR.** Adjuvant psychological therapy for patients with cancer: a prospective randomized trial. *Br Med J.* 1992;304:675–80.

31. **Capone MA, Good RS, Westie KS, Jacobson AF.** Psychosocial rehabilitation of gynecologic oncology patients. *Arch Phys Med Rehabil.* 1980;61:128–32.

32. **Linn MW, Linn BS, Harris R.** Effects of counseling for late-stage cancer patients. *Cancer.* 1982;49:1048–55.

33. **Speigel D, Bloom JR, Yalom I.** Group support for patients with metastatic cancer. *Arch Gen Psychiatry.* 1981;38:527–33.

34. **Cain EN, Kohron EI, Quinland DM, et al.** Psychosocial benefits of a cancer support group. *Cancer.* 1986;57:183–9.

35. **Speigel D, Bloom JR, Laemer HC, Gottheil E.** Effect of psychosocial treatment on survival of patients with metastatic breast cancer. *Lancet.* 1989;2:888–91.

36. **Fawzy FI, Fawzy NW, Hyun CS, et al.** Malignant melanoma: effects of an early structured psychiatric intervention, coping, and affective state on recurrence and survival 6 years later. *Arch Gen Psychiatry.* 193;50:681–9.

37. **Bursztajn HJ, Harding HP, Gutheil TG, Brodsky A.** Beyond cognition:role of disordered affective states in impairing competence to consent to treatment. *Bull Am Acad Psychiatry Law.* 1991;19:383–8.

38. **Lee M, Ganzini L.** Depression in the elderly: effect on patient attitudes toward life-sustaining therapy. *J Am Geriatr Soc.* 1992;40:983–8.

39. **Sullivan MD, Youngner SJ.** Depression, competence, and the right to refuse life-saving medical treatment. *Am J Psychiatry.* 1994;151:971–8.

40. **Uhlman RF, Pearlman RA.** Perceived quality of life and preferences for life-sustaining treatment in older adults. *Arch Intern Med.* 1991;151:495–8.

41. **Michelson C, Mulvihill M, Hsu MA, et al.** Eliciting medical care preferences from nursing home residents. *Gerontologist.* 1991;31:358–63.

42. **Garrett JM, Harris RP, Norburn JK, et al.** Life-sustaining treatments during terminal illness. *J Gen Intern Med.* 1993;8:361–8.

43. **Ganzini L, Lee MA, Heintz RT, et al.** The effect of depression treatment on elderly patients' preferences for life-sustaining medical therapy. *Am J Psychiatry.* 1994;151:1631–6.

44. **Gutheil TG, Bursztajn H.** Clinicians' guidelines for assessing and presenting subtle forms of patient incompetence in legal settings. *Am J Psychiatry.* 1986;143: 1020–3.

45. **Swartz CM, Stewart C.** Melancholia and orders to restrict resuscitation. *Hosp Community Psychiatry.* 1991;42:189–91.

46. **Appelbaum PS, Roth LH.** Competency to consent to research: a psychiatric overview. *Arch Gen Psychiatry.* 1982;39:951–8.

47. **Appelbaum PS, Grisso T.** Assessing patients' capacities to consent to treatment. *N Engl J Med.* 1988;319:1635–8.

48. **Drane JF.** Competency to give an informed consent: a model for making clinical assessments. *JAMA.* 1984;252:925–7.

49. **Marzuk PM, et al.** Increased risk of suicide in persons with AIDS. *JAMA.* 1988; 259:1333–7.

50. **Barraclough B, Bunch J, Nelson B, Sainsbury P.** A hundred cases of suicide: clinical aspects. *Br J Psychiatry.* 1974;125:355–73.

51. **Dorpat TI, Ripley HS.** A study of suicide in the Seattle area. *Compr Psychiatry.* 1960;1:349–59.

52. **Rich CL, Young D, Fowler RC.** San Diego suicide study. *Arch Gen Psychiatry.* 1986;43:577–82.

53. **Zaubler TS, Sullivan MD.** Psychiatry and physician-assisted suicide. *Psychiatr Clin North Am.* 1996;19:413–27.

54. **Brown JH, Henteleff P, Barakat S, Roew CJ.** Is it normal for terminally patients to desire death? *Am J Psychiatry.* 1986;143:208–11.

55. **Chochinov HM, Wilson KG, Enns M, et al.** Desire for death in the terminally ill. *Am J Psychiatry.* 1995;152:1185–91.

56. **Chochinov HM, Wilson KG, Enns M, Lander S.** Depression, hopelessness, and suicidal ideation in the terminally ill. *Psychosomatics.* 1998;39:366–70.

57. **Brody H.** Assisted death: a compassionate response to a medical failure. *N Engl J Med.* 1992;327:1384–8.

58. **Conwell Y, Caine ED.** Rational suicide and the right to die: reality and myth. *N Engl J Med.* 1991;325:1100–2.

59. **Bursztajn H, Gutheil TG, Warren MJ, Brodsky A.** Depression, self-love, time, and the "right" to suicide. *Gen Hosp Psychiatry.* 1986;8:91–5.

60. **Block SD, Billings JA.** Patient requests to hasten death. *Arch Intern Med.* 1994;154:2039–47.

61. **Quill T, Meier DE, Block S, Billings JA.** The debate over physician-assisted suicide: empirical data and convergent views. *Ann Intern Med.* 1998;128:552–8.

62. **Muskin PR.** The request to die: role for a psychodynamic perspective on physician-assisted suicide. *JAMA.* 1998;279:323–8.

63. **Hendin H, Klerman G.** Physician-assisted suicide: the dangers of legalization. *Am J Psychiatry.* 1993;150:143–5.

KEY REFERENCES

Block SD, Billings JA. Patient requests to hasten death. *Arch Intern Med.* 1994;154: 2039–47.

The authors discuss how clinicians should respond to patient requests for assistance in suicide. They focus on the importance of exploring with patients who are seeking assistance in suicide issues, such as poor pain control, problems in interpersonal relationships, perspectives on the dignity versus the sanctity of life, and depression.

Chochinov HM, Wilson KG, Enns M, et al. Desire for death in the terminally ill. *Am J Psychiatry.* 1995;152:1185–91.

This is one of the few studies to explore the association between suicidality and depression in the terminally ill. The authors discuss the prevalence of depression among patients who expressed a "serious and pervasive desire to die" (58% of these patients suffered from major depression).

Chochinov HM, Wilson KG, Enns M, et al. Prevalence of depression in the terminally ill: effects of diagnostic criteria and symptom threshold judgments. *Am J Psychiatry.* 1994;151:537–40.

The authors discuss the prevalence of depression in the terminally ill (13%–26% of patients). They address the impact of factors such as the stringency of the criteria used for depression on the prevalence rate of depression.

Ganzini L, Lee MA, Heinttz RT, et al. The effect of depression treatment on elderly patients' preferences for life-sustaining medical therapy. *Am J Psychiatry.* 1994;151: 1631–6.

This is one of the few studies to explore the effect of depression treatment on patients' desires for life-sustaining treatment. Depression treatment did not seem to alter the desire to forego life-sustaining treatment in patients with mild to moderate depression. However, in patients with severe depression, there was an increased desire for life-sustaining treatment.

Sullivan MD, Youngner SJ. Depression, competence, and the right ro refuse lifesaving medical treatment. *Am J Psychiatry.* 1994;151:971–8.

This paper contrasts psychiatric and medical perspectives on the refusal of life-saving treatment by patients with severe medical illness. It addresses 1) the impact that depression may have on patients' abilities to make competent treatment decisions, and 2) the importance of assessing competence in depressed patients who refuse life-saving treatment.

12

■   ■   ■

Practice Guidelines

Anthony L. Pelonero, MD

Practice guidelines are intended to assist practitioners and patients in making appropriate health care decisions in specific clinical circumstances. This chapter provides an overview of important principles from the depression guidelines and demonstrates that practical application of a guideline in everyday practice can be achieved and is, in fact, desirable for physicians because their patients ultimately benefit.

There are currently two major practice guidelines for major depressive disorder that have been systematically developed and published in the United States. In 1993, the American Psychiatric Association (APA) published *Practice Guideline for Major Depressive Disorder in Adults* (1), which is geared primarily toward psychiatrists, and the Agency for Health Care Policy and Research (AHCPR)—an agency of the U.S. Department of Health and Human Services that has since been renamed the Agency for Healthcare Research and Quality—published their own guidelines for the detection, diagnosis, and treatment of depression in primary care (2,3). This chapter focuses mainly on the AHCPR guidelines and their application in primary care practice.

Treatment Basics from the Guidelines

In general, there is a large amount of overlap between the APA and AHCPR guidelines. A side-by-side comparison of important topical areas of the guidelines can be found in Table 12.1. Treatment of depression in both guidelines

Table 12.1   Comparison of APA and AHCPR Treatment Guidelines for Major Depressive Disorder

	APA	AHCPR
Target audience	Mental health professionals	PCPs
Acute treatment	6–8 weeks	6–12 weeks
Medication		
Selection	√	√√
Dosage	√√	√
Side effects	√√	√√
Failure	√√	√√
Follow-up	Rely on clinical	Severe: weekly for 6–8 weeks
		Less severe: every 10–14 days
Psychotherapy	√√	√ (suggests trained therapist)
Drugs and psychotherapy combined	√	√√
ECT	√	√
Light therapy	√	√
Continuation treatment	4–5 months after acute treatment completed	4–9 months after acute treatment completed
Follow-up	Rely on clinical judgment	Full responders: every 1–3 months; symptoms are more frequent
Maintenance treatment	5 months to ? (Individualize)	9 months to ? (Reevaluate)
Follow-up	Rely on clinical judgment	*See* Continuation follow-up
Special topics		
Drug discontinuation	√	√
Referrals	Not discussed	√√
Suicidal patients	√	√√
Hospitalization	√√	√
Comorbid medical disorders	√√	√
Comorbid psychiatric disorders	√√	√

√ = general coverage; √√ = detailed coverage; AHCPR = Agency for Health Care Policy and Research; APA = American Psychiatric Association; ECT = electroconvulsive therapy; PCPs = primary care physicians.

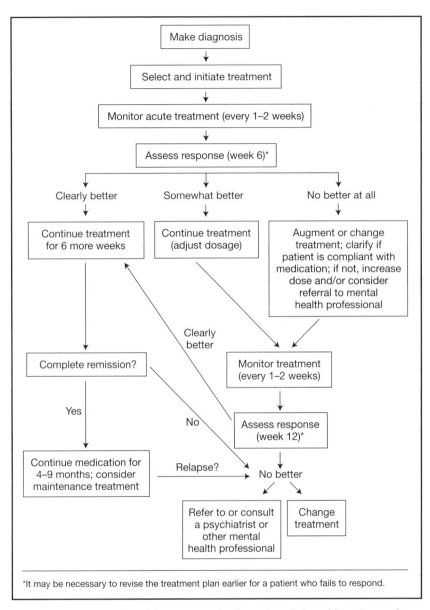

Figure 12.1   An overview of the treatment for depression. (Adapted from Agency for Health Care Policy and Research [2,3].)

is divided into three phases: acute, continuation, and maintenance. The length of time that each phase is expected to last is approximate, with generally longer estimates in the AHCPR compared with the APA guidelines. Both sets of guidelines state that effective treatments to achieve symptom resolution for depression include medication, psychotherapy, or both. Each set of guidelines stresses that the goal of treatment is not just the improvement of symptoms but complete symptom resolution. A flow chart overview from the AHCPR depression guidelines is reproduced in Figure 12.1.

After a diagnosis of depression has been made, the goal of the initial or *acute phase* of treatment is to achieve full remission of symptoms using one or both of the recommended modalities. The acute phase may last between 6 and 12 weeks, taking into consideration the typical delay between the initiation of antidepressant therapy and symptom resolution. The second or *continuation phase* of treatment is essentially the follow-up that should occur to monitor the patient and prevent a relapse or recurrence of symptoms. The continuation phase may last between 4 and 9 months. During continuation, any antidepressant medication prescribed should be continued at the full dose at which symptoms improved, and patient compliance should be monitored and encouraged. The final or *maintenance phase* (≥5 months) is intended to prevent depression from recurring, especially in patients with previous episodes of depression. Individuals with a history of depressive episodes are at higher risk for recurrence. As in the continuation phase, maintenance medication at an effective dose is important to prevent a relapse or new episode of depression. Both sets of guidelines list recommended medications and doses; however, there are minor differences in the dose ranges of medications listed in the full texts of the guidelines. The phases of treatment are represented graphically in Figure 12.2.

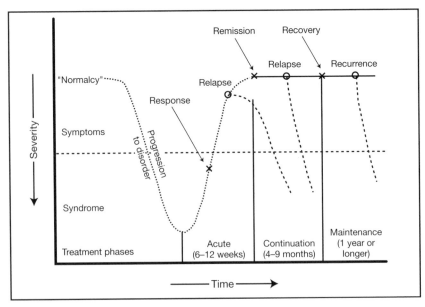

Figure 12.2   Phases in the long-term treatment of depression. (Adapted and reprinted with permission from Kupfer DJ. Long-term treatment of depression. *J Clin Psychiatry.* 1991;52(Suppl):28–34. © 1991 Physicians Postgraduate Press.)

"Usual Care" or Guideline Care?

Barriers to Diagnosis and Treatment of Depression

It is well established that the majority of treatment for depression occurs in the nonpsychiatric medical care system, especially primary care, whereas a minority occurs in specialty mental health settings. However, primary care providers had been criticized in the past for both underrecognition and undertreatment of depression (*see* Chapter 3). With this in mind, the AHCPR practice guidelines for depression were developed for and promoted to practitioners. Although the guidelines are not controversial, it became apparent after publication that there were a number of barriers to the appropriate care of depression and that medical practice was not modified easily. The physician's lack of time and the patient's lack of recognition of their own depression have been identified as barriers to the appropriate identification of patients with depression (4,5). Variability in clinical presentation, patient reluctance to admit psychological symptoms, and physician reluctance to inquire about depression are additional barriers to identification. Recently, it also was demonstrated that the knowledge of diagnostic criteria for major depression and the objective application of criteria to recognize depression are highly variable among primary care physicians (6).

Once depression is diagnosed, there are a number of frequently identified deviations to guideline-recommended care. For example, inadequate antidepressant dose is a commonly found deviation from guideline recommendations (7). Additionally, the recommended need to monitor patients every 1 to 2 weeks in the acute phase differs significantly from the common practice of having a patient return in 1 to 3 *months*. The guidelines emphasize that dose adjustment, assessment of compliance, side-effect monitoring, and measurement of response cannot be accomplished effectively with long intervals between appointments.

Another key deficit in "usual care" is a failure to educate the patient about depression and its treatment, including the risk of relapse. The typical busy pace of primary care practices and subsequently brief appointments may make patient education less likely to occur. There is a significant risk of relapse with depression, and lack of patient education may explain the common occurrence of early treatment discontinuation. A number of studies report that patient education improves adherence to treatment, and the AHCPR guidelines recommend that all depressed patients (and their families, when appropriate) receive education on the illness, treatment options, importance of compliance, and warning signs of recurrence (3). Lin and coworkers (8) demonstrated that educational messages could be "simple and specific" and "easily integrated into primary care visits."

A number of external barriers also exist for many patients and their physicians. Behavioral health care insurance benefits are commonly "carved out" and treated as specialty care and may require pre-authorization, primary care referral, or both for coverage. It has been reported that the substitution of an alternative diagnosis for major depression is a widespread practice; the most likely reasons for this are an uncertainty about the diagnosis and problems with reimbursement (9). Also, specialist visits often have a higher copayment for the insured. These requirements may discourage patients or their physicians from referral to behavioral health care specialists when it would be helpful.

Creative approaches to reimbursement problems potentially may reveal methods to facilitate guideline care and achieve improved outcomes. A primary care capitation-payment methodology may encourage an up-front investment of time in depressed patients to avoid higher expenditures later. Because most primary care physicians understand the benefits of stabilizing a patient with asthma, why not use the same approach for patients with depression? From a survey of primary care physicians, highly capitated physicians reported fewer insurance restrictions or instances of inadequate reimbursement. However, Williams and coworkers (6) also noted that there are organizational barriers to adequate depression care in both capitated and noncapitated settings (e.g., appointment times being too short for an adequate history or to provide counseling).

It is important to acknowledge the difficulty of keeping patients in treatment and the real-life complexities of adhering to guidelines (10). Most guidelines recognize that the final judgement and the responsibility for treatment decisions rest with the treating physician. Guidelines are not meant to be rigid and should allow the clinician to consider individual patient characteristics and to adjust treatment planning accordingly. However, even with built-in flexibility, dissemination of guidelines by publication alone or with "academic detailing" of physicians by other physicians or pharmacists unfortunately have not been effective in achieving enduring guideline compliance (11,12).

Poor adherence with guideline recommendations is particularly distressing in light of the improved outcomes that have been demonstrated using guideline-recommended care compared with "usual care." A randomized controlled study demonstrated that standardized treatment using the AHCPR's depression guidelines resulted in superior outcomes in a primary care practice after 8 months compared with a control group (13). Seventy percent of patients recovered from depression at 8 months compared with 20% in a control group that received a primary care physician's "usual care." The study's authors emphasized the AHCPR recommendation, which states that depressed patients receive an adequate dose and duration of antidepressant throughout the acute and continuation phases of treatment. They concluded that "pharmacotherapy and psychotherapy consistent with the AHCPR guidelines are markedly superior to a physician's UC [usual care] in resolving an episode of major depression." It is noteworthy that the standardized treatment group consisted of family practitioners and internists "trained in pharmacotherapy protocol procedures through a written manual and didactic sessions." In view of the convincingly improved outcomes, one primary care journal editorialized, "the 'usual care' of depression is not good enough." (14).

Because the following of guidelines improves outcomes in depression, actions to assist practitioners in providing guideline care should be encouraged. Continuing medical education is important but inadequate. Collaborative models of care (*see* Chapter 4) and collaboration with health plan case managers could assist in following guideline standards as well as in reducing care variation.

The monitoring of care and outcomes with feedback to providers and patients can be particularly powerful. Recently, the National Committee for Quality Assurance (NCQA) announced a new three-part measure for health plans to report that is designed to assess facets of depression management. The measure looks at the following (15):

1. **Optimal provider contacts for medication management:** The percentage of patients with a new episode of depression and treated with antidepressant medication who had at least three follow-up contacts with a primary care provider or mental health provider during the 12-week acute-treatment phase

2. **Effective acute-phase treatment:** The percentage of patients having a new episode of depression and treated with antidepressant medication who remained on an antidepressant drug during the entire 12-week acute-treatment phase

3. **Effective continuation-phase treatment:** The percentage of patients having a new episode of depression and treated with antidepressant medication who remained on an antidepressant drug for at least 6 months.

Although this NCQA health plan employer data and information set (HEDIS) measure is for health plans, the plans will likely share their expectations for providers to deliver this level of care and may share performance data with individual provider or practice groups. Some plans are currently providing data to practitioners about their antidepressant prescribing, patient medication discontinuation, breaks in therapy, drug interactions, and other data. For example, using prescription-claim data, one insurer had letters sent to physicians prescribing antidepressants for depression to a cohort of adult commercial health maintenance organization (HMO) members. Potential nonadherence to the prescription was identified for each specific patient by physician, highlighting breaks in therapy (late refills) or early discontinuation (no refills). This intervention improved compliance (defined as a subsequent prescription renewal) by 68% (Pelonero AL, Unpublished data).

Using Guidelines Directly with Patients

Treatment options should be discussed with the patient at the time of diagnosis and during ongoing treatment modifications. After concluding that a patient is suffering from major depression, the patient can be told that there is a nationally endorsed set of guidelines for the treatment of depression based on a cumulative body of research and that following these guidelines is a way to deliver the care that is most likely to be effective. Patients play a large role in getting effective treatment and therefore should be educated about their role in following the instructions of their physician to adhere to therapy and follow-up. To encourage patient participation and compliance further, the risk of recurrence and the major causes of recurrence (e.g., an inadequate dose of medication, an insufficient duration of treatment) can be emphasized.

The patient is encouraged to participate at a number of decision points. For example, preference for medication or psychotherapy is the first major decision they should consider. For those entering the maintenance phase, they must consider whether to taper and discontinue antidepressant or continue it beyond 9 to 12 months. At times, patient preferences may transcend the guidelines, especially on the issue of discontinuation after a single episode. Many patients will report that they would rather stay on medication than risk a relapse into another severe major depression. Likewise, there are patients who would clearly benefit from medication but who refuse even to consider using them. There are many pamphlets and other educational resources developed for patients on depression, and patients are encouraged to learn about the illness and become invested in their own treatment and recovery (*see* Chapter 4).

As discussed in the following section, the depression guidelines will not answer every question that a practitioner may confront during a course of treatment. Although the AHCPR guidelines offer an overview of "special situations" (e.g., suicide risk, geriatric depression, co-existing medical disorders) the practitioner may need to look elsewhere for guidance in certain situations (e.g., pregnancy).

Advantages and Limitations

The use of guidelines can have a number of advantages for both the patient and practitioner, including the enhancement of patient confidence in their doctor, their health care, and the doctor-patient relationship itself. Discussion of depression and guideline-recommended treatment also may reduce the stigma that accompanies psychiatric illness. The physician can reassure the patient with confidence that the care recommended is evidence-based medicine or, in other words, a practical approach supported by scientific data. As described above, routinely explaining the guidelines to the patient will help include him or her in the decision-making process. Whether treating a new patient with a single episode of depression or a person with recurrent depression, physicians who review guideline recommendations with their patients can help reframe an understanding of the treatment into a larger picture encompassing the entire treatment process, which may encourage continued compliance.

Practice guidelines that are effective (i.e., those that aid decision-making and produce desired clinical outcomes) improve a physician's value to his or her patients and to the health care delivery system of which they are a part. It is also reassuring to physicians to know their recommendations are supported by expert consensus. Delivering effective and useful treatment and service contributes to job satisfaction.

Guideline-based practice may reduce practice variation, improve the quality of treatment, and help reduce health care costs by improving efficiency. The depression guidelines have distilled expert consensus from a large amount of critically reviewed scientific data (16) and also can be used as a valuable educational tool.

Any weaknesses of the guidelines seem to stem from their target audience. The weakness of the APA guideline for major depression is that it is designed primarily for mental health professionals, especially psychiatrists, and it is not as useful outside of the field of psychiatry. Interestingly, the AHCPR's focus on primary care perhaps has led to less attention to the issue of when to refer to a specialist, especially regarding the role of psychotherapy. Some authors argue that both the APA and AHCPR guidelines understate the value of psychotherapy (17).

The development of guidelines is an expensive and time-consuming process. Given the continual clinical developments and research findings, keeping guidelines up to date is a concern (17,18). Since the publication of the APA and AHCPR depression guidelines, new antidepressants have been introduced, and there is much new data on continuation of therapy, treatment-resistant depression, and light therapy. To date, only AHCPR has offered an update (19,20).

Guidelines that are unduly restrictive may breed resentment and ultimately resistance among physicians to their recommendations. Despite the acknowledgement that not all patients will fit neatly into a guideline because of varying individual characteristics and comorbidities, clinicians may find themselves explaining clinical approaches that deviate from guidelines (21). An ironic outcome for patients and society is that rigid guideline compliance may lead to an inhibition of clinical creativity. Practice guidelines for depression should support physicians in their decision-making, not make the decision for them. Ultimately, the clinician must consider guideline decision points and recommendations in the larger context of his or her individual patient.

Conclusions

Many managed-care organizations have endorsed practice guidelines to promote successful treatment of patients with major depression through a process of accurate assessment, effective intervention, and appropriate maintenance treatment. This makes sense because care must be effective and efficient before it can be cost effective. Although following guideline recommendations may require practitioners to modify some aspects of their practice or individual interactions with their patients, it seems clear that better patient outcomes will be the result.

■   ■   ■

Key Points

- Using a practice guideline in the treatment of depression has a number of important advantages.

- There are two major sets of guidelines for the treatment of depression (APA and AHCPR).

- The AHCPR guidelines are most useful in primary care practice.

- Studies have shown that using a depression guideline results in better patient outcomes.

- Treatment of depression is divided into three phases: acute, continuation, and maintenance.

- Common mistakes in treating depression can be corrected by incorporating guideline recommendations into primary care practice.

■   ■   ■

REFERENCES

1. **American Psychiatric Association.** Practice guideline for major depressive disorder in adults. *Am J Psychiatry.* 1993;150(Suppl 4):1–26.

2. **Depression Guideline Panel.** Detection and diagnosis. *Depression in Primary Care*, vol. 1, no. 5. Rockville, MD: USDHHS, PHS, Agency for Health Care Policy and Research; 1993 [AHCPR publication 93-0551].

3. **Depression Guideline Panel.** Treatment of major depression. *Depression in*

Primary Care, vol. 2, no. 5. Rockville, MD: USDHHS, PHS, Agency for Health Care Policy and Research; 1993 [AHCPR publication 93-0551].

4. **Rost K, Humphrey J, Kelleher K.** Physician management preferences and barriers to care for rural patients with depression. *Arch Fam Med.* 1994;3:409–14.

5. **Docherty JP.** Barriers to the diagnosis of depression in primary care. *J Clin Psychiatry.* 1997;58 (Suppl 1):5–10.

6. **Williams JW, Rost K, Dietrich AJ, et al.** Primary care physicians' approach to depressive disorders. *Arch Fam Med.* 1999;8:58–67.

7. **Simon GE.** Can depression be managed appropriately in primary care? *J Clin Psychiatry.* 1998;59(Suppl 2):3–8.

8. **Lin EHB, Von Korff M, Katon W, et al.** The role of the primary care physician in patients' adherence to antidepressant therapy. *Med Care.* 1995;33:67–74.

9. **Rost K, Smity GR, Matthews DB, Guise B.** The deliberate misdiagnosis of major depression in primary care. *Arch Fam Med.* 1994;3:333–7.

10. **Schulberg H, Block MR, Madonia MJ, et al.** Applicability of clinical pharmacotherapy guidelines for major depression in primary care settings. *Arch Fam Med.* 1995;4:106–12.

11. **Goldberg HI, Wagner EH, Fihn SD, et al.** A randomized controlled trial of CQI teams and academic detailing: Can they alter compliance with guidelines? *Jt Comm J Qual Improv.* 1998;24:130–42.

12. **Lin EHB, Katon WJ, Simon GE, et al.** Achieving guidelines for the treatment of depression in primary care: Is physician education enough? *Med Care.* 1997;35: 831–42.

13. **Schulberg H, Block MR, Madonia MJ, et al.** Treating major depression in primary care practice: eight-month clinical outcomes. *Arch Gen Psychiatry.* 1996;53: 913–9.

14. **Higgins ES.** The "usual care" of depression is not "good enough." *Arch Fam Med.* 1997;6:340–1.

15. **National Committee for Quality Assurance.** *Health Plan Employer Data and Information Set (HEDIS),* ver. 3.0, vol. 2; 1999.

16. **Hetznecker W.** Are practice guidelines useful in managed care? In Lazarus A (ed). *Controversies in Managed Mental Health Care.* Washington, DC: American Psychiatric Press; 1996.

17. **Persons JB, Thase ME, Crits-Christoph P.** The role of psychotherapy in the treatment of depression. *Arch Gen Psychiatry.* 1996;53:283–90.

18. **McIntyre JS, Zarin DA, Pincus HA.** The role of psychotherapy in the treatment of depression: review of two practice guidelines. *Arch Gen Psychiatry.* 1996;53: 291–3.

19. **Agency for Health Care Policy and Research.** *Treatment of Depression: Newer Pharmacotherapies,* evidence report/technology assessment no. 7; 1999 [AHCPR Publication No. 99-E014].

20. **Schulberg HC, Katon W, Simon GE, Rush AJ.** Treating major depression in primary care practice: an update of the agency for heath care policy and research practice guidelines. *Arch Gen Psychiatry.* 1998;55:1121–7.

21. **Nathan PE, Gorman JM.** Treatments that work and what convinces us they do. In Nathan PE, Gorman JM (eds). *A Guide To Treatments That Work.* New York: Oxford University Press; 1998.

KEY REFERENCES

American Psychiatric Association. Practice guideline for major depressive disorder in adults. *Am J Psychiatry.* 1993;150(Suppl 4):1–26.

These detailed guidelines were developed for mental health professionals. They cover diagnosis and management, including medications, ECT, and psychotherapy.

Agency for Health Care Policy and Research. *Treatment of Depression: Newer Pharmacotherapies,* evidence report/technology assessment no. 7; 1999 [AHCPR Publication No. 99-E014].

This report supplements the guidelines with the AHCPR update. For more information, see the AHCPR (now AHRQ) Web site at http://www.ahcpr.gov or http://www.ahrq.gov.

Depression Guideline Panel. Detection and diagnosis. *Depression in Primary Care,* vol. 1, no. 5. Rockville, MD: USDHHS, PHS, Agency for Health Care Policy and Research; 1993 [AHCPR publication 93-0551].

Depression Guideline Panel. Treatment of major depression. *Depression in Primary Care,* vol. 2, no. 5. Rockville, MD: USDHHS, PHS, Agency for Health Care Policy and Research; 1993 [AHCPR publication 93-0551].

These depression guideline publications can be obtained from the AHCPR. They provide the clinician with an easy-to-read, scholarly review of depression assessment and treatment along with a supporting bibliography.

13

▦ ▦ ▦

Drug Interactions

Douglas Dale Brink, BS Pharm, PharmD, BCPP
Michele Lynn Thomas, BS Pharm, PharmD

*"Where there is much desire to learn, there of necessity will be
much arguing, much writing, many opinions; for opinion in
good men is but knowledge in the making."*

—*John Milton*, Areopagitica, *1644*

Pharmacotherapy for depression has changed significantly since the marketing of fluoxetine, the first selective serotonin-reuptake inhibitor (SSRI), in 1988. The introduction of additional SSRIs and other types of antidepressants has resulted in improvements in the treatment of this common psychiatric disorder. However, along with the availability of new medications has come recognition of new potential drug interactions. Much has appeared in the literature about interaction risks, but valid scientific data are limited and published opinions are varied. Experts' interpretations of the same data differ, and the line between science and marketing has sometimes become blurred. Drug-interaction profiles have been an area in which manufacturers have tried to demonstrate advantages for their agent over the competitors, especially for the SSRIs. In these marketing efforts, the difference between statistically and clinically significant interactions is sometimes obscured. Many drug interactions have no clinically apparent effect; they merely increase the intrinsic variability of patient response to drugs. However, some drug interactions are potentially dangerous. This chapter focuses on the interactions that warrant the most concern.

Types of Drug Interactions

Drug interactions generally are classified as being one of two types, pharmacodynamic or pharmacokinetic. *Pharmacodynamic* interactions occur when the pharmacologic response of one drug is modified by another drug without a change in either drug's plasma levels. These interactions occur at the drugs' site of action. For example, drugs that produce sedation often produce an additive effect when administered together; however, as with many interactions, the amount of additive sedation can be difficult to measure and study. A potentially fatal pharmacodynamic interaction is the serotonin syndrome, which results from the combination of two or more highly serotonergic medications. Because many of the new antidepressants are potent serotonin agonists, the risk for this potential interaction has increased in recent years. Its clinical features are discussed later in this chapter.

Pharmacokinetic interactions occur when one drug changes the plasma or tissue levels of another drug. Pharmacokinetic interactions can occur during any phase of the drug's passage through the body: absorption, distribution, protein binding, metabolism, or elimination. The subsequent change may result in clinically significant effects or merely contribute to the intrinsic individual variability in drug response. For example, antidepressants are all fat soluble and are weak bases; thus, they are subject to various factors that influence absorption (e.g., fat content in the diet, use of antacids or laxatives). Although these factors may produce significant changes in an individual who is stable on a chronic regimen, in general the effects are no greater than the normal variability in absorption seen from person to person. As for protein binding, although some antidepressants are highly protein bound, they do not bind tightly enough to albumin to displace other protein-bound drugs. Most clinically significant pharmacokinetic interactions result from changes in metabolism or elimination. Whether pharmacodynamic or pharmacokinetic in nature, drug interactions can be beneficial (e.g., augmenting the effect of one agent with the addition of another) or detrimental (e.g., producing toxic levels/effects of one agent when another is added). Most of this chapter focuses on detrimental pharmacokinetic interactions.

Cytochrome P450 System

The cytochrome P450 (CYP450) isoenzyme system is a group of heme-containing enzymes found primarily in hepatocytes (1). They also are found in the enterocytes of the small intestine as well as in other tissues such as the kidneys, lungs, and brain (2). Their primary biological functions seem to be twofold: metabolism of endogenous compounds (e.g., steroid hormones, prostaglandins) and detoxification of exogenous compounds, including many prescribed medications (1,2). It is estimated that they collectively participate in the metabolism of more than 80% of all drugs used (2,3).

Substrates, Inhibition, and Induction

Pharmacokinetic interactions involving drug metabolism may involve inhibition or induction of the responsible processes. Knowledge of inducers, inhibitors, and substrates of CYP450 isoenzymes can assist in predicting clinically significant pharmacokinetic drug interactions. Inhibition of CYP450 isoenzymes most often occurs as a result of competitive binding at the enzyme's binding site. Competitive inhibition depends on the concentration of the inhibiting agent and therefore is influenced by the agent's half-life and time to steady state (4). For antidepressants with a long half-life (e.g., fluoxetine), inhibitory interactions may not be apparent for weeks. Enzyme induction also is dependent on the half-life of the responsible agent. However, induction is further influenced by being dependent on the time required to synthesize new CYP450 enzymes (4). Also complicating these issues are the facts that a single isoenzyme may metabolize many drugs and a particular drug may be metabolized by several isoenzymes (2,5). For example, tricyclic antidepressants (TCAs) are metabolized by CYP2D6, CYP1A2, and CYP3A4.

In addition, many drugs exist as stereoisomers and their different forms may be metabolized by different isoenzymes. For example, the R-form of warfarin is metabolized by CYP1A2 and 3A4, whereas the more potent S-form is metabolized by CYP2C9 (5). Therefore, when one enzyme system is inhibited or induced by an interacting drug, a clinically significant interaction may or may not occur (4). It is also important to recognize that genetic polymorphism exists in the functional expression of some CYP450 isoenzymes, such as CYP2D6 (2, 6). This means that a percentage of the population possesses mutant genes that alter the activity of the enzyme, usually diminishing its activity. This contributes to marked interpatient variability in drug metabolism, leading to "poor metabolizers" and "extensive metabolizers" (5,6). In addition to genetic influences, CYP450 activity is influenced by age, nutritional status, and hepatic disease (2,7). To complicate matters even further, another major metabolic system recently has been proposed: a flavin-containing mono-oxegenase system (known as the FMO family) that has five members to date (5,8). Both the FMO family and the CYP450 system may be involved in the metabolism of the same drugs and may interact in as yet undefined ways. Because so little is known about the FMO family, this section concentrates on the CYP450 isoenzyme system.

Overview of Individual Enzymes

Nomenclature

The nomenclature widely used today to label CYP450 isoenzymes employs a three-tier system consisting of the family, subfamily, and individual gene (9). A family shares less than 40% homology in amino acid sequence and is designated by an Arabic number (e.g., CYP1). A subfamily shares more than 50% sequence homology and is designated by a capital letter (e.g., CYP1A). An Arabic number is used for designating individual enzymes within a subfamily (e.g., CYP1A2) (2). Although hundreds of CYP450 isoenzymes have been identified to date in living organisms, fewer than 50 have been identified in humans (2,5) and fewer than 10 are responsible for the metabolism of most drugs: CYP1A2, CYP3A4, CYP2D6, and the CYP2C subfamily (2,4) (Table 13.1). This limited number is as likely to be a reflection of our current state of knowledge as it is an accurate reflection of all the isoenzymes responsible for drug metabolism.

Table 13.1   Human Cytochrome P450 Enzymes Classified by Family, Subfamily, and Gene

1A1	2A6	3A3/4*	4A9	5A1	7A1	8	11A1	17	19	21	27	51
1A2*	2A7	3A5	4A11				11B1					
1B1	2A13	3A7	4B1				11B2					
	2B6	3D6	4F2									
	2B7		4F3									
	2C*											
	2C8											
	2C9*											
	2C10											
	2C17											
	2C18											
	2C19*											
	2D6*											
	2E1†											
	2F1											
	2G											
	2J2											

* Major isoenzymes responsible for drug metabolism.
† Major isoenzyme responsible for alcohol metabolism.

CYP1A2

The CYP1A2 isoenzyme has been of clinical interest in part because of its role in the metabolism of xanthine compounds such as caffeine and theophylline (4). It also is involved in the metabolism of the *R*-isomer of warfarin and several benzodiazepines and in the conversion of tertiary amine TCAs to their secondary-amine active metabolites. It comprises approximately 13% of the total CYP450 content of the human liver (2,3). CYP1A2 is induced by components of cigarette smoke and charbroiled food (3,4,7). Although no genetic polymorphism has been proven, the observation of a trimodal pattern of caffeine metabolism suggests the presence of genetic influences (4,10), and 12% of people may be "poor metabolizers" of CYP1A2 substrates (11). Table 13.2 shows a more complete list of potential substrates.

CYP3A4

Enzymes of the CYP3A subfamily seem to be responsible for the metabolism of the widest range of drugs and endogenous compounds in humans. These enzymes account for 30% to 60% of the CYP450 isoenzymes in the liver and 70% of those in the gut wall; hence, they are probably the most clinically important of the CYP450 isoenzymes in terms of the metabolism of drugs (2,3,4,10). The isoenzymes CYP3A3 and CYP3A4 are 97% identical in structure and are sometimes referred to as CYP3A3/4, but expression of CYP3A4 seems to be more significant in the human liver (7). There is no evidence that CYP3A4 exhibits genetic polymorphism (4,10). Significant interest in the inhibition of this isoenzyme has occurred secondary to potentially life-threatening interactions with nonsedating antihistamines and cisapride. Other common substrates of CYP3A3/4 are listed in Table 13.3 and include calcium-channel blockers, protease inhibitors, and benzodiazepines.

Table 13.2   CYP1A2 Isoenzyme: Substrates

Acetaminophen	Ondansetron
Amitriptyline	Phenacetin
Chlordiazepoxide	Propafenone
Clomipramine	Propranolol
Desipramine	*R*-warfarin
Diazepam	Sertraline
Haloperidol	Tacrine
Imipramine	Theophylline
Olanzapine	Verapamil

Table 13.3   CYP3A3/4 Isoenzyme: Substrates

Alfentanil	Cyclosporine	Lansoprazole	Pravastatin
Alprazolam	Dapsone	Lidocaine	Prednisone
Amiodarone	Dextromethorphan	Losartan	Progesterone
Amitriptyline	Diazepam	Lovastatin	Propafenone
Amlodipine	Diltiazem	Methadone	Quinidine
Astemizole	Disopyramide	Metoprolol	Quinine
Atorvastatin	Donepezil	Mexilitene	Rifampin
Bupropion	Doxorubicin	Mibefradil	Ritonavir
Buspirone	Dronabinol	Miconazole	R-warfarin
Busulfan	Erythromycin	Midazolam	Saquinavir
Cannabinoids	Estradiol	Navelbine	Sertraline
Carbamazepine	Ethosuximide	Nefazodone	Sildenafil
Cisapride	Etopside	Nelfinavir	Tacrolimus
Clindamycin	Felodipine	Nicardipine	Tamoxifen
Clomipramine	Fentanyl	Nifedipine	Temazepam
Clonazepam	Fexofenadine	Nimodipine	Testosterone
Cocaine	Haloperidol	Nisoldipine	Timolol
Codeine	Ifosfamide	Nitrendipine	Triazolam
Colchicine	Imipramine	O-desmethylvenlafaxine	Verapamil
Cortisol	Indinavir	Omeprazole	Vinblastine
Cyclobenzaprine	Isradipine	Ondansetron	Vincristine
Cyclophosphamide	Ketoconazole	Paclitaxel	Zileuton

CYP2D6

The isoenzyme CYP2D6 is prominent in the psychiatric literature as being responsible for the metabolism of many psychotropic medications. Although it comprises a small percentage (1.5%–2.5%) of the total CYP450 isoenzyme content of the human liver (2,3), it is one of the most intensely studied of the CYP450 isoenzymes since the identification of a genetic polymorphism 15 years ago (7). This polymorphism results in a bimodal distribution of CYP2D6 activity in humans, with approximately 5% to 10% of whites and 1% to 3% of blacks and Asians being "poor metabolizers" (PMs) or genetically deficient in this enzyme (4). PMs will exhibit greater plasma concentrations, prolonged elimination half-lives, and possible exaggerated pharmacologic response from standard doses of drugs that are metabolized by CYP2D6. For example, there have been reports of PMs experiencing TCA-induced cardiotoxicity and neuroleptic-induced adverse effects (4,10). Substantial inhibition of this isoenzyme can convert "extensive metabolizers" into PMs, whereas people who are initially PMs will not show significant effects if given a CYP2D6 inhibitor (10). Because we currently do not have the ability to predict *a priori* who is a PM and who is not, all patients should be managed as if they were PMs when any drug is administered that may inhibit CYP2D6. Table 13.4 shows a listing of common substrates, including several beta-blockers and antidepressants.

CYP2C Subfamily
The CYP2C subfamily consists of the isoenzymes 2C9, 2C10, 2C19 and others. It comprises approximately 18% of the total CYP450 isoenzyme content of the human liver (2,3) and as such is probably the second most important isoenzyme in terms of drug metabolism (2). There has been considerable confusion in the literature as to which members of the CYP2C subfamily are involved in the metabolism of particular substrates because they are so close in their amino acid sequencing (6). CYP2C19 exhibits genetic polymorphism, with 20% of blacks and Asians and 3% to 5% of whites reported as being PMs (3,4,10). The CYP2C subfamily is involved in the metabolism of phenytoin, S-warfarin, and several nonsteroidal anti-inflammatory agents. Other potentially significant substrates are listed in Table 13.5.

Table 13.4   CYP2D6 Isoenzyme: Substrates

Alprenolol	Donepezil	Meperidine	Propafenone
Amitriptyline	Doxepin	Methadone	Propranolol
Bisolprolol	Encainide	Methamphetamine	Risperidone
Chlorpheniramine	Flecainide	Metoprolol	Thioridazine
Chlorpromazine	Fluoxetine	Mexiletine	Timolol
Citalopram	Fluphenazine	Morphine	Tramadol
Clomipramine	Haloperidol	N-desmethylclomipramine	Trazodone
Clozapine	Hydrocodone	Nortriptyline	Trimipramine
Codeine	Imipramine	Ondansetron	Venlafaxine
Cyclobenzaprine	Indoramin	Oxycodone	
Desipramine	Maprotiline	Paroxetine	
Dextromethorphan	m-CPP*	Perphenazine	

* Metabolite of nefazodone and trazodone.

Table 13.5   CYP2C Subfamily: Substrates

Amitriptyline	Moclobemide
Citalopram	Omeprazole
Clomipramine	Phenytoin
Diazepam	Propranolol
Imipramine	S-warfarin
Losartan	Tolbutamide
Mephenytoin	Topiramate

CASE 13.1

An obese man 50 years of age presents with symptoms of a major depressive episode. He has a 30-year history of tobacco use, a 1-year history of congestive heart failure, and chronic renal insufficiency. His medications include digoxin, metoprolol, aspirin, and lisinopril. You prescribe the TCA nortriptyline. What potential problems may arise?

Nortriptyline and metoprolol are substrates for cytochrome P450 isoenzyme 2D6 (CYP2D6). Substrate competition for metabolism is expected, and plasma levels of both substrates are likely to be higher, potentiating the cardiac effects of the TCA. Among the TCAs, nortriptyline is a superior choice because of 1) its reduced risk for causing orthostasis, 2) the fact that decreased renal function does not affect the excretion of nortriptyline significantly, and 3) the advantage of measurable serum concentrations that correlate with efficacy.

Tricyclic Antidepressant Interactions

Tricyclic antidepressants (TCAs) are not commonly responsible for producing pharmacokinetic interactions because they do not inhibit or induce the CYP450 system significantly. When they do produce such interactions, it is because they are competing for metabolism with another substrate for the same isoenzyme (see Case 13.1). It is important to be aware of such competitive interactions, but they are usually not as clinically significant as the interactions produced by inhibitors or inducers of isoenzymes responsible for TCA metabolism. Tertiary-amine TCAs (e.g., amitriptyline, doxepin, imipramine) are demethylated by CYP1A2, CYP3A4, and CYP2C and secondary-amine TCAs (e.g., nortriptyline, desipramine) are hydroxylated by

CYP2D6 (3). Pharmacokinetic interactions involve potentially significant increases in TCA levels when they are combined with cimetidine (3) or any of the SSRIs. SSRI interactions with TCAs also include serotonin syndrome. All SSRI interactions with TCAs will be discussed in more detail later in this chapter. Pharmacokinetic interactions that induce TCA metabolism and decrease their plasma levels have been reported with barbiturates, carbamazepine, and phenytoin (18,19).

When TCAs are responsible for producing interactions, they are usually pharmacodynamic. Potential development of hypertensive crisis, severe seizures, and possible death are well known when TCAs are combined with monoamine oxidase inhibitors (MAOIs) (3). Another clinically significant potential pharmacodynamic interaction with TCAs may occur with antihypertensive agents that have adrenergic mechanisms. Published reports include decreasing the hypotensive effects of clonidine, reserpine, methyldopa, guanethidine, and related agents (12). Concomitant administration of TCAs with sympathomimetic agents such as epinephrine, norepinephrine, or phenylephrine may result in additive sympathomimetic activity. After intravenous administration of sympathomimetics, such reactions have been fatal (13). Additive sympathomimetic effects also may be seen with combinations of TCAs and amphetamines or methylphenidate, but these reactions are less severe. Methylphenidate also may inhibit the metabolism of TCAs so that resulting interactions with this combination may be both pharmacokinetic and pharmacodynamic (14).

Another combination that may result in both pharmacokinetic and pharmacodynamic interactive effects involves the use of quinidine along with TCAs. Quinidine may inhibit the metabolism of TCAs as well as have additive anti-arrhythmic effects (15,16). Such additive anti-arrhythmic effects are possible with all Type I anti-arrhythmics, because of likely pharmacodynamic interactions and significant prolongation of cardiac conduction that result in arrhythmias. Other situations when additive effects may be seen with TCAs include when they are given with other anticholinergic agents, possibly resulting in ileus or delirium (17). Anticholinergic TCAs may antagonize the cholinomimetic memory-enhancing effects of acetylcholinesterase inhibitors like donepezil or tacrine. Additive sedative effects are common when TCAs are combined with other sedating medications such as antihistamines or narcotics. Table 13.6 shows further information about TCA interactions.

Second-Generation Antidepressants

Second-generation antidepressants, especially the SSRIs, overshadowed the TCAs in the pharmacologic management of depression during the 1990s.

Table 13.6   Clinically Significant Drug Interactions with Tricyclic Antidepressants

Substrate*	Interacting Drug	Effect
TCAs (tertiary amines)	Fluvoxamine (inhibition 1A2)	Increased TCA levels
TCAs	Fluoxetine (inhibition 2D6), paroxetine (inhibition 2D6), sertraline (inhibition 2D6), citalopram (inhibition 2D6)	Increased TCA levels; wait 2–4 weeks for fluoxetine washout period
TCAs	Cimetidine (inhibition 2D6)	Increased TCA levels
TCAs	Ritonavir (inhibition 2D6)	Increased TCA levels
TCAs	Saquinavir (inhibition 3A4)	Increased TCA levels
TCAs	Type I anti-arrythmics, quinidine	May prolong cardiac conduction time; increased TCA levels
TCAs	MAOIs	Hypertensive crisis/serotonin syndrome
TCAs	Clonidine, reserpine, methyldopa, guanethidine	Antagonize antihypotensive effects
TCAs	Phenylephrine, epinephrine, norepinephrine	Additive sympathomimetic activity
TCAs	Donepizil, tacrine	Antagonizes cholinergic effects
TCAs	Anticholinergics	Additive anticholinergic effect, may lead to delirium
TCAs	Antihistamines	Additive anticholinergic effect, increased sedation
TCAs	Phenytoin, carbamazepine, barbiturates	Increased TCA levels
TCAs	Amphetamine, methylphenidate	Additive sympathomimetic activity; methylphenidate may increase TCA levels

MAOIs = monoamine oxidase inhibitors; TCAs = tricyclic antidepressants.
* Interaction not demonstrated with all TCA agents; however, based on chemical and pharmacologic similarities, extrapolation within the class is appropriate.

They are not more effective than the TCAs, but their side effects generally are tolerated better, and they are significantly safer in overdose. The SSRIs are not superior to TCAs in all respects, however, and one disadvantage is in drug interactions (Table 13.7).

Table 13.7   Clinically Significant Drug Interactions with Selective Serotonin-Reuptake Inhibitors*

Interacting Drug and Isoenzyme	Citalopram	Fluoxetine	Fluvoxamine	Paroxetine	Sertraline
P450 1A2	W	W	P	W	W
Clozapine			XXX		X
TCAs (tertiary amines)			XXX		X
Theophylline			XXX		X
P450 3A4	—	M	M	W	M
Alprazolam		XX	XX		XX
Astemizole		XX	XX		XX
Carbamazepine		XX	XX		XX
Cisapride		XX	XX		XX
Cyclosporine			XX		XX
Midazolam		XX			XX
Nelfinavir					XX
Tacrolimus			XX		XX
Triazolam		XX	XX		XX
P450 2D6	W–M	P	W	P	W–M
Codeine	†	XXX		XXX	†
Cyclobenzaprine	†	XXX		XXX	†
Encainide	†	XXX		XXX	X
Flecainide	†	XXX		XXX	X
Indecainide	†	XXX		XXX	X
Metoprolol	XX	XXX	X	XXX	†
Mexiletine	†	XXX		XXX	X
Pimozide	†	XXX		XXX	†
Propafenone	†	XXX		XXX	X
TCAs	X	XXX		XXX	X
Timolol				XXX	
P450 2C	W	M	P	W	M
Phenytoin		XX	XXX		XX
TCAs	XX	XX	XXX		XX
S-warfarin	X	XX	XXX	X	XX
Pharmacodynamic-serotonin syndrome					
MAOIs	XXX	XXX	XXX	XXX	XXX
Meperidine	XX	XX	XX	XX	XX
Selegiline	XX	XX	XX	XX	XX
Sibutramine	XXX	XXX	XXX	XXX	XXX
St. John's wort	X	X	X	X	X
TCAs (tertiary amines)	XX	XX	XX	XX	XX
Venlafaxine	XX	XX	XX	XX	XX

M = moderate inhibition of isoenzyme; MAOIs = monoamine oxidase inhibitors; P = potent inhibition of isoenzyme; TCAs = tricyclic antidepressant; W = weak inhibition of isoenzyme; X = possible interaction; XX = probable interaction; XXX = extremely likely interaction.
* See specific isoenzyme tables (13.2, 13.3, 13.4, and 13.5) for a more complete list of substrate drugs.
† Interaction not demostrated with all agents; however, extrapolation to all isoenzymes is appropriate.

Selective Serotonin-Reuptake Inhibitors

Each of the currently available SSRIs is an inhibitor of different clusters of CYP450 isoenzymes. The resulting profiles of drug interactions are individual but also show some overlap (10). Keeping in perspective the real and perceived differences between the SSRIs, they may be more similar in terms of risks of drug interactions than they are different. For example, all of the available SSRIs have been shown to be inhibitors of CYP2D6 (10,28). Although some are clearly more potent in this activity than others, clinicians treat individuals, not averages. For example, if eight of 10 people develop clinically significant enzyme inhibition on one SSRI and only 2 of 10 develop it on another, then there is only a clinical advantage for the latter agent if we can identify the two patients who are at risk. For CYP450 isoenzyme activity, we do not have the ability to make such clinical risk predictions. In the absence of such a prediction, we must consider that all patients in both groups might experience the interaction and, thus, there is no advantage in terms of clinical management. Clinically, the important question is "Does a drug inhibit a specific isoenzyme or not?" rather than "Is one agent a potent inhibitor, whereas another is only moderately potent?" Based on current science, the latter question leads only to a perceived difference in terms of averages, not a real difference in terms of an individual patient's risk management. In the absence of studies that directly compare the SSRIs head to head in terms of their ability to inhibit the CYP450 isoenzymes, it is not possible to rank them precisely with regard to their potential to cause clinically significant drug interactions.

How common are such potential interactions? One study that attempted to look at that issue found that of 544,309 patients who were receiving SSRIs, 25.5% also were prescribed one of the 33 potentially interacting drugs on the study list. All 33 of the potentially interacting drugs were metabolized by CYP3A4 or CYP2D6. These SSRI-treated patients were more than twice as likely to be prescribed a potentially interacting agent metabolized by CYP3A4 (19.5%) as they were one metabolized by CYP2D6 (9.1%) (20). Unfortunately, this study did not address whether people who were prescribed potentially interacting drugs actually experienced significant interactions. Before moving on to consider the specific drug-interaction profiles of individual SSRIs, we review the serotonin syndrome.

Serotonin Syndrome

The serotonin syndrome (SS) is a rare but potentially fatal iatrogenic drug-related disorder that has been of increasing concern in recent years as more medications with potent serotonergic pharmacology become available. Theoretically, SS can be produced by any drug or combination of drugs that increase serotonergic activity in the central nervous system. In practice, it is most often seen when two or more serotonergic agents are combined. The most common mechanism by which drugs increase serotonin activity is by inhibiting serotonin reuptake into presynaptic neurons—an activity of many antidepressants, including all the SSRIs. Other mechanisms for increasing serotonin activity include stimulating the release of presynaptic serotonin (e.g., amphetamine derivatives such as phenteramine or sibutramine) or by directly stimulating postsynaptic serotonin receptors (e.g., the triptan class of antimigraine agents). Although the agents in the triptan class of medications predominately stimulate postsynaptic serotonin 1D receptors (21,22), the risk of developing SS is associated with stimulation of postsynaptic serotonin 1A receptors in the brain stem (23). Therefore, the risk for SS would seem to be low with triptan-class agents; however, at least one case has been reported involving the combined use of sumatriptan and fluoxetine (24).

The clinical presentation of SS is characterized by abnormal function in three areas: cognitive and behavioral, autonomic nervous system, and neuromuscular. Neuromuscular dysfunction is the one most commonly reported and includes myoclonus, hyperreflexia, and muscle rigidity. Cognitive and behavioral changes include confusion and agitation, progressing to seizures and coma in severe cases. Autonomic disturbances, including hyperthermia, diaphoresis, tachycardia, and hypertension, may represent the most frequent disturbances seen in SS (23). Despite potentially fatal outcome, SS usually has a favorable prognosis if it is recognized and if the offending agents are stopped. Symptoms rarely last longer than 96 hours, and many patients experience complete resolution in 24 hours (23). There are no specific antidotes for treating SS, but nonspecific serotonin antagonists such as cyproheptadine or propranolol have been employed in some cases. Cyproheptadine has been the most frequently reported treatment for SS, with 4- to 8-mg doses repeated every 1 to 4 hours to therapeutic improvement or a maximum dose of 32 mg in adults or 12 mg in children (23).

Clearly, the best strategy is to avoid the development of SS by minimizing the combined use of serotonergic medications. The most dangerous combinations involve the infrequently prescribed nonspecific MAOIs, such as phenelzine, and any other serotonergic agent. Less dangerous but now more commonly prescribed is the selective MAOI selegiline, which has been implicated when prescribed with serotonergic antidepressants (25). The herbal medicine St. John's wort also has been characterized as an MAOI, but the magnitude of this activity does not seem to be clinically significant. Inhibition of serotonin reuptake also has been postulated as its mechanism of action. Until its pharmacology has been better characterized, it is unwise to prescribe a serotonin agonist to people who are using this over-the-counter herbal agent (26). Among commonly prescribed medications, those with the most serotonergic activity are SSRIs, tertiary amine TCAs (e.g., amitriptyline, doxepin, imipramine), venlafaxine, meperidine, selegiline, and sibutramine. Agents with weaker serotonergic activity but those that still present some risk for SS include buspirone, lithium, trazodone, nefazodone, mirtazapine, L-dopa, tramadol, and agents in the triptan class (23). Although SS is rare (27) and monitoring for a rare adverse interaction is difficult, the risk of SS rises with the number and potency of simultaneously prescribed serotonergic drugs. For the purposes of illustrating other potential interactions with the newer antidepressants, each agent is discussed separately below.

Citalopram

Citalopram (Celexa) is the newest of the SSRIs available in the United States, and its drug-interaction profile is not well characterized despite it having been available in European countries for several years. It is metabolized to an active metabolite, N-desmethylcitalopram, by CYP3A4, CYP2C19, and CYP2D6 (28–30). Citalopram is a weak inhibitor of CYP1A2 and CYP2C19, and case reports of interactions related to this activity generally are lacking (31–33). It also is described frequently as a weak inhibitor of CYP2D6, but it may have clinically significant activity inhibiting this isoenzyme. When citalopram was combined with imipramine in healthy volunteers, there was an approximate 50% increase in the area under the blood-level curve of desipramine—the secondary-amine active metabolite of imipramine—which indicates potentially significant inhibition of CYP2D6 (35). Therefore, it probably is classified better as a weak to moderate inhibitor of CYP2D6. Based on *in vitro* and limited *in vivo* data, citalopram seems to be a weaker inhibitor of CYP450 isoenzymes than other currently available SSRIs, but further *in vivo* research is needed to determine the true potential impact of its drug-interaction profile. Clinically significant drug interactions may become more apparent as the drug is used more widely in different populations (3,29). The manufacturer indicates that administration of citalopram with warfarin for 21 days did not alter the pharmacokinetics of warfarin but did increase prothrombin times by an average of 5% (29). This interaction may occur because of changes in serotonin and in the serotonin receptors in platelets (36) and, thus, may be a pharmacodynamic rather than a pharmacokinetic interaction.

Fluoxetine

Fluoxetine (Prozac) is metabolized to an active metabolite (norfluoxetine) primarily by CYP2D6, but other isoenzymes also may contribute to its metabolism (28,37). Fluoxetine is also a potent inhibitor of CYP2D6 (3,10,28, 37,38). Inhibiting the isoenzyme responsible for its metabolism results in nonlinear pharmacokinetics in which dose increases result in disproportionate increases in plasma concentrations (28,38). The potent inhibition of CYP2D6 also may result in clinically significant interactions with narrow therapeutic index drugs metabolized by this isoenzyme (e.g., TCAs, flecainide and other Type I anti-arrhythmics), thus causing enhanced toxicity from the TCAs (31,38). However, with careful monitoring of plasma concentrations and/or adverse effects, these classes of medications can be used simultaneously. In addition, CYP2D6 is responsible for the metabolism of codeine, a prodrug that requires metabolism to morphine to be an active analgesic. Therefore, the analgesic efficacy of codeine may be diminished substantially by fluoxetine (3,10,28,37).

The active metabolite of fluoxetine, norfluoxetine, is a moderately potent inhibitor of CYP3A3/4 (10,11,28). Because this metabolite has a longer half-life than fluoxetine and accumulates to higher plasma levels than the parent drug, this inhibition is clinically significant. In particular, adverse interactions are possible with cisapride or astemizole, although none have been reported. Although fluoxetine has not been reported to produce pharmacokinetic interactions with warfarin, exercise caution when these two drugs are used together. There are numerous reports of increased international normalized ratios (INRs) resulting from the combination (4,10,36,39), and the manufacturer has received reports of increased bleeding (38). As with citalopram, this may be a pharmacodynamic interaction via serotonin's effect on platelet aggregation. Fluoxetine seems to be a mild inhibitor of the CYP2C subfamily of isoenzymes (37), but case reports indicate clinically significant interactions at this isoenzyme, such as with phenytoin (3,4,10,11,28). Fluoxetine is a weak inhibitor of CYP1A2, and significant interactions with this isoenzyme are unlikely (10,28,37). It is important to recognize that the prolonged half-lives of fluoxetine and its active metabolite norfluoxetine (2–4 days and 7–14 days, respectively) mean that drug interactions may be an ongoing risk or may persist for weeks after cessation of the agent.

Fluvoxamine

Fluvoxamine (Luvox) is metabolized by CYP1A2 and CYP2D6 to inactive metabolites (28). Nonlinear pharmacokinetics are possible depending on the polymorphic CYP2D6 status of the individual. Fluvoxamine is a potent inhibitor of CYP1A2 (40) and is the only SSRI that has been shown *in vitro* to inhibit this enzyme significantly (3,4,10,11,28,37). Thus, it is the SSRI most likely to interact with several narrow therapeutic index drugs, including warfarin and theophylline. Fluvoxamine has been reported to increase warfarin concentrations by 65% to 95%, and bleeding complications have been reported (4,36,40,41). Theophylline levels were found to increase threefold when even low doses of fluvoxamine were added (40). CYP1A2 is also the isoenzyme primarily responsible for the metabolism of tertiary-amine TCAs to their secondary-amine active metabolites. As an inhibitor of this isoenzyme, fluvoxamine may increase significantly the plasma levels of tertiary-amine TCAs such as amitriptyline, doxepin, and imipramine (10,28). CYP3A3/4 also is inhibited by fluvoxamine, and case reports indicate that significant interactions involving this isoenzyme may occur (3,10,11,28,31). Careful monitoring should be employed if fluvoxamine is used in combination with cisapride or astemizole because significant prolongation of the corrected Q–T interval (QTc) is possible (40). Fluvoxamine has been reported to cause toxicity with cyclosporin, which also is metabolized by CYP3A4 (42). Furthermore, fluvoxamine is a potent inhibitor of CYP2C19, as exemplified by reports of increased phenytoin levels with resultant toxicity (3,10,11,28); however, it is a weak inhibitor of CYP2D6, and reported interactions with this isoenzyme are limited (10,37).

CASE 13.2

A woman 71 years of age returns 5 weeks after being placed on paroxetine for depression. She reports increased bruising, dizziness, weakness, and fatigue. Current medications include warfarin 5 mg/d, paroxetine 20 mg/d, and sustained-release propranolol 80 mg/d. Her heart rate is 62 bpm, blood pressure is low (90/60), and INR is elevated (>5).

There are two potential drug interactions occurring. Pharmacodynamically, paroxetine's effect on platelet aggregation has caused an increase in INR and bleeding. Pharmacokinetically, paroxetine's inhibition of CYP2D6 isoenzyme accounts for probable increased plasma concentrations of propranolol, causing bradycardia and hypotension.

Paroxetine

Paroxetine (Paxil) is metabolized to inactive metabolites primarily by CYP2D6, but other isoenzymes also may contribute to its metabolism (28,37). Paroxetine is also a potent inhibitor of CYP2D6 (10,28,37), and *in vitro* data indicate that it is the most potent SSRI at inhibiting this isoenzyme (11). This potency also is accompanied by some specificity because it is only modestly active at inhibiting other CYP450 isoenzymes, and interactions with them do not seem to be clinically significant (11,43). The activity of inhibiting CYP2D6—the isoenzyme responsible for its metabolism—results in a profile of nonlinear pharmacokinetics in which dose increases result in disproportionate increases in plasma concentrations (28,37,44). The potent inhibition of CYP2D6 also may result in clinically significant interactions with narrow-therapeutic-index drugs metabolized by this isoenzyme (e.g., TCAs, flecainide) and other Type I anti-arrhythmics (44). As with fluoxetine, inhibitory activity at CYP2D6 may decrease the analgesic efficacy of codeine (3,10,28,37). Paroxetine has minimal inhibitory effects at CYP1A2, CYP3A3/4, and the CYP2C subfamily, and interactions at these isoenzymes do not seem to be of clinical significance (10,28). However, case reports have indicated that paroxetine interacts with warfarin and causes increased bleeding (4,36,39,45). As with citalopram and fluoxetine, this may be a pharmacodynamic interaction due to the drug's effect on platelet aggregation rather than a pharmacokinetic interaction (44) (Case 13.2).

Sertraline

Sertraline (Zoloft) is metabolized by unidentified CYP450 isoenzymes to desmethylsertraline, an active metabolite (28,37). Sertraline is a moderate inhibitor of CYP2D6, but desmethylsertraline is a potent inhibitor. Although some references refer to sertraline as a weaker inhibitor of this isoenzyme than fluoxetine or paroxetine (4,11,37), this remains controversial. In general, the evidence to date supports the view that sertraline does cause clinically significant interactions at this isoenzyme (3,10,28,31,43), and the effects may be greatest in those with higher baseline activity (34). The manufacturer acknowledges that such interactions are possible (46), and, as with the other SSRIs, care should be taken if sertraline is co-administered with TCAs or Type I anti-arrhythmics. The analgesic effects of codeine may be decreased. Case reports in the literature also indicate that sertraline may cause clinically significant inhibition of the CYP2C subfamily of isoenzymes (10,11,28). It is also a moderate inhibitor of CYP3A3/4, and case reports in the literature indicate that significant interactions may occur (10,11,28). The manufacturer recently changed the package insert to reflect a potential concern with the co-administration of sertraline and astemizole (46). Sertraline is a weak inhibitor of CYP1A2, and clinically significant interactions at this isoenzyme are unlikely (10,28). As with the other SSRIs, sertraline has been reported to interact with warfarin and to increase bleeding time (4,36,39).

Non-SSRI Second-Generation Antidepressants

Bupropion

Bupropion is metabolized by CYP2B6, CYP3A4, and other CYP450 isoenzymes to several active metabolites (28,47). It does not seem to be a significant inhibitor of any CYP450 isoenzyme systems (28); however, animal data suggest that it may have weak inducing ability. Adequate human studies of its enzyme-inducing properties are lacking, and its plasma levels are linear in relationship to dose, which indicates that it does not influence the enzymes responsible for its metabolism (47). Information about clinically significant pharmacokinetic interactions with bupropion is limited, but it has been listed as being contraindicated with ritonavir due to that agent's ability to inhibit numerous CYP450 isoenzymes (48). Given the lack of systematic data about concomitant use of bupropion and many other medications, clinicians should monitor for possible adverse interactions (Table 13.8). Pharmacodynamic interactions with additive dopaminergic effects have been reported when bupropion is used in combination with levodopa (47). Because bupropion may lower the seizure threshold significantly, it

Table 13.8   Clinically Significant Drug Interactions with Bupropion

Substrate	Interacting Drug	Effect
TCAs	Bupropion	Decreased seizure threshold
Antipsychotics	Bupropion	Decreased seizure threshold
Theophylline	Bupropion	Decreased seizure threshold
Levodopa	Bupropion	Increased levodopa levels
Bupropion	Ritonavir	Increased plasma levels

TCAs = tricyclic antidepressants.

should be combined cautiously with other drugs that do the same (e.g., theophylline, neuroleptics, TCAs). In addition, rapid withdrawal of benzodiazepines may be more likely to induce seizures in combination with bupropion use (3).

Mirtazapine

Mirtazapine is metabolized by CYP1A2, CYP2D6, and CYP3A4 to clinically inactive metabolites (28,49). It does not seem to be a significant inhibitor or inducer of any CYP450 isoenzyme systems (11,28), and its plasma levels are linear in relationship to dose (49). Specific studies of drug interactions with mirtazapine are limited, and case reports are lacking (50); however, because it is highly sedating, mirtazapine is expected to have additive effects with other central nervous system depressants (3). Clinically significant drug interactions are given in Table 13.9.

CASE 13.3

A woman 32 years of age, stable for 5 years after a renal transplant, presents with complaints of symptoms of depression. The patient already has started taking some of her husband's prescribed antidepressant, nefazodone. Her other medications include tacrolimus, mycophenolate, and trimethoprim-sulfamethoxazole.

Nefazodone is a potent CYP3A4 substrate and inhibitor. There have been reports of toxicity from immunosuppressants (cyclosporin and tacrolimus) with the administration of nefazodone. An alternative agent, such as a SSRI without the significant CYP3A4 activity (e.g., paroxetine, sertraline, citalopram) or an atypical antidepressant (e.g., bupropion, venlafaxine), should avoid any significant interactions with the immunosuppressant therapy. Additionally, close monitoring of immunosuppressant plasma levels is recommended after each new added drug to prevent adverse drug reactions, toxicity, or both.

Table 13.9   Clinical Significant Drug Interactions with Mirtazapine

Substrate	Interacting Drug	Effect
MAOIs	Mirtazapine	Increased risk of serotonin syndrome
St. John's wort	Mirtazapine	Increased risk of serotonin syndrome

MAOIs = monoamine oxidase inhibitors.

Nefazodone

Nefazodone is metabolized to two active metabolites (m-CPP and hydroxy-nefazodone) by as-yet-unidentified CYP450 isoenzymes (28). Although the isoenzymes responsible for its metabolism remain unidentified, its pharmacokinetics are nonlinear, with plasma levels showing more than proportional increases per dose increase (28,51). Nefazodone is a potent inhibitor of CYP3A4 (3,10,11,28,50,51); thus, it may cause clinically significant interactions with triazolam and alprazolam (increasing their levels as much as 75%), and adverse effects have been reported (50). It also may produce significant prolongation of the QTc if combined with astemizole or cisapride (3,50,51). Toxicity also has been reported in transplant patients when nefazodone was added to regimens containing cyclosporin or tacrolimus (42,52). Although the inhibitory effect on CYP3A4 is theoretically capable of indirectly increasing S-warfarin levels, there are currently no published reports of such interactions (36). Nefazodone is a weak inhibitor of CYP2D6 (10,11). Its inhibitory activity at this isoenzyme is 100-fold less than that of the SSRIs, and interactions have not been reported (50). It is also a weak inhibitor of CYP1A2 and CYP2C (11,50). Nefazodone has been reported to increase digoxin levels in healthy volunteers (51), but the clinical significance of this is unclear (see Case 13.3). Clinically significant drug interactions are shown in Table 13.10.

Table 13.10   Clinically Significant Drug Interactions with Nefazodone

Substrate	Interacting Drug	Effect
Cisapride, astemizole	Nefazodone [inhibition 3A4]	Increased risk of QT prolongation
Cyclosporin, tacrolimus	Nefazodone [inhibition 3A4]	Increased plasma levels; case reports of toxicity
Digoxin	Nefazodone [inhibition 3A4]	Increased plasma levels
Carbamazepine	Nefazodone [inhibition 3A4]	Increased plasma levels
Triazolam, alprazolam, midazolam	Nefazodone [inhibition 3A4]	Increased plasma levels
MAOIs	Nefazodone	Increased risk of serotonin syndrome
St. John's wort	Nefazodone	Increased risk of serotonin syndrome

MAOIs = monoamine oxidase inhibitors.

CASE 13.4

A man 30 years of age who has tested positive for hepatitis C, but who is asymptomatic, is now complaining of fatigue, decreased energy, difficulty concentrating, loss of interest, and depressed mood. Laboratory tests are within normal limits, with the exception of liver enzymes. The patient already is being treated for panic disorder, which has been well controlled. The patient's current medications include interferon-alpha, acyclovir, and alprazolam. A diagnosis of major depressive disorder with symptoms of anxiety is made after an evaluation reveals no significant changes in his medical condition. The patient self-prescribed St. John's wort and has been taking it for approximately 3 weeks.

Antidepressant choices in this individual are limited by the potential adverse drug reactions. St. John's wort should be tapered and discontinued before initiating any antidepressant, because hepatic dysfunction may increase the risk of serotonin syndrome. Fluoxetine, fluvoxamine, and sertraline are likely to interact with alprazolam secondary to their moderate inhibition of CYP3A4 (*see* Table 13.7). Additionally, fluoxetine's long half-life may be prolonged further in a patient with hepatic dysfunction. During the initial stages of treatment, interactions at the CYP3A4 isoenzyme may occur, so close monitoring of the patient is warranted. Ideally, alprazolam should be tapered when the patient is stable on an SSRI (e.g., paroxetine or citalopram).

The atypical antidepressant venlafaxine may be a good initial choice because venlafaxine has low protein-binding properties and primarily is eliminated renally. In this patient with liver dysfunction, however, a dose reduction of approximately 25% should be made as the parent drug (venlafaxine) and its major metabolite (*O*-desmethylvenlafaxine) are metabolized. The dose should be increased cautiously as the patient is being monitored closely for any signs of adverse effects.

Venlafaxine

Venlafaxine is metabolized to an active metabolite (*O*-desmethylvenlafaxine) primarily by CYP2D6, but other isoenzymes also may contribute (28). Venlafaxine is a weak inhibitor of CYP2D6 (10,11); its inhibitory activity is approximately threefold less than that seen with the SSRIs, and *in vivo* drug interactions related to this activity seem to be uncommon (50). Although the manufacturer indicates that its pharmacokinetic profile is linear (53), nonlinearity in pharmacokinetics with increasing doses has been reported (28). Venlafaxine has received limited study in relation to other CYP450 isoenzymes, but there is no reported evidence that it either inhibits or induces other isoenzymes (10,11,53) (*see* Case 13.4). Being a potent inhibitor of serotonin reuptake, its use in combination with other serotonergic agents may result in serotonin syndrome. Clinically significant drug interactions are shown in Table 13.11.

Table 13.11   Clinically Significant Drug Interactions with Venlafaxine

Substrate	Interacting Drug	Effect
Cimetidine	Venlafaxine	Increased plasma levels
MAOIs	Venlafaxine	Increased risk of serotonin syndrome
St. John's wort	Venlafaxine	Increased risk of serotonin syndrome

MAOIs = monoamine oxidase inhibitors.

Conclusion

Our knowledge of and ability to predict drug interactions has improved with growing understanding of substrates and inhibitors of CYP450 isoenzymes. When viewed with an understanding of the mechanisms of interactions, drugs can be combined with a degree of confidence as to the possible consequences. There is the potential for drug interactions between any agent metabolized by a CYP450 isoenzyme and another drug that inhibits that enzyme, regardless of whether that level of inhibition is potent, moderate, or weak. The degree of potency influences how likely you are to see the interaction, not necessarily how significant it will be if it is seen. In certain individuals, even a moderate or weak inhibitor may produce substantial increases in another substrate's levels.

Although CYP2D6 has received the most attention in the psychiatric literature, other isoenzymes—particularly CYP3A4—may be more important in the mediation of drug interactions. In addition, an erroneous perception has been fostered, in part by drug company promotions, that inhibition of CYP2D6 reflects the interactive potential with all CYP450 isoenzymes. This is clearly inaccurate, as demonstrated by this review of the literature. Although none of the newer antidepressants can be prescribed without consideration of drug interactions, the interactive potential of each agent must be considered individually. All SSRIs, except fluvoxamine, are inhibitors of CYP2D6, but fluvoxamine is the only SSRI that potently inhibits CYP1A2. CYP2C isoenzymes are inhibited by fluvoxamine, fluoxetine, and sertraline. CYP3A isoenzymes—possibly the most important in terms of potential drug interactions—are inhibited by fluvoxamine, nefazodone, fluoxetine, and sertraline.

During therapy, substrates of various isoenzymes with narrow therapeutic indices (e.g., TCAs, theophylline, phenytoin, astemizole, warfarin, Type 1 anti-arrhythmics) should be administered cautiously with any of the newer antidepressants known or suspected to inhibit metabolism of that drug. The clinical consequences of interactions may be minimized or avoided by reducing the dose of the substrate or that of the inhibiting agent, although the latter intervention may be less effective. Marked inter-patient variability, due in part to genetic polymorphism in many CYP450 isoenzyme systems, precludes the accurate prediction of the risk of drug interactions in clinical practice, and caution is recommended in relying on any type of summary data in routine clinical use. Although a few absolute contraindications exist about the co-administration of drugs and the resulting interactions, available research data remain inconclusive and clinical outcomes seem variable for most combinations. Until definitive *in vivo* studies are performed with phenotyped patients (if they are ever performed), erring on the side of caution seems to be good advice. When potentially interacting drugs are introduced at minimal doses and titrated slowly, keen patient observation along with measurement of plasma concentrations, if available, may make their concomitant use safe.

Recommendations

- Pharmacodynamic drug interactions are relatively predictable based on the pharmacologic effects of the agents being used concurrently. They are usually additive, and agents with overlapping clinical effects generally should be avoided, such as multiple serotonergic agents (which may result in serotonin syndrome) or TCAs and Type I anti-arrythmics (which may cause cardiac conduction abnormalities). Less commonly, the pharmacodynamic interactions are antagonistic, as with TCAs and cholinomimetic agents used to treat dementia.

- Pharmacokinetic drug interactions are less predictable due to individual variability in metabolic enzyme activity in the liver. Some interactions have been well characterized, and combinations of potent inhibitors of various CYP450 isoenzymes with specific substrates should be avoided. Combinations with fewer potent inhibitors cause effects that are less consistent but that still may result in clinically significant problems. Whenever multiple medications that are metabolized in the liver are combined, the potential for an interaction is present and close patient observation is warranted.

Key Points

- TCAs are most likely to produce pharmacodynamic drug interactions; the most common consequence is additive effects with agents with similar pharmacologic effects.

- SSRIs are most likely to produce pharmacokinetic drug interactions, with each agent having an individual but overlapping profile.

- Serotonin syndrome can occur with any drug or combination of drugs that increase serotonergic activity in the central nervous system.

- Of all the SSRIs, fluvoxamine is the most likely to interfere with other drugs that are eliminated hepatically.

- Non-SSRI second-generation antidepressants have fewer drug interactions, with the exception of nefazodone.

REFERENCES

1. **Brouwer KRL, Dukes GE, Powell JR.** Influence of liver function on drug disposition. In Evans WE, Schentag JJ, Jusko WJ (eds). *Applied Pharmacokinetics.* Spokane, WA: Applied Therapeutics; 1993:1–59.

2. **Rendic S, Di Carlo FJ.** Human cytochrome P450 enzymes: a status report summarizing their reactions, substrates, inducers, and inhibitors. *Drug Metab Rev.* 1997; 29:413–580.

3. **DeVane CL, Nemeroff CB.** 1998 guide to psychotropic drug interactions. *Prim Psychiatry.* 1998;5:36–75.

4. **Michalets EL.** Update: clinically significant cytochrome P-450 drug interactions. *Pharmacotherapy.* 1998;18:84–112.

5. **Jefferson JW.** Drug interactions: friend or foe? *J Clin Psychiatry.* 1998;59(Suppl 4):37–47.

6. **Meyer UA, Zanger UM, Grant D, Blum M.** Genetic polymorphisms of drug metabolism. *Adv Drug Res.* 1990;19:197–241.

7. **Slaughter RL, Edwards DJ.** Recent advances: the cyctochrome P450 enzymes. *Ann Pharmacother.* 1995;29:619–24.

8. **Ring BJ, Catlow J, Lindsay TJ.** Identification of the human cytochrome P450 responsible for the in vitro formation of the major oxidative metabolites of the antipsychotic agent olanzapine. *J Pharmacol Exp Ther.* 1996;276:658–66.

9. **Nebert DW, Adesnick M, Coon MJ, et al.** The P450 gene superfamily: recommended nomenclature. *DNA.* 1987;6:1–11.

10. **Nemeroff CB, DeVane CL, Pollock BG.** Newer antidepressants and the cytochrome P450 system. *Am J Psychiatry.* 1996;153:311–20.

11. **Richelson E.** Pharmacokinetic drug interactions of new antidepressants: a review of the effects on the metabolism of other drugs. *Mayo Clin Proc.* 1997;72:835–47.

12. **White AG.** Methyldopa and amitriptyline. *Lancet.* 1965;2:441.

13. **Boakes AJ.** Interactions between sympathomimetic amines and antidepressant agents in Man. *Br Med J.* 1973;1:311–3.

14. **Flemenbaum A.** Hypertensive episodes after adding methylphenidate (Ritalin) to tricyclic antidepressants. *Psychosomatics.* 1972;8:265–7.

15. **Steiner E.** Inhibition of desipramine 2-hydroxylation by quinidine and quinine. *Clin Pharmacol Ther.* 1988;43:577–61.

16. **Bigger JT.** Cardiac antiarrhythmic effect of imipramine hydrochloride. *N Engl J Med.* 1977;296:206–9.

17. **Janowsky D.** Combined anticholinergic agents and atropine-like delirium. *Am J Psychiatry.* 1972;33:304–8.

18. **Burrows GD, Davies B.** Antidepressants and barbiturates. *Br Med J.* 1971;4:113–8.

19. **Nawishy S, Dawling S.** Antidepressant drugs, convulsions, and epilepsy. *Br J Clin Pharmacol.* 1982;13:612–9.

20. **Gregor KJ, Way K, Young CH, James SP.** Concomitant use of selective serotonin-reuptake inhibitors with other cytochrome P450 2D6 or 3A4 metabolized medications: How often does it really happen? *J Affect Disorders.* 1997;46:59–67.

21. **Blier P, Bergeron R.** The safety of concomitant use of sumatriptan and antidepressant treatments. *J Clin Psychopharmacol.* 1995;15:106–9.

22. **Smith DA, Cleary EW, Watkins S, et al.** Zolmitriptan (311c90) does not interact with fluoxetine in healthy volunteers. *Int J Clin Pharmacol Ther.* 1998;36:301–5.

23. **Mills KC.** Serotonin syndrome. *Crit Care Clin.* 1997;13:763–83.

24. **Joffe RT, Sokolov STH.** Co-administration of fluoxetine and sumatriptan: the Canadian experience. *Acta Psychiat Scand.* 1997;95:551–9.

25. **Weiss DM.** Serotonin syndrome in Parkinson disease. *J Am Board Fam Pract.* 1995;8:400–2.

26. **Miller LG.** Herbal medicinals: selected clinical considerations focusing on known or potential drug-herb interactions. *Arch Intern Med.* 1998;158:2200–11.

27. **Spigset O.** Adverse reactions of selective serotonin reuptake inhibitors: reports from a spontaneous reporting system. *Drug Saf.* 1999;20:277–87.

28. **DeVane CL.** Translational pharmacokinetics: current issues with newer antidepressants. *Depression Anxiety.* 1998;8:64–70.

29. Celexa (citalopram) package insert. St. Louis, MO: Forrest Pharmaceuticals; 1998.

30. **Scates AC, Doraiswamy PM.** Focus on citalopram: a selective serotonin-reuptake inhibitor for the treatment of depression. *Formulary.* 1998;33:725–40.

31. **Baumann P.** Pharmacokinetic-pharmacodynamic relationship of the selective serotonin-reuptake inhibitors. *Clin Pharmacokinet.* 1996;31:444–69.

32. **Sproule BA, Naranjo CA, Bremner KE, Hassan PC.** Selective serotonin-reuptake inhibitors and CNS drug interactions. *Clin Pharmacokinet.* 1997;33:454–71.

33. **Sproule BA, Otton V, Cheung SW.** CYP2D6 inhibition in patients treated with sertraline. *J Clin Psychopharmacol.* 1997;17:102–9.

34. **Gram LF, Hansen MGJ, Sindrup SH.** Citalopram: interaction studies with levomepromazine, imipramine, and lithium. *Ther Drug Monit.* 1993;15:18–24.

35. **Duncan D, Sayal K, Taylor D.** Antidepressant interactions with warfarin. *Int Clin Psychopharmacol.* 1998;13:87–94.

36. **Harvey AT, Preskorn SH.** Cytochrome P450 enzymes: interpretation of their interactions with selective serotonin-reuptake inhibitors. *J Clin Psychopharmacol.* 1996; 16:273–85,345–55.

37. Prozac (fluoxetine) package insert. Indianapolis: Dista Products; 1997.

38. **Fineley PR.** Selective serotonin-reuptake inhibitors: pharmacologic profiles and potential therapeutic distinctions. *Ann Pharmacother.* 1994;28:1359–69.

39. Luvox (fluvoxamine) package insert. Marietta, GA: Solvay Pharmaceuticals; 1997.

40. **Wagner W, Vause EW.** Fluvoxamine: a review of global drug-drug interactions data. *Clin Pharmacokinet.* 1995;29:26–32.

41. **Vella JP, Sayegh MH.** Interactions between cyclosporin and newer antidepressant medications. *Am J Kidney Dis.* 1998;31:320–3.

42. **Jefferson JW.** Drug and diet interactions: avoiding therapeutic paralysis. *J Clin Psychiatry* 1998;59(Suppl 16):31–9.

43. Paxil (paroxetine) package insert. Philadelphia: SmithKline Beecham; 1997.

44. **Bannister SJ, Houser VP, Hulse JD, et al.** Evaluation of the potential for interactions of paroxetine with diazepam, cimetidine, warfarin, and digoxin. *Acta Psychiatr Scand.* 1989;80(Suppl 350):102–6.

45. Zoloft (sertraline) package insert. New York, NY: Pfizer; 1997.

46. Wellbutrin (bupropion) package insert. Research Triangle Park, NC: Glaxo Wellcome; 1997.

47. **Tseng AL, Foisy MM.** Significant interactions with new antiretrovirals and psychotropic drugs. *Ann Pharmacother.* 1999;33:461–73.

48. Remeron (mirtazapine) package insert. West Orange, NJ: Organon; 1997.

49. **Owen JR, Nemeroff CB.** New antidepressants and the cytochrome P450 system: focus on venlafaxine, nefazodone, and mirtazapine. *Depression Anxiety.* 1998; 7(Suppl 1):24–32.

50. Serzone (nefazodone) package insert. Princeton, NJ: Bristol-Meyers Squibb; 1997.

51. **Campo JV, Smith C.** Tacrolimus toxic reaction associated with the use of nefazodone: paroxetine as an alternative agent (Letter). *Arch Gen Psychiatry.* 1998; 55:1050–2.

52. Effexor (venlafaxine) package insert. Philadelphia: Wyeth-Ayerst Laboratories; 1997.

KEY REFERENCES

DeVane CL. Translational pharmacokinetics: current issues with newer antidepressants. *Depression Anxiety.* 1998;8:64–70.

Currently the only published review that includes information about citalopram along with the previously available SSRIs; includes information about non-SSRI second-generation antidepressants.

Michalets EL. Update: clinically significant cytochrome P450 drug interactions. *Pharmacotherapy.* 1998;18:84–112.

Comprehensive review of the CYP450 isoenzyme system; includes tables of substrates, inducers, inhibitors, management strategies, and potential alternative agents.

Mills KC. Serotonin syndrome. *Crit Care Clin.* 1997;13:763–83.

Comprehensive review of this important drug-related complication; includes discussion of potential causative agents, recognition of syndrome, and management strategies.

Nemeroff CB, DeVane CL, Pollock BG. Newer antidepressants and the cytochrome P450 system. *Am J Psychiatry.* 1996;153:311–20.

A review evaluating the in vitro *and* in vivo *evidence for inhibition of CYP450 isoenzymes by the newer antidepressants; provides clinical recommendations for avoiding and managing drug interactions.*

Richelson E. Pharmacokinetic drug interactions of new antidepressants: a review of the effects on the metabolism of other drugs. *Mayo Clin Proc.* 1997;72:835–47.

A review of potential drug interactions with all second-generation antidepressants except citalopram; includes tables comparing inhibitor constant values at various CYP450 isoenzymes.

Clinical
Vignettes

A Man with HIV Infection Complicated by Major Depression

A male lawyer 49 years of age with AIDS presents for evaluation due to increasing fatigue. He has been maintained successfully on a triple combination of antiretroviral therapies for the past year, with resulting nondetectable viral load in his plasma and a CD4 count of approximately 200 cells/mm^3. He has noticed recently that he is having trouble managing his law practice due to fatigue and difficulty in concentrating. On the day before his office visit, he called in sick to rest.

On physical examination, the patient seems well and his vital signs are normal. He has no focal neurological deficits. His laboratory testing reveals a moderate decrease in CD4 count (125 cells/mm^3) from his last visit, with evidence of a viral load increase (5000 copies/mL). A magnetic resonance imaging (MRI) scan of the patient's brain is normal. On mental status examination, the patient admits feeling sad most of the time, experiences frequent crying spells, and has isolated himself from friends and loved ones. He expresses difficulty in experiencing pleasure and is preoccupied with the worry that his fatigue means that his HIV disease is progressing. He also talks of difficulty sleeping, decreased appetite, diminished libido, and difficulty concentrating for several weeks. His Mini-Mental Status Examination is normal, with no evidence of cognitive impairment. On direct questioning, he also confides that he has not been taking his antiretroviral regimen as prescribed because he has lacked the motivation required to maintain it rigorously.

▪ QUESTION

What are the implications of failing to recognize and treat this patient's depression?

▪ COMMENT

Based on the findings, this patient is likely experiencing an episode of minor depression. The fact that some of his symptoms (e.g., fatigue) are physical can be misleading if taken out of context with his full syndrome of depression. (e.g., depressed mood, anhedonia, fatigue, insomnia, diminished appetite and libido, social withdrawal, poor concentration, preoccupation with death). The critical step in this patient's evaluation is establishing rapport with him in such a way that he confides his feelings of depression, including how these feelings have altered his motivation regarding treatment adherence. His lack of medical adherence and the resulting immunologic changes may yield subtherapeutic antiretroviral dosing and subsequent disease progression and viral resistance.

Depression in patients with HIV infection may be associated with a range of adverse consequences, including treatment nonadherence, increased use of health care services, and impaired functional abilities. Research also has documented that depressed HIV-positive patients may be at increased risk for engaging in high-risk behaviors (e.g., unsafe sexual practices, injection-drug use). Moreover, depression and stress have been linked to more rapid physical decline and greater mortality in patients with HIV infection. Finally, depressed HIV-positive patients are at increased risk for suicide.

▨ CONCLUSION

Diagnosis and treatment of major depression in patients with HIV infection is critically important due to well-documented negative consequences that affect a range of parameters from survival to treatment adherence.

Evans DL, Leserman J, Perkinds DO, et al. Severe life stress as a predictor of early disease progression in HIV infection. *Am J Psychiatry.* 1997;154:630–634.

Kelly JA, Murphy DA, Koob JJ, et al. Factors associated with severity of depression and high-risk sexual behavior among persons with HIV infection. *Health Psychol.* 1993;12:215–9.

Mayne TJ, Vittinghoff E, Chesney MA, et al. Depressive affect and survival among gay and bisexual men infected with HIV. *Arch Intern Med.* 1996;156:2233–8.

Stober DR, Schwartz JAJ, McDaniel JS, Abrams RF. Depression and HIV disease: prevalence, correlates, and treatment. *Psychiatr Ann.* 1997;27:372-7.

J. Stephen McDaniel, MD

A Colleague with
Depression and Alcohol Abuse

A male physician 56 years of age who is on staff at the same community hospital as you, his treating physician, presents for a "yearly check-up." His last contact with the treating physician was 6 years ago for a similar visit. He reports displeasure with his work and dissatisfaction with the changes in medical care that have occurred in his career. He goes on to note a recent 12-lb weight loss, a decrease in energy, problems paying attention to his tasks, a feeling of being "too busy" for any fun, and difficulty sleeping. He says that he helps his insomnia with "a cognac." He is evasive with further questioning about his alcohol consumption, although he admits that his father was an alcoholic. He also reports that his paternal uncle committed suicide. The results from the remainder of his history and physical examination are negative.

The next evening, when you call him about the results of his laboratory work-up (slightly elevated AST and ALT), his speech is slurred. You briefly, awkwardly approach the topic of drinking, but again he is evasive. Feeling uncomfortable, you stop questioning him on the issue and the conversation ends.

Two months pass, and several of your other patients have reported dissatisfaction with your colleague (patient) because he has canceled and rescheduled appointments erratically. You also notice that he is absent at committee and hospital staff meetings, which is unusual for him. He approaches you in the hall and says that he needs to talk to you after hours that day. In your office, he reports that his wife has asked him for a separation; he has "had enough," he says, and wants a "break from all this." He inquires if you would like to take over his practice. He seems tired, speaks softly, shows signs of psychomotor retardation and has poor eye contact. You ask about his drinking. He says that it is the only thing that helps. When asked directly about "hurting himself," he does not answer. After an awkward silence he stands up and asks you to consider his offer but leaves before you can respond.

■ QUESTION

What are the risk factors for suicide in this case?

■ COMMENT

At this juncture, you as the treating physician are in a difficult situation. First, the patient has escalating symptoms of depression (e.g., decreased energy and concentration, poor sleep, isolation, hopelessness, weight loss, cessation of pleasurable activities, psychomotor retardation). Second, he has indications of significant substance abuse (e.g., erratic work schedule, self-medicating with alcohol, evasiveness when discussing alcohol, elevated hepatic enzymes, positive family history). Third, the patient has significant risk factors for suicide (e.g., escalating symptoms, alcohol abuse, male gender, pending divorce, positive family history, giving away his practice). You have adequate information to believe that your patient has both major depression and alcohol abuse and that he is at significant risk to commit suicide.

▣ QUESTION

When should a treating physician break confidentiality?

▣ COMMENT

The next step in treating this patient involves breaking your confidential relationship with him to access other resources on his behalf. However, you feel uncomfortable doing so because he is your colleague and professional peer. Despite your discomfort, it is appropriate and indicated to break confidentiality to get further information.

You call the patient's wife and she confirms that he drinks to intoxication nightly. She says she is leaving him because he has repeatedly denied "the problem" and flatly refuses treatment; she says she "can't take it anymore." She also says that she is worried because he has been acting "very strangely." She describes that he has been in the garage late at night the last few nights and "does not seem like himself anymore." He has not come home tonight, she says, and this is unusual. You inform her of your concerns, and that you are going to activate emergency measures to find him and have him evaluated and treated.

▣ QUESTION

How is an emergency referral made?

▣ COMMENT

You contact the mental health crisis service in your area and they explain to you the steps needed to have him located and brought in for evaluation. Two hours later, the psychiatrist in the emergency room calls and reports that the Sheriff found him in a rest area, intoxicated, with a gun on the seat next to him. He still refuses treatment. The psychiatrist reports that the patient is going to be admitted involuntarily for treatment. After being hospitalized and completing an outpatient alcohol treatment program, the patient returns to work 3 months later with the help of the impaired physicians program in your state.

■ CONCLUSION

This case illustrates the complex mixture of escalating depression and alcohol abuse in an impaired colleague. As with any patient suspected of imminent danger due to suicidality, the treating physician may break confidentiality to assess and treat the patient further. In this case, the information received from the patient's wife confirmed the suspicions of the treating physician, who then appropriately activated an emergency referral to mental health services. The patient was found and treated before any harm occurred.

Gabbard GO, Nadelson C. Professional boundaries in the physician-patient relationship. *JAMA.* 1995;273:1445–9.

Green SA. The ethical limits of confidentiality in the therapeutic relationship. *Gen Hosp Psychiatry.* 1995;17:80–4.

Harris EC, Barraclough B. Suicide as an outcome for mental illness. *Br J Psychiatry.* 1997;170:205–28.

Hassin DS, Tsai WY, Endicoff J, et al The effects of major depression on alcoholism: 5-year course. *Am J Addict.* 1996;5:144–55.

Mausley PA. Alcohol and drug abuse: physician health programs and the potentially supervised physicians with a substance abuse disorder. *Psychiatr Serv.* 1996;47.

Robert K. Schneider, MD
Robert N. Glenn, PhD
James L. Levenson, MD

CASE 3

A Woman with Depression, Prominent Fatigue, Mild Obesity, and a History of Seizure Disorder

Mrs. A, 35 years of age, presents to the clinic with a 4-month history of low mood and loss of interest in her work and hobbies (e.g., playing the piano). She has become more irritable and notes she has been having arguments with her coworkers and husband, which is what prompted her to make an appointment. Associated symptoms include an increased amount of sleep (11 hours per night), prominent fatigue, poor concentration, and an increased appetite (especially for sweets), with an 8-lb weight gain. She says that when she goes out with her friends she is able to feel better for a brief amount of time, but "it never lasts, and I end up feeling depressed again even before the evening is over." She reports that she frequently has thoughts about wishing she could go to sleep and never wake up, but denies specific suicide plans or an intent to harm herself. Although she recently changed jobs (as a bank manager), she denies any particular losses or stresses over the past several months.

Mrs. A has never been treated for depression but reports a similar, milder episode that lasted for approximately 6 months when she was in college. She has no history of periods of abnormally elevated or euphoric mood, decreased need for sleep, or racing thoughts. She also denies a history of alcohol or other substance abuse. Her older sister also has a history of depression and by report has done well on bupropion (Wellbutrin) 150 mg bid.

She has a history of an idiopathic seizure disorder, which has been well controlled on phenytoin 250 mg/d, with a therapeutic blood level. She has no other medical problems and has no medication allergies.

Mrs. A's physical examination is unremarkable except for mild obesity. Her mental status examination is remarkable for significant psychomotor retardation, depressed mood with a congruent and restricted affect, passive suicidal ideation, and no evidence of psychosis or cognitive deficits.

Complete blood count and a chemistry panel are within normal limits. A thyroid panel shows a free T_4 (FT_4) of 1.1 ng/dL (0.7–2.0) and a thyroid stimulating hormone (TSH) of 4.8 ng/nL (0.4–5.4).

Mrs. A is prescribed fluoxetine (Prozac) 20 mg every morning with a follow-up appointment in 1 month. She calls the office after 3 days complaining of intolerable jitteriness and restlessness. The fluoxetine is discontinued, and sertraline (Zoloft) 25 mg every morning is prescribed, with instructions to increase after 1 week to 50 mg every morning. Four weeks later she presents with little change in her signs or symptoms of depression. The sertraline is increased to 100 mg every morning for 2 weeks without significant change, and then increased to 150 mg every morning. After 2 weeks at this dosage, she notices a substantial reduction in her symptoms, with improvements in mood, sleep, irri- ˙ tability, and a reduction in thoughts of death. However, she reports that her mood has not yet reached her baseline, and she continues to have moderate fatigue, concentration problems, difficulty enjoying activities, and elevated appetite. In addition, she has begun to notice mild diarrhea and an increase in sweating, which coincided with the most recent increase in sertraline.

At this point L-tri-iodothyronine (T_3) is added at 25 μg/d. Three weeks later, Mrs. A reports that she feels much better, with near complete resolution in her depressive symptoms. The diarrhea has resolved, and the increased sweating, although persistent, is mild and tolerable according to the patient. She is maintained on the sertraline and T_3 at the same dosages. A thyroid panel 3 months later shows a FT_4 of 0.9 ng/dL and a TSH of 2.4 ng/nL.

▣ COMMENT

Mrs. A is a woman 35 years of age who presents with signs and symptoms of a major depressive episode. Her symptom cluster suggests the atypical subtype (reversed neurovegetative symptoms and preservation of mood reactivity). We would consider her current episode to be moderate to severe because of the degree of functional impairment and passive suicidality.

Before prescribing a medication for her symptoms, it is important to make the proper diagnosis. Depression can be part of a bipolar mood disorder (e.g., manic depression), can be secondary to substance abuse or dependence, or can be secondary to a general medical illness (e.g., an endocrinopathy). Mrs. A's physician has ruled out these other causes of depression with a medical and psychiatric history, physical examination, and appropriate laboratory studies.

Given that Mrs. A has never been treated with antidepressants before and that no antidepressant has been shown convincingly to have a higher efficacy than any other, the initial choice of medication is influenced by family history of response, concomitant medications or medical problems, and the varying side-effect profiles of the different classes of agents. In general, a selective serotonin-reuptake inhibitor (SSRI) or another of the newer-generation agents would be first-line treatment because their safety, tolerability, and ease of administration are superior to that of the tricyclic antidepressants (TCAs) and monoamine oxidase inhibitors (MAOIs). In addition, bupropion (Wellbutrin) is avoided, despite Mrs. A's sister's history of response, because it is contraindicated in patients with seizure disorders. Mirtazapine (Remeron) is not used as a first-line agent because its potential weight-gain side effect is undesirable in an overweight patient.

The SSRI fluoxetine is a reasonable choice for Mrs. A because it tends not to be sedating, and Mrs. A is experiencing prominent fatigue. Mrs. A unfortunately experiences excessive activation to this medication, which is seen occasionally. Instead of switching to another medication at this point, her physician could have considered lowering the dose to see if it would be better tolerated. However, switching to another agent also is common in this situation; sertraline is an appropriate alternative SSRI for Ms. A because it, too, is not particularly sedating. Other reasonable alternatives available to her physician include citalopram (Celexa), venlafaxine (Effexor), and paroxetine (Paxil) because of their comparably benign side-effect profiles and lack of serious interaction with her other medications.

Because Mrs. A tolerated sertraline well at the 50-mg dose, it was appropriate to wait 4 weeks for response. Lack of response after an appropriate time period (usually 4–6 weeks) should be followed generally by a tapering upward of the dose of antidepressant, unless side effects are excessively burdensome. In Mrs. A's case, her depressive symptoms partially remitted on the 150-mg dose, but side effects precluded a further dose increase. In this situation, we often consider pursuing an augmentation strategy as opposed to discontinuing the partially effective antidepressant and beginning a new trial. There are few data to guide the choice between the various augmentation strategies; T3 is a reasonable choice for Mrs. A given that she has prominent fatigue and psychomotor retardation. As in Mrs. A's case, T3 may be used even when a patient's thyroid function tests (TFTs) are within normal limits. However, her physician instead could have chosen lithium or one of several less-studied alternatives, which are reviewed in Chapter 7.

We generally maintain our patients on the same regimen that leads to the most complete response, as did Mrs. A's physician. When using T3, it is undesirable to make the patient iatrogenically hyperthyroid and, thus, is important to recheck TFTs approximately 3 months after a patient has begun this agent, adjusting the dose if necessary.

Charles DeBattista, MD
David L. Smith, MD
Alan F. Schatzberg, MD

A Man with Physiologic and Psychological Symptoms of Depression Who Is a Candidate for Psychotherapy

At the request of his wife, a man 37 years of age comes to see the physician because of his low energy and poor appetite. He has difficulty getting out of bed in the morning, has lost interest in playing with his children on the weekends, and has stopped exercising because "it's just too difficult to get started." When the physician observes that the patient seems irritated, the patient agrees and apologetically notes that nothing seems to make him happy these days. He has not wanted to burden anyone with his feelings. He has lost interest in being intimate with his wife and wonders why she puts up with him. When questioned about work, the patient indicates that he does not think he has been doing a good job and would not be surprised if they let him go. The physician confirms the suspected diagnosis, noting that these symptoms have persisted for several months. When the physician suggests a referral for psychotherapy, the patient angrily replies that he is feeling a bit down but that he is not crazy.

▦ QUESTION

Is this patient a good candidate for psychotherapy? If so, how can the referral be facilitated?

▦ COMMENT

This patient does seem to be a good candidate for psychotherapeutic treatment of depression. He is able to identify not only physiologic symptoms but also psychological symptoms. He states that he has motivational deficits, has been experiencing strong negative emotions, and notes that nothing is enjoyable at this time. In addition, there is a strong sense of a negative perception of himself. Although not always apparent in a brief interview, the emergence of a pattern of negativistic thinking, apparently self-defeating behaviors, and problems in relationships suggests that the patient would benefit from psychotherapeutic intervention. However, it is also important to note that a presentation dominated by physiologic symptoms does not preclude a referral for psychotherapy. For example, some patients may think that it is inappropriate to discuss nonphysical symptoms with their physicians.

The referral can be facilitated by discussing with the patient any apparent misconceptions he has about psychotherapy. A discussion about why the patient is reluctant to accept a referral for psychotherapy can be accompanied by clarifying that psychotherapy is an effective treatment for depression that targets symptoms and provides tools to fight their re-emergence. A clear, confident presentation of information will communicate to the patient that the physician does not see him as "weak" or "crazy" but that the physician is genuinely concerned for his well-being and is prescribing an effective treatment.

Following a discussion about depression and the nature and effectiveness of psychotherapy, the patient reluctantly accepts a referral to a local psychologist who practices cognitive-behavioral therapy for depression. During the initial phase of therapy, it becomes apparent that the patient has a particularly harsh view of himself. More specifically, he tends to attribute poor outcomes at home and work and in his personal life to himself, whereas he attributes positive outcomes to others or to "luck." Further investigation reveals that he is sure his children do not want to be around him when he is "a grump."

■ QUESTION

How does cognitive-behavioral therapy address the depressive symptoms?

■ COMMENT

During the initial phase of therapy, the therapist will target both the psychological and behavioral symptoms of depression. During therapy sessions, the patient and therapist will work to identify those thoughts that apparently lead to feeling depressed. Simultaneously, the therapist will address symptoms like low motivation and fatigue through behavioral prescriptions. For example, the patient may be assigned homework to return to his exercise regimen (with the approval of his physician) 2 days per week or keep a food diary of what he is eating during the week. These activities are intended to break patterns of depressed behavior through both awareness and behavioral activation. As therapy progresses, the patient and therapist will begin to identify what situations elicit the negative patterns of thinking identified in the early phase of therapy. It then becomes the task of the therapist and patient to identify methods to counter that thinking, to remain vigilant in situations that may prompt a return to depressed behaviors or thinking, and to develop strategies to continue this progress after the termination of therapy.

■ CONCLUSION

Psychotherapy is an effective front-line treatment for clinical depression. Although patients initially may be reluctant, the long-term benefits of psychotherapy make an initial time investment in supporting such a referral worthwhile to physician and patient alike.

DeGood DE. Reducing medical patients' reluctance to participate in psychological therapies: the initial session. *Prof Psychol Res Prac.* 1983:570–9.

Fava GA, Rafanelli C, Grandi S, et al. Prevention of recurrent depression with cognitive behavioral therapy. *Arch Gen Psychiatry.* 1998;55:816–20.

Sacco WP, Beck AT. Cognitive theory and therapy. In Beckham EE, Leber WR (eds). *Handbook of Depression.* New York: Guilford Press; 1995:329–52.

John W. Klocek, PhD

CASE 5

A Young Woman with Treatment-Resistant Depression

A woman 33 years of age presents with major depression. Her symptoms began 5 years ago when she separated from her husband. She has had multiple medication trials at therapeutic doses and adequate duration. These included sertraline, fluoxetine, venlafaxine, amitriptyline, fluvoxamine, and bupropion. She continues to experience dysphoric mood, hypersomnia, hyperphagia with weight gain, helplessness, hopelessness, crying spells, anhedonia, anergy, passive suicidal ideation, and a feeling of her limbs being "weighed down." Her past medical history, review of systems, physical examination, and laboratory data were unremarkable. She denied any psychotic or manic symptoms.

▪ QUESTION

What therapy would you recommend?

▪ COMMENT

The patient has no evidence of a bipolar or psychotic depression. Given her symptoms of hypersomnia, hyperphagia, and leaden paralysis, a diagnosis of atypical major depression is most likely. Although monoamine oxidase inhibitors (MAOIs) have been demonstrated to be effective in treating atypical depression, this patient has had to endure her symptoms for a prolonged period of time; an additional MAOI trial would take at least 6 more weeks. At this point, rapid treatment with electroconvulsive therapy (ECT) (right unilateral) was recommended and initiated. She began to experience relief following her sixth treatment (i.e., within 2 weeks).

▪ CONCLUSION

MAOIs may be effective for the treatment of atypical depression. However, following a prolonged period of depression, rapid improvement can be achieved through the use of ECT.

McGrath P, Stewart J, Harrison W. Predictive value of symptoms of atypical depression for differential drug treatment outcome. *J Clin Psychopharmacol.* 1992;12:197–202.

Prudic J, Sackeim HA, Devand DP. Medication resistance and clinical response to ECT. *Psychiatr Res.* 1990;31:287–96.

Quitkin FM, Stewart JW, McGrath PJ. A subgroup of depressives with better response to MAOI than to tricyclic antidepressants or placebo. *Br J Psychiatry.* 1993;163:30–4.

Yvonne M. Greene, MD
William M. McDonald, MD

CASE 6

An Elderly Female Caregiver with Symptoms of Major Depression

Before entering the examination room, the clinic nurse informed the physician that the patient, a woman 76 years of age, was not her usual self. She had lost 15 pounds since her last visit and was tearful. When asked why she was upset, the patient reported that her 77-year-old husband, who suffered a stroke several years ago, was "not doing well, and I don't think I can care for him any more." The patient's previous medical problems were stable and included hypertension, osteoarthritis, osteoporosis, and hypothyroidism. Her current medications were thyroxine, nifedipine, and ibuprofen.

The patient began to cry before the physician could ask a question. After reassurance, she reported feelings of depression for at least 6 weeks. She stated, "I can't stop worrying about placing my husband into a nursing home." She confirmed that she had lost her appetite, had increasing problems with early morning awakening, difficulty with concentration, forgetfulness, and felt useless because she was not doing her housework. She had become more irritable with her husband and no longer had patience for his many needs, creating a tremendous amount of guilt. Although she denied suicidal ideation, she felt her situation was hopeless. All of her children lived out of state.

She scored four out of four on the Four-Item Geriatric Depression Scale (*see* Chapter 8), indicating a fairly severe level of distress. After promising the patient that he would order in-home chore-provider services, the physician and patient discussed various medication options for her depressive disorder. They mutually agreed on a trial of citalopram, 10 mg/d. He also drew blood to check her thyroid-stimulating hormone levels. The physician scheduled a follow-up appointment in 3 weeks and informed the patient that his nurse would be calling her within several days to check for medication side effects and to gauge how she was doing.

The patient returned to the physician's office in 3 weeks and reported some improvement. She appreciated the in-home assistance from the chore-provider service, stating that this had given her an opportunity to have personal time away from home. Her Four-Item Geriatric Depression Scale score was now 1 out of 4, indicating improvement; however, residual symptoms remained, especially guilt and sleep disturbance. The physician increased the citalopram to 20 mg/d and asked her if he could refer her to a psychiatrist to discuss some of the stresses that she was experiencing. The patient initially balked at the suggestion but agreed to take the name of the psychiatrist. When she returned to the office at the end of another 3 weeks, her symptoms were substantially better. Her appetite had returned, and she had gained 2 lb. Her demeanor and sleep patterns had improved substantially. In an off-handed manner, she acknowledged that she had made an appointment with the psychiatrist. She added, "Although I didn't really feel I needed to see her, the psychiatrist has helped me look at things differently." The Four-Item Geriatric Depression Scale score now was 0 out of 4.

■ QUESTION

What is the best approach to the diagnosis and treatment of an ambulatory geriatric patient with moderately severe major depression?

■ COMMENT

This case illustrates several points about diagnosing and treating geriatric depression in ambulatory primary care settings. Many elderly patients with mild to moderate major depression present to primary care offices for initial evaluation and treatment. The patient's profile, an elderly woman with considerable caregiver responsibilities and burden without a great deal of social support from her family, is not unusual. The patient's vulnerability to depression is largely a result of her caregiving responsibilities. Importantly, cognitive impairment was minimal, consisting primarily of diminished attention and concentration.

The physician's approach to evaluating and treating this patient followed a biopsychosocial model. First, the physician allowed sufficient time during the interview to determine the symptoms, the psychosocial stressors, and time course required to make a diagnosis of major depression. The use of a brief depression-screening instrument assisted the physician in measuring and monitoring the patient's level of distress during treatment. Importantly, the physician did not dismiss her symptoms as just being attributable to fatigue or caregiver burden. Rather, he actively considered a diagnosis of depression. Because the elderly are sensitive to the stigma of mental illness and may be reluctant to seek psychiatric services, the physician's open and engaging approach enabled her to receive needed treatment.

The physician's treatment plan was multidimensional. To address the patient's psychosocial stressors, he ordered in-home chore-provider services. He also checked for possible medical causes of her depression by evaluating her thyroid function. The choice of a selective serotonin-reuptake inhibitor (SSRI) with once-per-day dosing and reduced side-effect profile improved the likelihood of patient compliance with pharmacotherapy. It also should be noted that the starting and final therapeutic dosage was lower than that typically used for middle-aged adults. The physician reinforced the legitimacy of her illness by scheduling a series of follow-up appointments and insisting that his nurse call the patient in the interim to check on "how she was doing." This approach not only fostered reassurance but also helped ensure patient compliance with the treatment plan.

During the scheduled return, the patient experienced some improvement in her symptoms, but remission was not complete. The physician titrated the dosage of the SSRI to a higher level and, importantly, made a referral to a psychiatrist. He explained the referral as a means of helping the patient deal with the stresses of caregiving for her disabled husband. This approach reduced stigma and framed the referral from the perspective of learning new skills to help deal with stress. Combining pharmacotherapy and problem-focused therapy has been shown to improve compliance and treatment outcomes and helps to prevent relapse for patients with late-life depression in ambulatory settings.

Christopher C. Colenda, MD, MPH
Lon S. Schneider, MD
Ira R. Katz, MD, PhD
George S. Alexopoulos, MD
Charles F. Reynolds III, MD

CASE 7

A Woman with
Premenstrual Dysphoric Disorder

A woman 31 years of age presents for evaluation of premenstrual symptoms. She describes significant irritability with angry outbursts toward her husband and children, low mood, anxiety, mood swings, breast tenderness, bloating, headaches, and food cravings. She also notes decreased efficiency and productivity at work. She reports that her symptoms occur during most menstrual cycles; they typically begin 7 to 10 days before menses and remit by the third day of the next cycle. Her symptoms began 5 years ago after an episode of postpartum depression after the birth of her daughter.

■ QUESTION

What is the appropriate management for this patient?

■ COMMENT

A diagnosis of premenstrual dysphoric disorder (PMDD) is suggested by the regular recurrence of symptoms during the week preceding menses, abrupt remission of symptoms shortly after the start of menses, prominent mood disturbance, impairment in functioning, and history of postpartum depression. However, this preliminary diagnosis requires confirmation with prospective daily ratings of symptoms for two cycles. To verify a diagnosis of PMDD, the charting should demonstrate significant symptoms during the luteal phase of the menstrual cycle and little to no symptoms during the follicular phase. Importantly, the clinician must rule out a premenstrual exacerbation of another psychiatric disorder, such as major depression or an anxiety disorder; in such a case, the symptoms also would be present during the follicular phase, with worsening premenstrually.

Given the severity of this patient's mood symptoms and the level of functional impairment, a trial of a selective serotonin-reuptake inhibitor (SSRI) would be most appropriate. Fluoxetine (20–60 mg/d) and sertraline (50–150 mg/d) have both been proven effective for PMDD in large multicenter trials. Paroxetine and clomipramine also have demonstrated efficacy in double-blind studies. Preliminary data suggest similar improvement with antidepressant use restricted to the luteal phase. Although the required duration of treatment for PMDD is unknown, initial studies have shown high relapse rates on discontinuation of the antidepressant after 6 to 12 months.

If residual symptoms remain, consideration should be given to adding a symptom-specific or hormonal treatment. For example, diuretics may be used to control bloating on symptomatic days. Irritability and anxiety may respond to alprazolam. Bromocriptine may be prescribed for breast tenderness. Nonsteroidal anti-inflammatory drugs (NSAIDs) or estrogen patches may be used premenstrually for headaches. Based on anecdotal experience, the addition of an oral contraceptive agent to the SSRI also may enhance response. For severe cases that are unresponsive to SSRIs, the use of gonadotropin-releasing–hormone agonists may be considered, with the addition of low-dose hormone replacement therapy to prevent the medical consequences of hypoestrogenism.

▣ CONCLUSION

PMDD is a disabling condition that should be treated aggressively. Antidepressants, particularly the SSRIs, are currently the first-line therapy.

Freeman EW. Premenstrual syndrome: current perspectives on treatment and etiology. *Curr Opin Obstet Gynecol.* 1997;9:147–53.

Kornstein SG. Premenstrual syndrome: an overview. *Prim Psychiatry.* 1997;14:56–60.

Yonkers KA. Antidepressants in the treatment of premenstrual dysphoric disorder. *J Clin Psychiatry.* 1997;58(Suppl 14):4–10.

Susan G. Kornstein, MD
Barbara A. Wojcik, MD

CASE 8

A Boy with Symptoms of Depression

BJ is a boy 11 years of age who was referred by the school guidance counselor and brought in by his parents. Both parents have advanced degrees and work full time. BJ had received five A's and one B with little effort but looks fatigued in class. He seems unmotivated, and the teacher and parents fear he is beginning to slip academically. Recently, the teacher has noted that he is avoiding work, talking out of turn, and acting as the "class clown." In the past, he has complained that others make fun of him. He needs frequent redirection and supervision, which is a big change. If corrected, he pouts and sulks. His parents report that he looks lethargic at home and is turning into a "couch potato." He eats well and acknowledges that when something bothers him he runs to the refrigerator. He loved playing baseball with neighborhood friends every evening until 3 months ago. He now claims to be too tired and frequently complains of headaches and looks preoccupied. His parents are especially surprised by the recent emergence of explosive anger. He is variably and unpredictably happy, moody, and furious. There is no history of suicidality. Tested IQ puts him in the superior range, but there is a marked discrepancy between performance and verbal IQ. His parents deny any stressors in the past year.

His paternal grandfather and great uncle have bipolar disorder, and a paternal uncle had depression and committed suicide. Another uncle had depression and anxiety as a young adult. His paternal grandmother had depression and anxiety. One sibling has a learning disability. His perinatal course was unremarkable. BJ was born when the family had significant financial problems. All milestones were achieved on time. His mother recalled him to be a fussy, sensitive, temperamentally difficult child who often would withdraw from any stressful situation. She always suspected he had depressive tendencies but had been avoiding considering this because of the strong family history.

On mental status examination, BJ is a mildly obese, casually dressed boy with a tendency to slump into the sofa when not directly addressed. He clearly looks fatigued. Halfway through the interview he reluctantly agrees with the history his parents give and says that most of the time he feels angry. On a scale of one to 10, with 10 being the best, he rates his own mood as a four. He denies any suicidal feelings.

■ QUESTION

How should this patient be managed?

▨ COMMENT

This 11-year-old boy presents with a recent history of irritability, mood lability, fatigue, sensitivity to criticism, headaches, hyperphagia, and declining interest in school work. He has a strong family history of affective disorders. His moodiness cannot be attributed to normal developmental regression because his symptoms are too pervasive. Depression also must be considered to be highly likely because there are no stressors to explain his symptoms as a temporary reaction. Physical causes of fatigue should be ruled out with a physical examination and routine laboratory workup, including a thyroid profile.

A selective serotonin-reuptake inhibitor (SSRI) would be a good choice because of his weight gain and fatigue, and he has no other comorbid disorder responsive to tricyclic antidepressants (TCAs). A low dose (e.g., 10 mg of fluoxetine) should be started with reassessment in 2 to 4 weeks. In this case, because of the strong family history of bipolar disorder, there is a significant risk of antidepressant-induced hypomania (e.g., increased irritability, hyperactivity, overly happy, excited or "giddy" behavior). Parents should be informed about this risk. As part of the overall management, both child and parents should be educated about 1) why depression occurs, 2) the natural course of untreated depression, and 3) how to recognize stressors that could precipitate an episode. There seems to be a need for psychotherapy to address peer- and family-related problems. Cognitive-behavioral psychotherapy should be utilized in BJ because of his age and verbal abilities, with exploration of anger, poor self-image, and parental expectations. Although the decline in school performance and the wide discrepancy between verbal and performance IQ suggest the need for a psychoeducational assessment, the assessment should be deferred until depressive symptoms abate to provide more accurate and valid information.

Birmaher B, Ryan ND, Williamson DE, et al. Childhood and adolescent depression: a review of the past 10 years. Part I. *J Am Acad Child Adolescent Psychiatry.* 1996;35:1427–39.

Birmaher B, Ryan ND, Williamson DE, et al. Childhood and adolescent depression: a review of the past 10 years. Part II. *J Am Acad Child Adolescent Psychiatry.* 1996;35:1575–83.

Kovacs M. Presentation and course of major depressive disorder during childhood and later years of the lifespan. *J Am Acad Child Adolescent Psychiatry.* 1996;35:705–15.

Aradhana A. Sood, MD
Rakesh K. Sood, MD

CASE 9

A Man with Pancreatic
Cancer and Depression

A man 52 years of age with pancreatic cancer has been told by his physician that he has approximately 3 to 6 months left to live. Currently, he has occasional nausea and some lower back pain but says that his discomfort and pain are tolerable and fairly well controlled. For several weeks, he has been complaining of fatigue, poor appetite (with a 15-lb weight loss), insomnia, and poor concentration. He is living at home with his wife and children and says that he has been spending most of the time in bed watching television. When asked if he is depressed, he says that he is sad about his terminal illness and that there are few things about which he becomes enthusiastic; however, he does not think he is depressed. His wife says that he seems to be lacking in spontaneity, slowed down in his movements and activity level, and uninterested in his hobbies and socializing with friends and family.

■ QUESTIONS

Is this patient suffering from major depression? What is the appropriate treatment for this patient?

■ COMMENT

Diagnosis of depression in patients who are critically ill is often difficult. It is not uncommon for patients to deny significant psychological symptoms of depression while describing many physical symptoms that could be due to depression or the underlying medical illness. In this case, the patient denies being depressed, but both he and his wife note that he is less enthusiastic, much less active, and uninterested in activities that at one time had given him pleasure. Many patients with depression will not endorse a depressed mood, yet they or their family describe changes in behavior that are consistent with depression. The patient describes having several physical symptoms that may be due to depression or his cancer (e.g., fatigue, anorexia, weight loss, insomnia, and poor concentration). Because depression is more common in patients with critical illness and is widely underdiagnosed, it is generally preferable to be overinclusive rather than underinclusive of physical symptoms when making the diagnosis of depression. It may be difficult or impossible to determine to what extent this patient's physical symptoms are due to depression or to cancer. However, it is preferable to count the physical symptoms toward the diagnosis of depression, especially because this patient does endorse some psychological symptoms of depression (e.g., disinterest in pleasurable activities) and there are behavioral changes that also are consistent with depression (e.g., decreased activity level and social isolation). The patient also has had all of these symptoms for more than 2 weeks, thereby meeting the time frame criteria for major depression.

Given this patient's limited life span, it is critical to treat depression as expeditiously as possible. Although there are several treatments for depression in patients with critical medical illness, this patient is a particularly good candidate for a psychostimulant, such as methylphenidate (Ritalin) or dextroamphetamine (Dexedrine). A conventional antidepressant could take weeks to have an effect, whereas psychostimulants are likely to have an immediate effect, improving the patient's appetite, energy level, and general apathy. As an option in addition to the psychostimulant, the patient may be started on an antidepressant medication, which would facilitate tapering and discontinuing the psychostimulant after several weeks. The patient also may benefit from psychotherapy to help him with the depression and fears of death or dying. When appropriate, spiritual or religious counseling should be considered for terminally ill patients with depression. Attention also must be paid to providing maximal pain relief and involving the family in his care.

▓ CONCLUSION

This patient is suffering from major depression and should be started on a psychostimulant and possibly an antidepressant as well. The patient may benefit from a referral for psychotherapy, spiritual counseling, or both.

Chochinov HM, Wilson KG, Enns M, et al. Prevalence of depression in the terminally ill: effects of diagnostic criteria and symptom threshold judgments. *Am J Psychiatry.* 1994;151:537–40.

Fawzy FI, Fawzy NW, Arndt LA, Pasnau RO. Critical review of psychosocial interventions in cancer care. *Arch Gen Psychiatry.* 1995;52:100–13.

Masand PS, Tesar GE. Use of stimulants in the medically ill. *Psych Clin North Am.* 1996;19:515–47.

McDaniel JS, Musselman DL, Porter MR, et al. Depression in patients with cancer. *Arch Gen Psychiatry.* 1995;52:89–99.

Thomas S. Zaubler, MD, MPH

Achieving Symptom Resolution and Preventing Relapse in a Woman with Depression (Based on Recommendations of AHCPR Guidelines)

A female surgical nurse 43 years of age presented for physician consultation. She began by stating, "The nurse practitioner sent me to see you because paroxetine hasn't helped me." She reports difficulty coping, especially with her 9-month-old baby and her job. She was ill with a cold approximately 3 weeks ago and "things got worse." On further questioning, she admits her supervisor sent her home from the hospital because she was observed to be crying at work. She has concealed a number of crying spells from her husband and coworkers. She reported difficulty remembering things at work and is frightened she will make a medication error. She tearfully related that she realizes a patient in her care could be hurt or she could jeopardize her job, which is important to her.

She started taking paroxetine 10 mg 4 weeks ago but stopped due to side effects, including feeling "buzzed," "numbness," and a "tingling sensation." She endorses a depressed mood, sleep disturbance, loss of appetite, being irritable, and having decreased energy. She has lost weight below her pre-pregnancy baseline. During the review of systems, the patient revealed that 2 months ago she discovered she had unexpectedly become pregnant again. She did not believe she would be able to take care of a second child with her current child so young and decided to have an elective abortion. She stated that although she thought this was the right decision for her, she worried if "I would go to Hell." There was no suicidal ideation.

The patient had no other medical problems, was on no other medications, and did not use alcohol. She reported that her mother has bipolar disorder and takes lithium. The patient denies any current or past manic symptoms. She met the criteria for a diagnosis of major depression. Treatment options, including psychotherapy and antidepressant medication, were discussed, including the risk of a "switch" into mania from antidepressant medication.

The patient decided to wait to see if she responded to another antidepressant medication before committing to psychotherapy. Nefazodone was selected because its mildly sedating effects could improve her sleep and decrease her agitation. She was instructed to titrate to 300 mg qhs within a week or two, as tolerated. She was seen for follow-up 2 weeks later and reported "doing a lot better," noting improvement in sleep and mood. She was increased to 375 mg of nefazodone.

She returned in 1 month and reported that her depressive symptoms were much improved, including her cognition difficulties. There were no signs of hypomania. On questioning, the patient claimed the abortion issue did not have the emotional importance it had assumed when she was depressed. Over the next 9 months, she was seen every 2 to 3 months for brief appointments. Her physician discussed the guideline recommendations for continuing antidepressant treatment at the response dose for up to 9 months. She voiced her reluctance to discontinue medication, relating that being depressed was horrible and that she did not want to risk a relapse. A slow tapering of the dose was recommended, with monitoring for early signs of recurrence. At an appointment approximately 12 months after the initiation of treatment with nefazodone, the patient reported she had slowly tapered the dose of nefazodone over the last 5 weeks and discontinued it. She remained in remission and expressed her delight and gratitude over her outcome.

▪ COMMENT

Educating the patient about depression and the risk of relapse is recommended by the Agency for Health Care Policy and Research (AHCPR) guideline and can be a simple yet important intervention to improve adherence to therapy and to elicit a good outcome. As illustrated, explaining optimal care goals to the patient at important decision points brings the patient into the decision-making process.

The issue of abortion weighed on this patient and may have been a contributing factor in her depression. Counseling for unresolved feelings contributing to depression was important to offer. However, often there is no sharp distinction between cases appropriate for psychotherapy compared with antidepressants, and physicians should keep an open mind about when to use either or both.

There is a subtype of manic-depressive (bipolar) illness (bipolar type II) that is characterized primarily by depressive episodes and at least one hypomanic episode at some time (1). Some experts argue depression with irritability or agitation may be a clue to the type II variant of bipolar disorder (2). This patient's family history of a mother with bipolar disorder should make the clinician vigilant for symptoms of mood "switch" from depressed to euphoric on antidepressants. If this had occurred, it would have been appropriate to withdraw antidepressant medication and start a mood stabilizer like lithium or valproate.

1. **Michael B (ed).** *Diagnostic and Statistical Manual of Mental Disorders,* 4th ed. Washington, DC: American Psychiatric Press; 1997:327.
2. **Akiskal HS.** The prevalent clinical spectrum of bipolar disorder: beyond DSM-IV. *J Clin Psychopharmacol.* 1996;16(Suppl 1):32-47S.

Anthony L. Pelonero, MD

Misdiagnosis of a Case of Serotonin Syndrome in a Man 65 Years of Age

A man 65 years of age diagnosed with Parkinson's disease 6 months ago presented to the office with complaints of decreased sleep, decreased energy, difficulty concentrating, forgetfulness, loss of interest, a 15-lb weight loss over the past month, and depressed mood for the past 3 months. Laboratory tests were within normal limits, and the patient's Parkinson's disease had been stable on selegiline for the past 5 months. A diagnosis of major depressive disorder (secondary to Parkinson's disease) was made, and fluoxetine 10 mg/d was initiated. After 1 week, the patient reported no improvement, and the dosage of fluoxetine was increased to 20 mg/d. Three days later, the patient's wife called to report that her husband feels sleepy, achy in his joints, is shivering, and has a low-grade fever. The physician replied that this sounded like influenza and that she should urge her husband to drink plenty of fluids and take acetaminophen. The next day, the patient was brought to the hospital with the same complaints in addition to agitation, abdominal cramps, dizziness, and shortness of breath. The patient was found to be tachycardic, diaphoretic, and hypertensive. Appropriate laboratory tests were ordered, and a diagnosis of serotonin syndrome (SS) was made. Fluoxetine was discontinued immediately, and supportive care was initiated. Within 24 hours, the patient's symptoms improved, and by day 7 all symptoms had resolved.

▩ QUESTION

What are the antidepressants of choice for this patient?

▩ COMMENT

Selegiline is a partially selective, irreversible (monoamine oxidase-B) inhibitor. It is metabolized extensively in the liver and presumably in the gut. Selegiline has serotonergic activity secondary to its effects on monoamine oxidase and, in combination with serotonergic antidepressants, has been implicated in the development of SS. SS is characterized by a hyperserotonergic state within the central nervous system (CNS). Initially, this reaction develops quickly within hours to days and usually in relation to a change with a serotonergic drug. Minor symptoms such as gastrointestinal (e.g., abdominal cramping, diarrhea, bloating), neurological (e.g., headache), and an elevated temperature can be seen in the initial stages of the reaction. In light of the quick onset, the "flu-like" symptoms, and the fact that SS is actually a rare occurrence, confusion can arise in the diagnosis.

Psychopharmacologic choices in this patient are limited based on the increased susceptibility for SS. All antidepressants affect CNS serotonin neurotransmission. The agents that should be used first are those that have as their main mechanism of action less activity on serotonin or a mixed pharmacologic profile potentiating other neurotransmitters (or receptors), such as norepinephrine (noradrenergic pathways) and dopamine (dopaminergic pathways). Two examples are bupropion and mirtazapine. Although the possibility exists for development of SS, the potential is much lower based on the serotonergic properties (minimal) of these two agents. A less serotonergic tricyclic antidepressant also may be an option because the anticholinergic effects can benefit a Parkinson's disease patient. Low doses should be initiated and increases in dose should be made slowly and carefully as the patient is monitored closely for any signs of adverse effects. These patients may take longer to respond secondarily to normal physiologic changes and may need trials of up to 12 weeks before treatment response is noted.

▦ CONCLUSION

It is no longer appropriate to initiate a selective serotonin-reuptake inhibitor (SSRI) with the belief that adverse reactions are limited, because it has become clear that there are clinically significant interactions between SSRIs and many different medications. When adding an antidepressant to an established drug regimen, thorough investigation of potential drug interactions can minimize the likelihood of such complications and prevent such adverse reactions and events from occurring.

DeVane CL, Nemeroff CB. 1998 Guide to psychotropic drug interactions. *Prim Psychiatry.* 1998;5:36–75.

Mills KC. Serotonin syndrome. *Crit Care Clin.* 1997;13:763–83.

Tollefson GD. Selective serotonin-reuptake inhibitors. In Schatzberg AF, Nemeroff CB (eds). *Textbook of Psychopharmacology,* 1st ed. Washington, DC: American Psychiatric Press; 1995:161–82.

Weiss DM. Serotonin syndrome in Parkinson disease. *J Am Board Fam Prac.* 1995;8:400–2.

Douglas Dale Brink, BS Pharm, Pharm D, BCPP
Michele Lynn Thomas, BS Pharm, Pharm D

Index